Perspectives in Pragmatics, Philosophy & Psychology

Volume 3

Editor-in-Chief

Alessandro Capone, Barcellona, Italy

Consulting editors

Wayne Davis, Washington, USA
Igor Douven, Groningen, Netherlands
Franco Lo Piparo, Palermo, Italy
Louise Cummings, Nottingham, UK

For further volumes:
http://www.springer.com/series/11797

Louise Cummings

Pragmatic Disorders

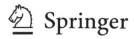 Springer

1424

KH

Louise Cummings
School of Arts and Humanities
Nottingham Trent University
Nottingham
UK

ISSN 2214-3807 ISSN 2214-3815 (electronic)
ISBN 978-94-024-0101-1 ISBN 978-94-007-7954-9 (eBook)
DOI 10.1007/978-94-007-7954-9
Springer Dordrecht Heidelberg New York London

Printed on acid-free paper

Springer is part of Springer Science+Business Media (www.springer.com)

2/4/23

For my siblings
Judith, Stewart, Edward
Victoria, Heather, Elizabeth

Preface

Clinical pragmatics has undergone a remarkable transformation in its relatively short history. From relative obscurity in early studies of language disorders in children, the field has developed into a thriving area of clinical language study which is on a par with clinical phonology and syntax. This development has been encouraged in large part by the expansion of pragmatics as a linguistic discipline, and also by the clinical imperative to develop assessments and interventions that better address the communication needs of clients. Clinicians now expect to assess and remediate pragmatic language skills as standard within the management of clients with a range of clinical conditions. So rapid have been the developments in clinical pragmatics that an examination of the state of the art in this discipline is now in order. Just such an examination is the aim of this book.

In capturing the state of the art in clinical pragmatics, this book addresses a number of predictable and not so predictable issues. With regard to the former, the reader needs to be introduced (or reintroduced) to the pragmatic concepts that are integral to the study of clinical pragmatics. No progress can be made in the absence of a clear understanding of notions such as speech act, implicature, presupposition and deixis. The reader must also have a sound appreciation of how clinical pragmatists have applied these concepts to the study of clients with clinical conditions as wide-ranging as schizophrenia and autism spectrum disorder. To this end, the full range of developmental and acquired pragmatic disorders will be examined in Chap. 2, with the discussion of each preceded by a characterization of the clinical populations in which these disorders are present.

Alongside these predictable issues, the book will also address a number of less predictable topics. It is often acknowledged that pragmatic disorders are uniquely sensitive to a range of cognitive deficits. These deficits, which include theory of mind impairments and executive dysfunction, have not been examined systematically to date. They will receive such a treatment in Chap. 3. Theoretical models, which have influenced clinical pragmatic studies, are only rarely explicitly discussed and evaluated. In Chap. 4, these models are analysed and evaluated at length. Clinicians and researchers have been almost exclusively preoccupied to date with the different ways in which pragmatics either fails to develop normally or becomes disrupted in children and adults. Until very recently, the impact of these disorders on the psychological wellbeing, social integration, and academic and vocational opportunities of clients had been largely overlooked. This book will examine this relatively new and important line of enquiry in the study of pragmatic disorders in Chap. 5. Several populations in which there are substantial pragmatic disorders have received little attention from clinicians and researchers. Three such populations—children with emotional and behavioural disorders, incarcerated youths and adults, and adults with one of the non-Alzheimer's dementias—will be examined in Chap. 6. Finally, in Chap. 7 the contribution of pragmatic disorders to social communication problems is considered. In short, there is much that is truly novel for the reader in the pages that follow.

So, how will the success of this book be measured? It will be measured in three ways. First, the book introduces readers to what I consider to be a necessary critical component to work in clinical pragmatics. To the extent that this critical component becomes well established (I hope it does), it should serve to reduce the overriding tendency of investigators to date to engage in largely descriptive studies which lack the capacity to explain pragmatic disorders. Second, the book develops in specific ways the cognitive character of clinical pragmatics. This is reflected in the discussion of the role of cognitive deficits in pragmatic disorders and in the analysis of pragmatic theories which have a 'strong' cognitive orientation. Third, the book explores a number of clinical conditions (e.g. non-Alzheimer's dementias) and topics (e.g. the impact of pragmatic disorders) which are likely to be significant in the future development of the field. In conclusion, if the study of pragmatic disorders can become more critical, cognitive and innovative as a result of this book, then it will have achieved some degree of success.

Acknowledgments

I wish to thank Ties Nijssen (Publishing Editor, History and Philosophy of Science & Logic, Springer) for his positive response to the proposal of a book in the area of pragmatic disorders. I would also like to acknowledge Alessandro Capone for prompting me to develop further my ideas on clinical pragmatics. The comments of Tim Wharton, who reviewed the manuscript, were particularly helpful to me, and I gratefully acknowledge his contribution. My sisters, Judith Heaney and Victoria Saunderson, assisted in the preparation of the manuscript and their attention to detail is truly appreciated. Finally, I have been supported by family members and friends who are too numerous to mention individually. I am grateful to them for their kind words of encouragement during my many months of writing.

Contents

Chapter 1
Pragmatics and Language Pathology

1.1 Introduction

The study of any language disorder requires a diverse knowledge base spanning several linguistic and medical disciplines (Cummings 2008). The student of language pathology must have an understanding of the neuroanatomical structures that support the production and comprehension of language. He or she must also appreciate how a range of pathologies including, but not limited to, head trauma, cerebrovascular accidents, cerebral infections and neoplasms, can disrupt these structures. Aside from the medical specialisms which inform the study of language pathology, students must also have a wide-ranging knowledge of linguistic disciplines from phonetics and phonology, through morphology, syntax and semantics to pragmatics and discourse (Cummings 2013b). This knowledge permits us to make sense of the child with phonological disorder who says [peɪn] for 'plane', the child with specific language impairment who utters 'He walking home' and the adult with Down's syndrome who cannot identify pictures of an apple, banana and pear as types of fruit.

These anomalies of phonology, morphosyntax and semantics, respectively, do not fully represent the many ways in which language can break down. The child with autism spectrum disorder, for example, may struggle to understand the idiomatic expression in 'Bill hit the sack', while the adult with schizophrenia may fail to use cohesive devices to link utterances with the result that spoken output can appear disjointed. These additional impairments of pragmatics and discourse are the focus of this book. In terms of the long history of the study of language pathology, pragmatic and discourse impairments are relative newcomers. Nevertheless, there is now a well-established academic and clinical literature on these impairments. The aim of this book is not only to capture the state of the art in our knowledge of these impairments, but also to address a number of topics in clinical pragmatics which have been inadequately examined to date.

In capturing the state of the art in the study of pragmatic disorders in Chap. 2, a lifespan perspective will be adopted. In this way, the chapter will

L. Cummings, *Pragmatic Disorders*, Perspectives in Pragmatics, Philosophy & Psychology 3, DOI: 10.1007/978-94-007-7954-9_1, © Springer Science+Business Media Dordrecht 2014

examine pragmatic disorders which have their onset in the developmental period and childhood, in the period extending from adolescence into adulthood and in later life, when neurodegenerative disorders can compromise pragmatic language skills. This survey will address a broad range of clinical conditions in which there are significant pragmatic impairments, including autism spectrum disorder (a neurodevelopmental condition), traumatic brain injury in adolescence and adulthood and the dementias, a group of disorders more commonly associated with increasing age. In recent years, investigators have begun to examine the link between cognitive deficits and pragmatic language disorders. Two groups of cognitive deficits in particular—theory of mind impairments and executive function deficits—have received increasing attention from investigators. However, studies have proceeded in a largely ad hoc fashion with the result that it is difficult to discern any general trends or to arrive at definitive conclusions about what these studies are revealing. Chapter 3 undertakes the first systematic examination of disorders on the pragmatics-cognition interface with a wide-ranging discussion that addresses empirical and theoretical issues.

More generally, theory has occupied a somewhat uneasy position in clinical studies of pragmatics. Many of these studies are not theoretically motivated, while others have employed theoretical frameworks which are not readily applied to the study of pragmatic disorders. Chapter 4 examines the role of theory in clinical pragmatics and discusses the reasons why theory has not always been successfully adopted by clinical investigators. Chapter 5 will examine the impact of pragmatic disorders on the lives of the children and adults who have these disorders. This is a neglected area of research, as evidenced by the paucity of clinical studies that have examined aspects of impact. Where studies of this type have been conducted, they have typically examined the psychosocial impact of pragmatic disorders. However, Chap. 5 will go further in its examination of impact by also considering the academic, occupational or vocational, behavioural and forensic impact of pragmatic disorders.

There are several clinical populations in which pragmatic disorders have been extensively investigated. They include clients who have sustained a traumatic brain injury or right-hemisphere damage. However, there are other populations whose pragmatic impairments have been overlooked by clinicians and researchers. They include incarcerated clients for whom societal and political prejudice has resulted in limited access to clinical language services (these clients form an 'underserved' population). These populations also include clients with emotional and behavioural disorders and one of the non-Alzheimer's dementias, in which pragmatic disorders occur in the presence of psychiatric disturbance and cognitive deficits, respectively (these clients form 'complex' populations). Chapter 6 will consider the pragmatic disorders of these largely overlooked populations. Finally, in Chap. 7, the relationship of pragmatic disorders to social communication is examined. Social communication has been variously defined, with different definitions attributing a more or less significant role to pragmatics within this form of communication. This chapter navigates the largely disparate strands of research in this area to arrive at a clearer understanding of this important relationship.

In laying the foundations for the rest of the book, the current chapter will attempt to do several things. Firstly, pragmatic concepts are often poorly understood and characterized by the clinicians and researchers who use them (Cummings 2012a). The result is the misapplication of these concepts, with linguistic behaviours which are not in any sense pragmatic in nature often incorrectly characterized as such (Cummings 2007a, b). To avoid the misapplication of these concepts in a clinical setting, their examination must become an essential part of the clinical education of students of language pathology (Cummings 2014c). To be clear from the outset on the nature and extent of the behaviours we are calling 'pragmatic', this chapter examines a range of pragmatic and discourse concepts which will be addressed throughout the book. A number of examples, including those taken from clinical subjects, will be used to demonstrate these concepts and to consolidate their understanding on the part of the reader.

Secondly, a 'pragmatic turn' in the study of language disorders has had a number of important implications for how these disorders are diagnosed, assessed and treated (Cummings 2010a, 2012b, 2014d). Formal language batteries that employ word- and sentence-testing formats are often wholly unsuited to the assessment of a client's pragmatic language skills. Increasingly, these batteries are being supplemented by assessments that emphasize the interactional nature of linguistic communication (e.g. conversation analysis) and that pursue linguistic analysis beyond the level of individual sentences (e.g. discourse analysis). By the same token, language interventions that train clients to use syntactic or semantic constructions with little consideration of whether these constructions are likely to bring about gains in everyday communication skills can appear somewhat naïve from a pragmatic perspective. The 'pragmatic turn' in language pathology has thus had implications for the study of language disorders beyond the introduction of new concepts such as implicature and speech acts. This turn has served to reshape every aspect of the clinical management of language disordered clients, and not just those with pragmatic disorders.

Thirdly, in an era of budgetary constraints and evidence-based health care, clinicians who treat clients with communication disorders are increasingly being required to demonstrate the effectiveness of speech and language therapy (SLT). This requirement has seen a proliferation of research which has examined and reviewed outcomes in clients in receipt of a range of speech and language treatments (e.g. the Cochrane Reviews). The outcome of treatment in these studies is often measured in terms of gains in functional communication. Moreover, on at least one significant outcomes measure—the National Outcomes Measurement System (NOMS) of the American Speech-Language-Hearing Association—a series of 15 functional communication measures has been developed for the purpose of determining the outcome of SLT intervention. The concept of functional communication has its origins in pragmatics. This chapter will conclude with a discussion of how pragmatics has also shaped the measures that are now used to demonstrate the effectiveness of SLT interventions.

1.2 Pragmatic Concepts

This section will examine a number of pragmatic and discourse concepts that are integral to the study of pragmatic disorders. These concepts will appear at various points in the following pages. A sound appreciation of these concepts on the part of the reader is thus essential for the discussions of later chapters to be fully understood. Four of the concepts to be discussed—speech act, implicature, presupposition and deixis—are core pragmatic concepts which are included as standard in introductions to pragmatics. A fifth class of concepts, which will be captured under the umbrella expression 'non-literal language', includes, amongst other things, idioms, metaphors and proverbs. A sixth concept, context, is more often alluded to than directly examined in introductions to pragmatics. The centrality of this concept to pragmatics in general, and to clinical studies of pragmatics in particular, requires that this concept be treated on a par with core concepts such as implicature. A seventh and eighth concept—discourse cohesion and coherence—will conclude the survey of concepts in this section. Although these concepts are premodified by the term 'discourse', it is the reliance of these concepts on pragmatic skills that warrants their examination alongside notions such as speech acts.

1.2.1 Speech Act

Until the latter half of the twentieth century, the dominant conception of meaning among philosophers of language was semantic in nature. According to this semantic conception, sentence meaning consists in a specification of the conditions that must exist in the world for a sentence to be true. That is, a sentence's meaning is given in terms of its truth conditions. This view of meaning applied to one type of sentence, the class of declaratives in language.

In the 1940s and 1950s, a group of philosophers at Oxford—among them John Austin—began to question this dominant conception of meaning. According to these philosophers, to reduce the meaning of any sentence to a set of truth conditions is to misrepresent the very large number of sentences in a language which are not intended to be true or false. Rather, sentences can be used to make promises and requests, issue threats, ask questions and much else besides. Even declarative sentences, it was argued, do not always report states of affairs and are not true or false for this reason. In the example 'I baptise this child John Brown', the speaker is not reporting an act of baptism but actually engaging in it. Utterances of this type led Austin to propose a distinction between constative utterances, which describe states of affairs in the world and are true or false, and performative utterances, which do not describe anything but whose uttering constitutes the performance of the act in question. These so-called speech acts are to be distinguished from the state of affairs that obtain when these acts are performed. So, while 'I baptise this child John Brown' is not something which is true or false, the fact that there is a child who has been baptised John Brown is something which is true or false.

While a criterion of truth (or falsity) cannot be applied to performative utterances, these utterances, Austin argued, can be performed felicitously or infelicitously. The so-called felicity conditions that attend the performance of a speech act describe the conditions which must hold for the act to be performed successfully. Austin identified three main categories of felicity condition: (1) a conventional procedure which has a conventional effect in the presence of appropriate people and circumstances; (2) the conventional procedure must be performed correctly and completely; and (3) the thoughts, intentions and feelings required by the conventional procedure are present in the people involved in the speech act. Applied to the utterance 'I baptise this child John Brown', the conventional procedure requires the presence of an individual who has the religious authority to perform an act of baptism. The conventional procedure is not performed correctly or completely if the priest or minister has forgotten to fill the font with water or overlooks placing some water from the font on the child's head. Finally, if the priest is really an imposter who is performing a baptism for some financial gain, there is a clear sense in which he is not entertaining the thoughts, feelings and intentions required by the ceremony.

In his book *How to Do Things with Words*, Austin (1962) examines grammatical and other criteria that may be used to identify performative utterances. He then rejects the distinction between constatives and performatives that he set out to defend. Rejection is necessary, Austin argues, because all utterances are performing speech acts, and not just those identified as performatives. Every utterance, Austin concludes, performs the following three acts: (1) a locutionary act, which is closest to the semantic or propositional meaning of an utterance and in the case of the utterance 'The river has burst its banks' is a description of a state of affairs; (2) an illocutionary act, which in the case of this same utterance may be a warning to local residents about an impending danger; and (3) a perlocutionary act, which results if the residents decide to heed the warning and leave their homes.

It was the work of John Searle which developed further the project initiated by Austin. In his book *Expression and Meaning*, Searle (1979) developed a taxonomy of illocutionary acts that included representatives (e.g. asserting), commissives (e.g. promising), expressives (e.g. thanking), directives (e.g. requesting), and declarations (e.g. appointing). Searle also advanced Austin's notion of felicity conditions. Specifically, it was Searle who argued that by questioning a felicity condition on the performance of a speech act, a speaker can perform an indirect speech act. For example, a preparatory condition on the performance of a directive is that the addressee can perform a certain action (in the case of 'Can you pass the salt?' that the addressee can actually pass the salt). By questioning that condition, the speaker is indirectly requesting that the salt be passed.

Speech acts are one of the most extensively examined pragmatic concepts in clinical studies. In Chap. 2, we will examine what these studies have revealed about the use and understanding of speech acts by language disordered children and adults. In the meantime, it is instructive to examine some examples of the use and comprehension of speech acts by clinical subjects. The exchange below takes place between a teacher (T) and a child (P) with pragmatic disorder. The teacher has issued a directive to the child, an indirect request to describe a TV programme. However, the child treats the teacher's utterance as a literal question about his or her ability to describe the TV programme and responds as such with 'yes'. A second, more direct utterance—a command—is then used by the teacher as a means of making this communicative intent clear to the child.

T: Can you tell me about it?
P: Yes (silence)
T: Well tell me about it. What's it like?

(adapted from McTear 1985, p. 132).

A similar failure to establish the communicative intent of the speaker is evident in the following exchange. The teacher's utterance is a command to the effect to take *and leave* the note with Mr. Smith. However, the child with pragmatic disorder fails to establish the illocutionary force of the teacher's directive and returns with the note.

T: Take this note to Mr. Smith's room
P: (obediently goes to Mr. Smith's room and returns still carrying the note)

(adapted from Crystal and Varley 1998, p. 179).

Even in the presence of severely compromised language skills, children and adults can still perform a range of speech acts. These speech acts are often realized through verbal and non-verbal means. In a study of adults with aphasia, Prinz (1980) used a number of elicitors to encourage the production of requests by three speakers with aphasia. The following requests were produced by adults with Broca's aphasia, Wernicke's aphasia and global aphasia (the elicitor used in each case is indicated):

59-year-old male with Broca's aphasia:

(1)   Need... (gestures writing)
       Elicitor: Patient is asked to sign his name on paper without being given a pen or pencil
(2)   No... pencil... pentil broke
       Elicitor: Patient is given a broken pencil to sign his name
(3)   (pointing to box) You... open box?
       Elicitor: Patient is shown a locked box

47-year-old male with Wernicke's aphasia (recovering to anomic aphasia):

(4)   Up here? Up here? (pointing to first X). Like this? Like that?
       Elicitor: Patient is asked to sign his name next to the X without indicating which of three X's on the page the experimenter intends
(5)   What'd you do—hurt yourself?
       Elicitor: Experimenter returns from getting a drink with a large bandage on his neck; no explanation is given

(6)   Don't they—don't you have something that you... (looking around room)
      Elicitor: Experimenter spills coffee on the paper without offering to clean it up

37-year-old male with global aphasia:

(7)   September... no... cold... (with experimenter assistance indicates
      lemonade)
      Elicitor: Patient is offered something to drink without indicating the selec-
      tion of drinks available in the vending machine
(8)   (looks at experimenter, quizzical looks, laughs—waves arms as if to say
      "forget it"—points to paper and pen and then writes "German").
      Elicitor: Experimenter starts speaking in a foreign language.

Requests are more or less successfully indicated in each case through a combination of verbal and non-verbal behaviours. The non-verbal behaviours on display
include facial expressions (the quizzical look in 8), eye gaze (looking around the
room in 6), pointing (such as in 4), hand gestures (such as writing in 1), and bodily
movements (the use of arm waving in 8). These behaviours are more often used in
support of a verbal response rather than in place of it (see 1 above) and are probably compensating for word-finding difficulties on the part of these patients.

   Verbal responses take both spoken and, less commonly, written form (see the
use of the written word 'German' in 8). A range of verbal strategies are used to
make requests of the experimenter. Sometimes, a speaker with aphasia describes
a condition that must obtain (but which does not hold) in order for an action to be
performed, e.g. in 2 when the patient with Broca's aphasia says 'pentil broke'. On
other occasions, the patient makes a request by using a declarative with questioning intonation (e.g. 'You... open box?' in 3) or by using an interrogative construction (e.g. 'What'd you do—hurt yourself?' in 5). (It should be noted that posing a
question is a conventional way of making a request in English, e.g. 'Do you know
the time?') On still other occasions, the speaker with aphasia makes extensive use
of deictic expressions such as 'here', 'this' and 'that' to indicate his request. In
only utterance 7 does the experimenter have to directly assist the patient in making
a request. Notwithstanding significant linguistic impairments, these patients are
able to use a range of quite sophisticated verbal and non-verbal strategies to fulfil
their performance of the speech act of request.

1.2.2   Implicature

Many utterances that speakers produce communicate meaning beyond what is said.[1]
In his landmark article 'Meaning', Paul Grice (1957) described this communicated
meaning as non-natural meaning (meaning$_{NN}$). The key characteristic of mean-
ing$_{NN}$, and the feature which distinguishes it from natural meaning (meaning$_{N}$), is
the emphasis placed on intentions in communication between speakers and hearers (see Wharton (2010a) for discussion of natural and non-natural meaning). Grice

(1989, p. 219) captures the role of intentions in meaning$_{NN}$ as follows: "'*A* meant something by *x*' is roughly equivalent to '*A* uttered *x*' with the intention of inducing a belief by means of the recognition of this intention". For the first time intentions were to play a central role in human communication, a Gricean insight that has had a profound influence on the development of the modern discipline of pragmatics.

Grice developed this view of communication through the establishment of a principle of cooperation and four maxims. Through its general prescription of the behaviours that can make a cooperative contribution to a conversational exchange, this principle sets in place certain rational expectations on the part of speakers and hearers. Grice (1989, p. 26) captures the cooperative principle as follows: 'Make your conversational contribution such as is required, at the stage at which it occurs, by the accepted purpose or direction of the talk-exchange in which you are engaged'. The four maxims which give effect to this principle are quality ('Do not say that which you believe to be false or that for which you lack adequate evidence'), quantity ('Do not contribute more information than is required but also do not contribute less information than is required'), relation ('Be relevant') and manner ('Be brief and orderly; avoid obscurity of expression and ambiguity').

The cooperative principle and maxims, Grice argued, can be employed by speakers in different ways to generate implicated meanings. Certain conversational implicatures can arise from the simple assumption that the speaker is observing the principle and maxims. In this way, the speaker who utters 'Jill collected the children and did the shopping' may be taken to implicate that Jill collected the children first and then did the shopping. In this case, the implicature arises because the speaker observes the manner maxim, a maxim which requires that the speaker report events in the order in which they occur. By the same token, the hearer can be expected to draw inferences about the order in which these events took place on the basis of the manner maxim. As well as implicatures that arise when speakers observe maxims, speakers can also generate implicatures through the overt flouting of maxims. In the exchange below, Fran may be taken to conversationally implicate that she did not wash the yard:

Jack: Did you wash the patio and the yard?
Fran: I washed the patio.

This implicature is generated by Fran's overt flouting of the quantity maxim. Even though Fran appears not to comply with the quantity maxim—she appears to provide Jack with less information than he requires—Jack can assume that Fran is still being cooperative in the exchange. He then uses this assumption of cooperation to derive the implicature that Fran did not wash the yard.

Grice made a further distinction between those implicatures that arise without the need for particular contextual conditions (*generalized* conversational implicatures) and those that do require particular contextual conditions (*particularized* conversational implicatures). The speaker who utters 'I've bought some of the books on the reading list' may be taken to produce a generalized conversational implicature to the effect that the speaker has not bought all the books on the list. Known as a scalar implicature, this generalized conversational implicature arises without the need for certain contextual conditions. Rather, there is a default interpretation from the use of 'some' to 'not all'. However, the implicature generated in the exchange below does depend on particular contextual conditions. If Frank knows that Patsy does not like her mother-in-law, he may derive the implicature that Patsy will join him for a drink later. If different contextual conditions obtain—for example, Frank believes that Patsy has a good relationship with her mother-in-law who visits only infrequently—then Frank may draw a quite different implicature, viz. that Patsy will not join him for a drink later.

Frank: Will you join me for a drink later?
Patsy: Bill's mother is visiting this evening.

Grice recognized a further class of implicatures. Known as conventional implicatures, these non-truth-conditional meanings arise not from a rational principle of cooperation but from conventional features attached to particular lexical items or linguistic constructions. For example, the word 'even' in the utterance 'Even Sally passed the linguistics exam' generates an implicature to the effect that it was not expected that Sally would pass the exam. Similarly, the word 'but' in the utterance 'Mike is obese but healthy' creates an implicature in which a state of good health is contrasted with obesity (in the sense of not being consistent with it). To the extent that conventional implicatures are attached by convention to certain linguistic expressions, they are not calculable (derivable) in the way that conversational implicatures are. For further discussion of the features of implicatures, the reader is referred to Cummings (2014c).

Like speech acts, implicatures have been investigated quite extensively in studies of clinical subjects. This said, most studies have examined the comprehension rather than the production of implicatures, and some types of implicatures (e.g. scalar implicatures) have only rarely been investigated. In the following example, a 9-year-old boy with Asperger's syndrome is shown a picture of a mother and a girl. The girl has a dress on and she is running on a road that has muddy puddles on it. The boy is then read a verbal scenario, at the end of which he is asked a question:

> The girl with her best clothes on is running on the dirty road. The mother shouts to the girl: "Remember that you have your best clothes on!" What does the mother mean? (Loukusa et al. 2007a, pp. 376–377).

Clearly, the mother is implicating by way of her utterance that she wants the girl to keep her dress clean. However, the boy with Asperger's syndrome fails to derive this implicature from the mother's utterance. Instead, he produces a response which is a verbatim repetition of (part of) that utterance: 'You have your best clothes on'. Other clinical subjects have difficulty adhering to Gricean maxims in their spoken output. For example, in this conversational exchange between a 36-year-old man (W) with AIDS dementia complex and a researcher (R), a relevant response to the researcher's question is followed by an extended turn that fails to adhere to maxims of relation and quantity:

R: What year were you born in?
W: 1964

R: 1964

W: The odd thing was, was I was filling out doctors' forms and hospital forms
      and all sort of things, putting down the date of birth as xxth of xxxx of 1964
      and my age was 34 but a diversional therapist in a nursing home was the
      only person who actually noticed that there was something wrong with this
      picture. I thought "well, it's fairly obvious I'm in it" so there's your problem
      (McCabe et al. 2008, p. 209).

The maxim problems evident in this short exchange were present in all three
interviews conducted with W over a period of 13 months.

1.2.3 Presupposition

Semantic and pragmatic definitions of presupposition abound. On a semantic
conception of this notion, presupposition is defined in terms of a proposition, the
truth of which must be taken for granted and without which a sentence's truth
value cannot be assigned. On a pragmatic conception, presuppositions may be
taken to be propositions that are assumed or taken for granted in an utterance.
Alternatively, they have been characterized in terms of the background, mutual
or shared knowledge of speakers and hearers. Marmaridou (2000, p. 141) states
that '[i]t has become obvious from the discussion of both semantic and pragmatic
approaches to presupposition that this phenomenon is related to some kind of
information that appears to be given, or is portrayed as given, in particular speech
situations in which sentences are used'.

Presupposition is distinct from entailment. In the utterance 'The doctor managed to save the baby's life', there is a presupposition to the effect that the doctor
tried to save the baby's life, and an entailment that the doctor *saved* the baby's
life. A test of constancy under negation can be used to distinguish the different
inferences generated by this utterance. For only the presuppositions of an utterance remain once the utterance is negated (the entailments are quickly cancelled
by negation). In this way, in the utterance 'The doctor did *not* manage to save the
baby's life', it is still the case that the doctor *tried* to save the baby's life (the presupposition still stands). However, it is no longer the case that the doctor *saved* the
baby's life (the entailment fails).

A further feature of presuppositions which distinguishes them from entailments
is their defeasibility or cancellability. In the utterance 'Jack managed to pass the
grammar exam without even trying to do so', the presupposition generated by
'managed'—that is, that Jack *tried* to pass the exam—is very quickly defeated by
the information in the rest of the utterance. However, the same information which
overturns the presupposition of this utterance has no effect whatsoever on its
entailment—it is still the case that Jack *passed* the grammar exam. For further discussion of these features of presupposition, the reader is referred to Marmaridou
(2010a).

It can be seen from the above examples that the implicative verb 'manage' generates a presupposition in which a person *tries* to do something. Implicative verbs
are one type of presupposition trigger. Other triggers include factive verbs (e.g.
'Mary *realized* that the situation was hopeless' presupposes a fact to the effect that
the situation was hopeless), change-of-state verbs (e.g. 'Have you *stopped* smoking?' presupposes that the addressee has been smoking), cleft constructions (e.g.
'*It was* the teenager who vandalised the bus shelter' presupposes that someone
vandalised the bus shelter), definite descriptions (e.g. '*The* castle on the hill is of
historic value' presupposes that there is a castle on the hill), comparisons of equal-
ity (e.g. 'Paul is *as sexist as* Fred' presupposes that Fred is sexist), counterfactual
conditionals (e.g. 'If I were the Prime Minister, I would cut taxes' presupposes that
the speaker is not the Prime Minister), iteratives (e.g. 'Fran failed her driving test
again' presupposes that Fran failed her driving test before), and temporal clauses
(e.g. '*After* he escaped from prison, the criminal fled to France' presupposes that
the criminal escaped from prison). These lexical items and constructions enable
the speakers of these various utterances to leave certain information implicit in
communication. Presupposition thus confers an economy on communication in
that not everything has to be explicitly stated by speakers.

Few clinical studies have examined the use and understanding of presuppositions by subjects. This lack of empirical investigation may be related to a misunderstanding of the concept of presupposition (intuitively, presupposition is somewhat
more difficult to grasp than either speech acts or implicatures). Alternatively, presupposition may be less amenable to investigation in a clinical context than other
pragmatic concepts. One can readily imagine how certain speech acts can be elicited from clients in a clinical setting. A favourite toy placed out of reach but within
view of a child can prompt request speech acts. However, it is less easy to imagine
how a researcher might investigate a client's use and understanding of certain presuppositions. Some studies have attempted to do this by means of so-called bar-
rier activities which require subjects to make assessments of their listeners' state
of knowledge and then tailor the informational content of their messages accordingly (see Wright and Newhoff (2005) for discussion of these activities). A client
who can foreground new information and background old or shared information in
utterances in accordance with the knowledge state of his listener may be said to use
presupposition effectively. The child (P) with pragmatic disorder in the following
exchange with a teacher (T) has clear difficulties with presupposition. The child's
second utterance presupposes that he has some knowledge of or familiarity with the
games mentioned by the teacher, when in fact he does not.

T: Do you want to see if you can play some games with me?
P: Yes
T: They're very easy games
P: They are indeed

                                                    (adapted from McTear 1985, p. 133).

The child with pragmatic disorder in the following conversational exchange
also exhibits problems with presupposition. His utterance 'I like to be in X at

the sports day' presupposes that X *has* a sports day. However, when the teacher directly interrogates this presupposition through the use of the question 'Is there a sports day in X?', the child's response 'There is not' indicates that he should not have couched this information as a presupposition of his earlier utterance. The teacher's continued questioning of the child indicates that he or she is aware of the presuppositional failure that has been introduced into the exchange by means of the child's first utterance and wishes to rectify it.

T: Which race would you like to be in?
P: I like to be in X at the sports day
T: In X?
P: Yes
T: What do you mean?
P: I mean something
T: Is there a sports day in X?
P: There is not. There is a sports day in Y
T: Then what's X got to do with it?
P: Nothing
T: Then why did you mention it?
P: Indeed I did mention it
T: Why did you mention it?
P: I don't know

(adapted from McTear 1985, pp. 135–136).

1.2.4 Deixis

Few pragmatic concepts so clearly demonstrate the way in which language relates to context as deixis. Marmaridou (2010b, p. 101) defines deixis as 'the use of certain linguistic expressions to locate entities in spatio-temporal, social and discoursal context'. These expressions include personal pronouns (e.g. '*I* am departing for Paris'), demonstratives (e.g. 'Mary arrives *this* week'), adverbs (e.g. 'Susan lives *here*'), adjectives (e.g. 'Stan is visiting *next* month') and verbs (e.g. '*Come* here'). To establish the referent of each of these expressions, a hearer must look to the context of an utterance. For example, in the case of the utterance 'Mary arrives *this* week', a hearer must know when the utterance has been produced (temporal context) in order to establish the particular week in which Mary will be arriving. Similarly, a hearer must look to the spatial context of the utterance 'Susan lives *here*' in order to establish the referent of the adverb 'here'.

Other linguistic expressions do not point to aspects of the spatio-temporal context of an utterance, but to (spoken or written) discourse that either precedes or follows an utterance. For example, in the utterance 'Moreover, the policy is likely to have an adverse impact on those with a low income', the term 'moreover' points to preceding discourse in which some other negative consequence of the policy has been described. Also, in the utterance 'I challenge this argument in the next chapter', the term 'next' points to an upcoming piece of written text.

A number of linguistic expressions can be used to perform two or more types of deixis. For example, the demonstrative determiner 'this' in the following utterances is used to perform temporal deixis in (1), spatial deixis in (2) and discourse deixis in (3):

(1)   Oscar arrives *this* week.
(2)   Bill walked home *this* way.
(3)   You raised strong points in *this* chapter.

Languages achieve deixis in different ways. French and German encode features of social context within their pronoun systems. For example, in the presence of a familiar addressee, the French speaker will utter 'Tu es beau' (the German speaker 'Du bist schön'). Different pronouns come into play when the addressee is unfamiliar to the speaker: 'Vous êtes beau' (French) and 'Sie sind schön' (German). This pronoun distinction does not occur in English. However, English speakers can still reflect aspects of the social context of an utterance in the linguistic choices that they make. For example, the mother who says to her 5-year-old daughter 'Is Sally going to be a good girl for mummy?' reflects the asymmetric power relationship between a caregiver and a child through the use of the noun phrases 'Sally' and 'mummy' as opposed to the pronouns 'you' and 'me'.

Like presupposition, deixis has received little investigation in clinical studies of pragmatics. When studies of deixis have been undertaken, they have largely involved children with autism. Autistic children are reported to display confusion of personal pronouns. This is how Kanner (1943, p. 244) characterized this difficulty in his first description of infantile autism: 'Personal pronouns are repeated just as heard, with no change to suit the altered situation. The child, once told by his mother, "Now I will give you your milk," expresses the desire for milk in exactly the same words. Consequently, he comes to speak of himself always as "you," and of the person addressed as "I." Not only the words, but even the intonation is retained'. Later clinical characterizations of autism have also emphasized the reversal of pronouns described by Kanner. Fay (1979, p. 247) describes how the autistic child uses 'You want biscuit' to mean 'I want biscuit'. Tager-Flusberg et al. (2005, p. 347) describes how an autistic child may ask for a drink by saying 'Do you want a drink of water?' Explanations of this pronoun confusion in autistic children have included echolalia. What is clear is that in the absence of further clinical studies of this deictic phenomenon, and of deixis in general in clinical subjects, little progress will continue to be made on this aspect of pragmatics.

1.2.5 Non-literal language

For convenience, a range of pragmatic phenomena may be grouped under the heading of 'non-literal language'. These phenomena include irony (e.g. 'What a delightful view!' uttered by a speaker who is looking out of a hotel window onto a building site), proverbs (e.g. 'A stitch in time saves nine'), idioms (e.g. 'He kicked the bucket'), metaphors (e.g. 'The children are angels'), hyperbole (e.g. 'I've got millions of things to do'), and understatement (e.g. 'It's rather windy' uttered during a hurricane). What each of these expressions has in common is that their intended meaning is not a sum of the meanings of the individual words contained within them. In fact, a compositional semantic approach to the meaning of these expressions is very often little or no guide to the meaning with which speakers use these expressions. In this way, there is not an obvious connection between sewing and the idea that problems should be dealt with early before they escalate, or the physical action of someone kicking a bucket and his or her death (although Gibbs (2010) argues that even in the case of a 'nondecomposable' or 'nonanalyzable' idiom such as *kick the bucket*, people appear to be using some aspects of word meanings to obtain the idiomatic meaning of the expression, e.g. the sudden action indicated by the verb 'kick' is appropriate in a context where someone died suddenly).

Of course, one's view of the analyzability of the meaning of these expressions determines one's view of how these expressions are stored and processed by language users. If the meaning of these expressions is stipulated in the same way that the meanings of words like 'dog' and 'house' are stipulated, then one is committed to a semantic view of these expressions in which they are stored in and retrieved from the mental lexicon. However, if a hearer actively builds the meaning of these expressions out of linguistic and world knowledge, then one will be more inclined to view the interpretation of these expressions as pragmatic in nature. For further discussion of these issues, the reader is referred to Gibbs (2010).

Non-literal forms have been studied extensively in a clinical context. In fact, some non-literal forms have been examined so routinely that they have come to have diagnostic significance in relation to certain disorders. In this way, proverb comprehension tests were for many decades believed to reveal hallmark features of schizophrenia, although they have been recently abandoned on the grounds of poor reliability (Brüne and Bodenstein 2005). When proverb understanding is tested in a clinical context, the typical testing format is to present subjects with a number of possible interpretations from which they select one. Alternatively, interpretations may not be provided by the examiner. Instead, subjects are asked to explain the meanings of proverbs. In the case of schizophrenia at least, these explanations are often irrelevant or bizarre in nature. For example, Halpern and McCartin-Clark (1984, p. 294) describe how an adult with schizophrenia in their study produced the utterance 'Take rags to junk yard' in explanation of the proverb *Don't put all your eggs in one basket*.

The use of metaphorical language can be symptomatic of pragmatic impairment in some clinical conditions (e.g. autism spectrum disorder). In the following conversational exchange between a researcher (R) and a male subject (W) with AIDS dementia complex, there is a metaphorical use of 'black duck'. W's use of this phrase may indicate inaccurate recall of the ugly duckling from the fairy tale written by Hans Christian Andersen. The ugly duckling in this tale was despised and rejected by the other ducklings, a sentiment possibly expressed by W through his use of the adjective 'common':

R: What would be the longest job you had?
W: Oh when I had the business, cleaning the building

R: mm and that was for how many years?
W: 8 years, like I said I was spoiled
R: And that was when you were in your twenties?
W: Twenty two. (Name) was the only person who had total faith in me. There
       was an intelligent person in there that, um, he said I've got more common
       sense. I like that idea 'cause there's nothing *common* about this little *black*
       duck and if I am on my way to prove that I'm not (McCabe et al. 2008,
       p. 214; *underlining* added).

1.2.6 Context

The notion of context has attracted the attention of theorists from a number of disciplines including psychology, philosophy and pragmatics (Cummings 2012c).
Illustrative of this broad theoretical approach is Clark's notion of common ground
which 'explicitly covers mutual knowledge, mutual beliefs, mutual assumptions,
and other mutual attitudes' (1992, p. 6). One aspect of this common ground,
mutual knowledge, is developed by Schiffer (1972). For Schiffer, mutual knowledge involves an infinite recursion of knowledge states: 'all "normal" people know
that snow is white, know that all normal people know that snow is white, know
that all normal people know that all normal people know that snow is white, and
so on *ad infinitum* (Likewise, I should think, for all or most of our common general knowledge…)' (1972, p. 32). Whatever the philosophical merits of Schiffer's
notion of mutual knowledge, an infinite recursion does not sit well with the types
of constraints that we recognize in normal cognitive processing. An approach to
context which has greater psychological plausibility is represented by the relevance-theoretic notion of mutual manifestness. This is how Sperber and Wilson
(1987, p. 699) define this notion:

> An individual's total cognitive environment consists not only of all the facts that he is
> aware of, but of all the facts that he is capable of becoming aware of at that time and
> place. Manifestness so defined is a property not only of facts but, more generally, of true
> or false assumptions. It is a relative property: Facts and assumptions can be more or less
> strongly manifest. Because *manifest* is weaker than *known* or *assumed*, a notion of mutual
> manifestness can be developed that does not suffer from the same psychological implausi-
> bility as mutual knowledge (italics in original).

Several aspects of context may be identified including (1) linguistic context (the
linguistic utterances that precede and follow a particular utterance); (2) physical
context (the setting in which a conversation takes place, the people present, and
the time at which a conversation occurs); (3) social context (the social relationship
between speaker and hearer); and (4) epistemic context (the speaker's and hearer's
knowledge and beliefs of the world and of how conversation is conducted). In an
important sense, linguistic, physical and social aspects of context are all subsumed
by epistemic context, in that they are part of the speaker's and hearer's *knowledge*

of a vast range of factors that play a role in the interpretation of utterances. (This idea lies at the heart of a relevance-theoretic notion of context.) Also, it is necessary to emphasize that although these different dimensions of context have been enumerated separately, no single aspect of context is more important than other aspects in the interpretation of utterances. This can be demonstrated in the following conversational exchange between two friends, Oscar and Felix. In this exchange, Oscar is attempting to get Felix's opinion of an art exhibition to which he (Oscar) is a significant contributor:

Oscar: What did you think of the exhibition in *The Riverside* last night?
Felix: The number of pieces on display was greater this year.

Like any witness to this exchange, Oscar is likely to conclude that Felix was not particularly impressed with the art exhibition. In deriving this particular implicature of Felix's utterance, Oscar will draw on several sources of information, or aspects of context. Felix's utterance is preceded by a question which is intended to elicit an opinion. This question, and the particular speech act which it performs (elicitation of opinion), forms the linguistic context of Felix's utterance. The physical context of that utterance includes the presence of two conversational participants (Felix and Oscar), and the fact that the conversation is taking place the day after the exhibition took place. The social context is one in which Oscar and Felix are friends. As such, there will be a high degree of familiarity (a lack of social distance) between the speaker and the hearer. In fact, it is a desire to maintain this close social relationship that leads Felix to indicate his negative evaluation of the exhibition indirectly to Oscar by way of implicature, rather than through the use of a direct reply (e.g. 'I thought the exhibition was terrible').

Finally, Oscar and Felix must both have shared world and conversational knowledge (epistemic context) in order to participate in this exchange. They must know, for example, that *The Riverside* is the name of an arts centre in town. They must also have knowledge of, and be able to put into practice, conversational rules such as the cooperative principle and maxims in order to participate competently in this exchange. The essential involvement of each of these different aspects of context is demonstrated by the fact that if any one of them is not present—imagine, for example, that Felix does *not* know that *The Riverside* is the name of an arts centre—then the entire conversational exchange, including the implicature, is unlikely to succeed.

Aspects of context can often be problematic for clients with pragmatic disorder. Difficulties with context can take several forms. In some cases, clients are unable to draw on context to arrive at an intended interpretation of a word or an utterance. It will be seen in Chap. 2, for example, that speakers with schizophrenia are poor at using preceding linguistic context to achieve the disambiguation or correct pronunciation of lexical items. (Unlike language intact individuals, adults with schizophrenia disregard context and operate with the dominant meaning or pronunciation of a lexeme.) In other cases, children and adults with pragmatic disorders are insensitive to features of context in their formulation of utterances. For example, the child (P) with pragmatic disorder in the following exchange fails to gauge the nature of his social relationship to Professor Crystal (C). As a result, he poses a question to Crystal about his marital situation which is inappropriately familiar:

P: [meeting the first author as he arrives at P's school] Hello. Are you Professor
     Crystal?
C: Yes
P: My name is J_K_. I have to take you to see the headmaster
C: Thank you. Which way is it?
P: Down here. [they begin to walk] Do you like being married?

(adapted from Crystal and Varley 1998, p. 179).

Another socially inappropriate conversational exchange, this time involving an adult with schizophrenia, is shown below. The patient has been asked by a doctor how he has come to be living in a certain US city. He responds as follows:

> Then I left San Francisco and moved to… where did you get that tie? It looks like it's left over from the 1950s. I like the warm weather in San Diego. Is that a conch shell on your desk? Have you ever gone scuba diving? (Thomas 1997, p. 11).

Amongst a number of pragmatic anomalies in this response, the patient's comments about the doctor's tie are inappropriate, given the socially distant relationship that normally obtains between doctors and their patients. The patient's failure to gauge politeness in conversation with the doctor suggests wider problems with his management of context.

1.2.7 Discourse Cohesion

The meaning relations that link sentences and utterances in spoken and written texts are studied within discourse cohesion. Notwithstanding the use of the term 'discourse', the ability to use and understand these relations is a key pragmatic skill. The dominant system for classifying these meaning relations, in clinical contexts and elsewhere, is that proposed by Halliday and Hasan (1976). These authors draw a distinction between grammatical and lexical cohesion. Reference is an example of the former type of cohesion. Through the use of the personal pronoun 'she', a speaker (or writer) is able to relate the second utterance (or sentence) in the following example to the first: 'Sally walked into town. *She* returned home in the afternoon'. This is an example of anaphoric reference. Personal pronouns can also relate (parts of) sentences and utterances to upcoming speech or a written text (cataphoric reference): 'Although *he* did not admit it, George was pleased the party was cancelled'. Another type of grammatical cohesion is ellipsis. This is the omission of elements required by the grammatical rules of the language. For example, in the following exchange between Betty and Susie, Susie's response makes use of ellipsis through its omission of 'like a gin and tonic':

Betty: Would you like a gin and tonic?
Susie: I would

There are also different types of lexical cohesion. In lexical reiteration, sentences and utterances are related through (1) the repetition of a word or phrase, (2) the use of a synonym or near-synonym, (3) the use of a superordinate term, or (4) the use of a general word:

(1)   The judge examined the Alsatian first. The Alsatian had great poise.
(2)   The judge examined the Alsatian first. The German shepherd had great poise.
(3)   The judge examined the Alsatian first. The dog had great poise.
(4)   The judge examined the Alsatian first. The animal had great poise.

In collocation, a second type of lexical cohesion, the speaker (or writer) weaves related words through successive utterances (or sentences). For example, collocation is achieved in the following example through the word sequence 'exam... test... assessment... paper':

> Students had been preparing for the grammar *exam* for many weeks. When the day of the *test* arrived, there was much anxiety. Although the students knew the *assessment* would be challenging, many had not anticipated such a difficult *paper*.

The management of cohesion in spoken and written discourse can pose problems for children and adults with pragmatic disorders. The following extract of narrative is produced by a girl aged 7 years and 4 months who has sustained a traumatic brain injury:

> Ummm, I, once, there was a, we went. There was a for. There was this umm fort. A tree fell down. And there was dirt, all kinds of stuff there. It was our fort. And one day, I have a friend named Jude. She's umm grown up. She has a kid. She has a cat named Gus, a kitten. It's so cute. But once, when she didn't have that kitten, one day, me, my brother, my cousin Matt, and her, and my dad, and one of his friends, went into the woods to see the fort, to show her (Biddle et al. 1996, p. 461).

This extract displays instances of cohesive strength and weakness. The speaker is able to use anaphoric reference to link utterances, e.g. 'I have a friend named Jude. *She*'s umm grown up'. Collocation is also used to good effect to link utterances, e.g. 'a cat... a kitten... that kitten'. However, there is also some evidence of problems on the part of this speaker in the use of cohesion. For example, the subject pronoun 'we' (we went), the demonstrative determiner 'this' (this fort) and the possessive determiner 'our' (our fort) are all used in the absence of a clear preceding referent for these expressions. The introduction of possible referents for 'we' and 'our' (e.g. Jude, Matt, the speaker's father) comes too late in the extract for cohesion among these utterances to be achieved.

Sometimes, the verbal output of clients can be difficult to follow even in the presence of relatively good use of cohesion. For example, the adult with schizophrenia, who produced the following extract in response to the question 'How did you come to be in the hospital?', displays considerable competence in his use of cohesion. An extensive series of proper nouns, pronouns and possessives underpins effective use of reference in this extract, e.g. 'Cliff Richard... he... him...

he... his... we'. However, it is still difficult for the hearer to glean any sense from this extract on account of its complete failure to maintain relevance to the original question:

> Somebody called Cliff Richard. He seems to project my image back to him. Whether he was born at the same time and I'm a twin of his is debatable. Because we have gone through quite a lot of things together over the years that have been quite extraordinary to me (Gordon 1990).

It should also be noted that another of Halliday and Hasan's grammatical cohesion categories, that of conjunction, is problematic for this adult with schizophrenia. He uses the subordinating conjunction 'because' in the absence of a main clause.

1.2.8   Discourse Coherence

As the above example of schizophrenic discourse demonstrates, language can contain many cohesive links and yet still fail to be coherent. Discourse coherence is that attribute of (spoken and written) texts which captures how well the component parts of a text come together as a whole or have thematic unity: it is 'a quality assigned to text by a reader or listener, and is a measure of the extent to which the reader or listener finds that the text holds together and makes sense as a unity' (Hoey 1991, pp. 265–266). While hearers and readers can often identify with ease when a text is incoherent, it is in general more difficult to say what linguistic feature or features contribute to a subjective impression of incoherence. This is because no single linguistic feature is the basis of the coherence of a text. Certainly, adjacency pair structure contributes to the coherence of conversational discourse. However, equally important to the coherence of discourse is the ability to manage topic, to establish causal and temporal relations between events, and to produce informative discourse which addresses questions about the goals and motivations of the characters in a narrative. If any one of these aspects of discourse is disrupted, the hearer or reader will be left with a sense that a text is unsatisfactory in some regard.

It is not difficult to find examples of children and adults with pragmatic disorder who have problems with discourse coherence. As will be discussed in Chap. 2, adults who sustain a traumatic brain injury often produce repetitive, uninformative discourse and have problems with topic management. Clients with schizophrenia and poverty of speech fail to address the informational needs of their listeners. The spoken output of clients with dementia can also reveal poor skills of topic management. These discourse deficits are evident in the following spoken extract produced by a female client, aged 41 years, who has sustained a traumatic brain injury:

> Well, I've gotten lost even coming here. It was probably the second time I came here. I, uh, went down, uh, 27, no 96, I think. And I came up... I remember they said 14 mile. I thought ended. Well, anyways, I just went around and around in circles. And uh... so I got lost there. And it does seem... I do drive myself when I came here but I still get confused. I don't get lost but I get scared. I see Southfield Road and then I just... Southfield and

Greenfield. And still, after coming since February, I'm still not sure whether for a few minutes, a few seconds there if I'm supposed to take Greenfield or Southfield, you know. And then I don't know Southfield, you know. And, uh… I did get lost the second time I came here (Biddle et al. 1996, pp. 461–462).

This speaker is recounting an occasion on which she got lost. However, her account is difficult to follow and confusing in several respects, that is, it is not a particularly coherent account. Several linguistic and discourse features contribute to this impression of incoherence. Firstly, the extract is highly repetitive with place names (e.g. Greenfield), verb phrases (e.g. came here, got lost), and noun phrases (e.g. second time) repeated on several occasions. The effect of this repetition is that the hearer does not achieve a sense that the speaker is making any progress in her account—the speaker keeps revisiting the same few points. Secondly, the information conveyed by the speaker is unclear on certain points (e.g. the number of the motorway) and contradictory on occasions (e.g. 'I got lost… I don't get lost'). Thirdly, the speaker fails to establish clear referents for a number of expressions including the personal pronoun 'they' and the adverb 'there'. This lack of reference will also contribute to the hearer's sense that the speaker is difficult to follow. Fourthly, there are several syntactic anomalies including the omission of subjects in embedded clauses (e.g. 'I thought ended') and incomplete constructions (e.g. 'And I came up…'; 'And it does seem…'). The combined effect of these various linguistic and discourse features is that the hearer will be left with many unanswered questions and much confusion, in fact, a sense that the speaker has not succeeded in presenting a *coherent* account.

While the above speaker has failed to give a coherent account of an occasion on which she got lost, she has at least been able to maintain topic relevance. On other occasions, discourse incoherence can be related to a lack of topic relevance. This is evident in a conversational exchange between a male client called Warren with AIDS dementia complex and a researcher. The researcher has asked Warren a series of questions about the longest job he has had. Although Warren produces a relevant response initially to these questions, he very quickly begins to digress from the topic. One digression resulted in the following extended turn:

My great grandmother was born into a family that was indentured to a castle near Salisbury, Newcastle. Well she was supposed to be a house servant. She sort of looked at then at the age of 17 and said "Do I look like a peasant girl to you? I don't think so, I'm jumping on a boat and going to Australia…" (continued in the same vein for six more utterances) (McCabe et al. 2008, p. 214).

Warren's verbal output is clearly cohesive. Through the use of the personal pronoun 'she', which refers to his great grandmother, Warren is able to link sentences together ('My great grandmother… she… she'). Unlike the previous speaker, Warren's spoken output does not contain syntactic anomalies. To the extent that his responses are relevant initially but then digress from the topic, Warren's difficulties lie squarely within topic maintenance. As Warren strays further and further from the topic established by the researcher, the hearer is left with the impression that Warren's contributions are not developing or addressing the purpose for which the conversational exchange was undertaken. It is this essential disconnection between the purpose of the exchange and Warren's contribution to it which generates a sense of conversational incoherence on the part of the hearer.

1.3 Pragmatic Assessment and Treatment

The 'pragmatic turn' in language pathology did more than introduce a rich array of new concepts into the study of language disorders. It also substantially revised how clinicians undertake assessment and treatment, and not just in relation to pragmatic disorders. This not the place to undertake a detailed review of techniques of pragmatic assessment and treatment (see Cummings (2009) and Wright and Newhoff (2005) for reviews). However, to the extent that I am claiming the emergence of pragmatics brought about a revolution in the management of language disorders, it is important to describe in specific terms what changes there have been.

Part of this discussion will touch on conceptual issues. This is not an indulgence on the author's part, but comes from a need to reflect the ramifications of a new way of thinking in the philosophy of language that went well beyond the boundaries of this discipline. Other parts of the discussion describe how pragmatics found itself uniquely able to address changing clinical priorities in health care in general and in speech-language pathology in particular. It will be argued that pragmatics was able to establish itself so effectively in a clinical context because it was better equipped than most linguistic disciplines to accommodate the types of communication skills that were becoming priorities for assessment and intervention. Moreover, changing agendas in health care have also necessitated that only those treatments which result in measurable gains in the daily activity and quality of life of clients should be priorities for funding. Of any aspect of linguistic study, pragmatics has a unique contribution to make to these outcome measures in efficacy research. This particular consequence of the 'pragmatic turn' in language pathology will be examined separately in the last section of this chapter.

Prior to the emergence of ordinary language philosophy in the 1940s and 1950s, the dominant semantic view of language meaning privileged declarative sentences. Meaning was defined in terms of the propositions expressed by these sentences, while propositions themselves described states of affairs in the world and were either true or false. Propositional meaning had a certain appeal and convenience about it. To the extent that the sentence was the focus of analysis, it meant that the emphasis on sentence-level analysis in disciplines such as syntax could be extended into the study of language meaning. Also, the emphasis on truth and falsity (truth conditions) in an account of language meaning was entirely consonant with the then dominant approach of analysing natural language using logical and formal languages (such languages used propositional logic and predicate calculus in which the concepts of truth and falsity are central).

This analytic predilection of certain 'ideal' language philosophers may seem at some remove from the study of language disorders. But it was not. For what was set in place at this time, and what took several decades to dispel, was an approach to the study of language, that went well beyond the abstract concerns of philosophers of language and many linguists. Specifically, the only aspects of language that were judged to be worthy of investigation were to be found within individual sentences. If a particular linguistic aspect fell outside of this boundary, it was either reanalysed in order to make it fall within this boundary (many aspects of meaning, which were subsequently analysed as pragmatic in nature, suffered this particular fate), or it was rejected as an anomaly which was not worthy of any further serious consideration.

So, the sentence had something of a privileged position in philosophy of language in the early part of the twentieth century. As its conceptual bedfellow, at least on issues of meaning, linguistics largely acquiesced in the more formal treatments of meaning that were philosophically dominant. To study language meaning was to engage in some form of truth-conditional semantics with all the logical and formal trappings that this entailed. Linguistics was shortly to embrace some new and radical ways of thinking about meaning, but in the meantime formal semantics was in the ascendance.

In the early part of the twentieth century, speech-language pathology in the US (speech and language therapy in the UK) was increasingly establishing itself both as a discipline of study and as a profession.[2] Speech-language pathology was not immune to developments in linguistics, and indeed drew upon linguistics as one of its foundational disciplines. To the extent that linguistic analysis appeared to be largely confined to the level of the sentence and its parts, it is not surprising that clinicians came to adopt a particular view of how a client's language skills should be assessed and treated. On this view, words and sentences were the only possible units of linguistic analysis. The publication of formal language assessments reinforced this view with tasks that required clients to demonstrate their use and understanding of individual words and sentences. Moreover, these tasks were undertaken in clinical conditions that bore little or no resemblance to the everyday environments in which children and adults experienced difficulty in their use of language. While these formal tests quickly became the standard way in which to assess language skills, their unit of linguistic analysis and testing format were largely insensitive to the types of difficulties with communication experienced by clients. The stage was thus set for a pragmatic revolution.[3]

One of the early signs of the influence of pragmatics on speech-language pathology was the appearance for the first time in the late 1970s and early 1980s of journal articles that investigated 'novel' communicative behaviours, principally in children. These behaviours included communicative intent in autistic children (Wetherby and Prutting 1984), the communicative functions of immediate and delayed echolalic behaviours in autistic children (Prizant and Duchan 1981; Prizant and Rydell 1984), the comprehension of metaphor by deaf children (Iran-Nejad et al. 1981), the marking of new and old information by language disordered children (Skarakis and Greenfield 1982) and presuppositional and performative abilities (Rowan et al. 1983), and use of revision behaviours (Gallagher and Darnton 1978) by language disordered children.

These studies indicated that clinicians were beginning to attribute significance to pragmatic notions such as communicative intentions, the functions of utterances, non-literal language, presuppositions and conversational repair strategies within an assessment of children's language skills.[4] Early pragmatic assessments were quick to embrace these communicative behaviours. Three pragmatics profiles which emerged in this period exemplify the new emphasis on pragmatics: Penn and Cleary's (1988) profile of communicative appropriateness; Prutting and Kirchner's (1987) pragmatic protocol; and Dewart and Summers' ([1988] 1995) pragmatics profile. Penn and Cleary's six categories capture a range of verbal and non-verbal pragmatic behaviours:

- response to interlocutor (e.g. clarification request)
- control of semantic content (e.g. topic initiation)
- cohesion (e.g. reference)
- fluency (e.g. repetitions)
- sociolinguistic sensitivity (e.g. polite forms)
- non-verbal communication (e.g. facial expressions)

Prutting and Kirchner's protocol recognized 30 so-called 'communicative acts' which were organized under the following three broad categories: verbal aspects (e.g. speech acts, topic, cohesion); paralinguistic aspects (e.g. prosody); and non-verbal aspects (e.g. gestures). Finally, Dewart and Summers ([1988] 1995) examined 33 communication behaviours under the following four broad headings: communicative functions (e.g. requesting), response to communication (e.g. understanding of speaker's intentions), interaction and conversation (e.g. conversational repair), and contextual variation (e.g. situation). Many of the pragmatic behaviours which were recognised for the first time in these early pragmatics profiles have persisted to the present day in similar checklists and protocols (e.g. Bishop's (2003) Children's Communication Checklist).

At around the same time as clinicians were beginning to acknowledge a new set of communicative behaviours in their assessments of children's language, therapy with aphasic adults was increasingly embracing insights from pragmatics. Early pioneers of a pragmatic approach to intervention in aphasiology were Martha Taylor Sarno (Sarno 1969) and Audrey Holland (1980). Holland (1991, pp. 197–198) recalls the very early emergence of pragmatics in aphasiology as a development that predated the appearance of pragmatics in child language disorders and that was almost contemporaneous with the philosophical work of Searle:

> It is no accident that concern for language pragmatics trickled down to speech-language pathology generally and to clinical aphasiology specifically. The discipline has always been a borrowing one […] In addition, although aphasiologists did not originally call it that, concern with functional and communicative aspects of language disorders predated the explosion of interest in other branches of speech-language pathology. Remember that Martha Taylor Sarno developed the Functional Communication Profile (Sarno 1969) quite near the time at which the work of Searle (1969) galvanized pragmatic concerns. The Functional Communication Profile also antedated by at least 7 years the publication of Bates' *Language in Context* (1976) which, at least for American therapists interested in children, served to crystallize pragmatic concerns.

A new pragmatic approach to aphasia therapy was evident in the following developments. The first significant development was that clinicians began to move away from a rather narrow concentration on linguistic competence, in which skills in phonology, syntax and semantics were emphasized, towards an acceptance of communicative competence as the target of clinical intervention. Communicative competence subsumes a broad range of considerations including knowledge of the social and conversational rules that apply to verbal interactions, the use of non-verbal behaviours in the communication of speaker intent, and the contribution of world knowledge, beliefs and cultural norms to language understanding through the application of scripts. These wider sociolinguistic and pragmatic concerns began to complement more traditional approaches to aphasia intervention in which the remediation of particular linguistic constructions was emphasized.[5]

A second significant development in aphasia therapy that was ushered in by pragmatics was the focus on the use of compensatory strategies to mitigate the effects of the aphasic language impairment. Many of these strategies are pragmatic in nature (e.g. the use of gesture to communicate intent, the use of background knowledge to decode syntactic constructions). Moreover, it was consistently observed by clinicians that pragmatic skills in aphasia are relatively spared compared to language skills. Pragmatic skills could, therefore, be employed to good effect to compensate for the (often severe) language deficits in aphasia.

A third significant development in aphasia therapy that was given impetus by the emergence of pragmatics was the move away from clinic-based therapeutic interactions in which the client and clinician were the only participants. Increasingly, clinicians started to acknowledge that clinic-based interactions were poor preparation for the different contexts in which clients were required to communicate with others in their daily lives. Also, the clinician was very far from being a typical conversational participant given his or her knowledge of the client's communication difficulties and of how best to address those difficulties during conversation. Gradually, therapy was opened up to include the spouses, carers and friends of clients with aphasia.[6] The presence of these additional conversational participants not only allowed aphasia therapy to more closely resemble the everyday settings in which clients with aphasia communicate, but with education and training from therapists, these participants could also serve as important communication facilitators of these clients.

At around the same time, group therapy also began to be used increasingly to treat clients with aphasia. As well as enabling therapy to be conducted in the presence of multiple conversational partners, group therapy had the additional benefit of providing these clients with much-needed psychosocial support. Pragmatic therapies also made it more likely that newly acquired communication skills would be generalized to contexts beyond the clinic. For a discussion of some early pragmatic therapies in the treatment of aphasia, the reader is referred to Holland (1991). An account of more recent pragmatic treatments can be found in Elman (2005) and in Chap. 6 of Cummings (2009).

1.4 Pragmatics, Treatment Efficacy and Disability

The emergence of pragmatics in speech-language pathology has done more than transform the assessment and treatment of language disorders. Such is the need to justify funding of health services nowadays that clinicians of all types are increasingly being required to demonstrate the efficacy of the interventions they offer clients. Speech-language pathology services have not been immune to this wider trend in health care. I will argue in this section that a pragmatic concept, that of functional communication, is typically the basis of the outcome measures that are used to assess the efficacy of interventions. The notion of functional communication embodies a range of communicative behaviours which are pragmatic through and through. As Wright and Newhoff (2005, p. 241) state, 'functional communication is a product of the effective use of several pragmatic behaviors'. Functional communication includes skills such as the ability to understand directions, to make one's needs known, to greet and take leave of others, to relate events, and to respond appropriately to requests. It is the type of communication which permeates our daily interactions with others and without which we are likely to experience considerable personal distress, social exclusion and occupational disadvantage.

The centrality of functional communication to measures of the efficacy of therapy will be demonstrated at three levels. Firstly, I examine studies in speech-language pathology that have used functional communication measures to assess the efficacy of interventions, and not just those interventions that have a pragmatic emphasis. Secondly, functional communication measures are also the basis upon which speech-language pathology as a profession is able to demonstrate the benefit of its interventions to clients and, in so doing, secure funding of its services through national health care budgets. In this regard, functional communication measures, as adopted by the American Speech-Language-Hearing Association (ASHA), will be examined. Thirdly, functional communication is also emphasized in international health frameworks which are used to assess disability in individuals who develop illness and sustain injury. One such framework employed by the World Health Organization (WHO) will be discussed. At all three levels, the distinctly pragmatic concept of functional communication can be seen to shape how we conceive of treatment gains and the disability which individuals continue to experience when treatment comes to an end.

Efficacy studies in speech-language pathology are now commonplace. Some of these studies have examined the outcome of interventions which have a pragmatic emphasis. Typically, these interventions are undertaken in clients who have pragmatic and social communication difficulties. For example, Adams et al. (2012a) assessed the effectiveness of a social communication intervention for children who have pragmatic language impairment with or without features of autism spectrum disorder. Other studies have examined the outcome of interventions which treat linguistic impairments often with a view to achieving measurable gains in clients' communication skills. Best et al. (2008) assessed the outcome of a therapy which targeted word retrieval in eight aphasic clients with anomia. Outcome measures examined communicative activity and participation of clients.

Regardless of the type of intervention examined in efficacy studies, outcome measures generally include an assessment of clients' functional communication skills. Dahlberg et al. (2007) used a functional communication measure—the Profile of Functional Impairment in Communication (Linscott et al. 1996)—to evaluate the efficacy of a replicable group treatment programme to improve social communication skills in 52 people with traumatic brain injury. Worrall and Yiu (2010) examined the effectiveness of a programme called Speaking Out in the treatment of aphasic stroke patients. Functional communication measures, including ASHA's Functional Assessment of Communication Skills (Frattali et al. 1995), were used to assess the outcome of intervention. Beyond language disorders, functional communication measures can also be used with clients who have speech disorders such as dysarthria (Ball et al. 2004) and to assess treatment outcomes in clients with fluency disorders (Yaruss 2000).

In 1997, the American Speech-Language-Hearing Association responded to calls to demonstrate the efficacy of speech-language pathology and audiology services by instituting the National Outcomes Measurement System (NOMS). NOMS uses ASHA's Functional Communication Measures (FCMs) to record changes in clients' functional communication skills over time. FCMs are a series of disorder-specific, seven-point rating scales which are scored at admission and again at discharge with a view to determining the outcomes of intervention. In 2008, the National Quality Forum (NQF) endorsed eight of the 15 FCMs from the Adult NOMS (NQF endorsement is considered to be the 'gold standard' for the measurement of health care quality).

Although there is a separate FCM for pragmatics, it is clear that pragmatics has shaped the view of functional communication that is the basis of each of ASHA's FCMs. Throughout ASHA's FCMs, there is an emphasis on communication effectiveness,[7] the use of compensatory strategies, the use of communication skills in conversation, the presence of communication partners, the ability of clients to identify and repair communication breakdown and the role of communication in vocational, avocational and social participation. FCMs acknowledge contextual factors through an assessment of how clients communicate with familiar and unfamiliar partners, and in conversations that are structured or spontaneous (spontaneous conversations provide clients with less contextual support). On the basis of these measures, it can be seen that pragmatics is not a separable component of ASHA's efficacy framework. Rather, pragmatics is integral to a demonstration of the efficacy of speech-language pathology services through its framing of functional communication.

When intervention ends, clients may be left with disability of varying degrees. The World Health Organization (2001) uses the *International Classification of Functioning, Disability and Health* (ICF) to characterize the functioning and disability associated with health conditions. (The ICF complements the World Health Organization's (1993) *International Classification of Diseases*, which is an aetiological framework of diseases, disorders and injuries.) The ICF contains a number of health domains, which are described from the perspective of the body, the individual and society. These domains are body functions, body structures, activities and participation. The individual with aphasia, for example, has impairment of the mental functions of language (body functions) as a result of damage in certain brain areas (body structures), while his or her difficulties with communication can result in restrictions in activities and participation.

The ICF's characterization of communication is revealing in terms of the significance it attributes to pragmatic behaviours. There is an emphasis on the comprehension and production of messages with implied meanings across different modalities (i.e. spoken, written and signed language). Specific communicative behaviours include understanding that a statement asserts a fact or is an idiomatic expression (comprehension) and telling a story (production). The ICF considers the use of facial expressions, hand movements and body postures in the comprehension and production of meaning. Pragmatic skills are considered in the context of daily communication activities such as writing a letter to a friend, following political events in the daily newspaper, and understanding the intent of religious scripture.

The ICF acknowledges that communication is played out in forms of dialogue beyond that of conversation. Discussion or debate, with arguments presented for or against an issue, is included in the activities and participation section of the framework. This may include discussion with one or more people who may be familiar or unfamiliar to the client as well as discussion conducted in formal and informal settings. These contextual features may reveal limitations in a client's communication skills. For example, the client who can engage in discussion of an issue with a single, familiar partner in an informal setting may struggle to do so in the presence of multiple partners or in a formal setting. Conversation is considered along these same parameters (number of partners, formality of setting, etc.), but is further characterized in terms of turn-taking behaviours and the ability to use customary greetings and termination statements.

Additionally, the ability to introduce, develop and bring closure to a topic during conversation is assessed. What this extensive list of pragmatic language skills demonstrates is the centrality of pragmatics to the ICF framework in terms of how that framework views disability and functioning in relation to communication. Pragmatics is at the heart of the activities and participation that one might expect to achieve by means of communication, and it is pragmatics which best captures the restrictions in those activities that are the essence of disability. The ICF represents the first formal recognition of this role of pragmatics in the context of an international health classification.

The acknowledgement of pragmatics by so influential an international classification system as the ICF represents the end point of a remarkable journey for this linguistic discipline. This journey has taken pragmatics from its origins in the philosophy of language to the point where it now defines notions such as disability and functioning in relation to communication. Along the way, pragmatics has substantially changed how clinicians assess and treat clients with communication disorders, and not just clients with pragmatic disorders. Pragmatics has also transformed how clinicians measure the outcome of intervention and demonstrate the efficacy of speech-language pathology services to national governments and private health care providers. Across these different clinical, social and economic domains, the achievement of pragmatics can be captured without overstatement as nothing short of a 'pragmatic revolution'.

1.5 Summary

This chapter has set the context for the clinical study of pragmatics which will be undertaken in the rest of this book. It has done this by surveying the main pragmatic and discourse concepts which will appear repeatedly in the following pages. This survey examined each pragmatic concept on its own terms, and then considered how it may be disrupted in children and adults with pragmatic disorders. Data were drawn from a wide range of clients with pragmatic disorders for this purpose. The chapter then considered how pragmatics made its way into speech-language pathology from its early beginnings in the language philosophies of Austin, Searle and Grice. The emergence of pragmatics in speech-language pathology brought about significant changes in the assessment and treatment of clients with language disorders. Pragmatics has also been integral to notions of disability and to studies of treatment efficacy through the emphasis on functional communication as a measurable outcome of intervention. The chapter examined each of these consequences of the 'pragmatic revolution' in speech-language pathology.

Notes

1. For Grice, 'what is said' is a technical notion which equates to the truth-conditional content of an utterance, or the proposition which is expressed by the utterance of a sentence on a particular occasion. See Huang (2010) and Wharton (2010b) for further discussion.
2. Milestones in the historical development of the discipline and profession of speech-language pathology include the following. The predecessor of the American Speech-Language-Hearing Association (ASHA)—known as the American Academy of Speech Correction—was established in 1925. The first issue of the Journal of Speech Disorders was published in March 1936. In the UK, the College of Speech Therapists—predecessor of the Royal College of Speech and Language Therapists (RCSLT)—was established in January 1945. Newcastle was the first university in the UK to award a degree in speech and language therapy in 1959.
3. The reader is referred to Duchan (2011) for an account of this revolution as it relates to speech-language pathology. Duchan (1984) describes the impact of the pragmatics revolution on language assessment. She urged a

'hot version' of the pragmatics movement: 'The hot version of the pragmatics movement is forwarded by the movement's revolutionaries, who opt for overthrowing our previous conceptions that language is what we are assessing, and propose that we move toward a new conceptualization which examines communication and context, and, if called for, the language within it. The hot view is the one that must be embraced if we are to take seriously what the literature in pragmatics has to tell us' (Duchan 1984, p. 178).

4. This is how two authors from the period characterized what they believed would be the impact of this new pragmatics on the assessment of children with language disorders: 'We predict that this pragmatics approach will not be just another addition to our evaluation techniques but that it will shake the very foundations of how we have been approaching children with language problems. Our notion that we can examine children's language by presenting them with controlled stimuli, such as sentences to imitate or formal tests, will come into question. Our idea that language in the clinic is the same as language outside the clinic will be suspect. Our hope that we can measure a child's language ability in one context in a two-hour diagnostic session will be demolished as results from the research in pragmatics become known to us' (Lund and Duchan 1983, p. 6).

5. The emphasis has to be on pragmatic therapies *complementing* more traditional language interventions, rather than *replacing* these interventions. As Holland (1991, p. 198) forcefully remarks, 'I am [...] aware that an overwhelming fascination with pragmatic issues, to the exclusion of concern about comprehension and production of words, phrases and sentences, as well as reading and writing, fails adequately to serve aphasic clients. Indeed, one of the most pervasive misperceptions about pragmatic treatment is that it precludes rigorous work on other aspects of language. If a patient with marginal comprehension for somewhat complex utterances can signal "yes" and "no" in some rudimentary way, let us fervently hope that he does NOT find himself under the care of a "pragmatically oriented" clinician who will term him "a functional communicator". This is not the case. Such a patient could hardly be a less functional communicator.'

6. I emphasize 'gradually' because it is clear that not all aphasiologists were equally quick to embrace new pragmatic therapies. In this way, Elman (2005, p. 41) describes how many clinicians continued to use traditional approaches to aphasia intervention long after the time when Sarno and Holland first began to advocate pragmatic and social approaches: 'Pioneers such as Sarno and Holland were early and vocal advocates of real life and functional assessments as well as the psychosocial impact of aphasia. However, the majority of clinicians and researchers continued to concentrate on impairment-level linguistic treatment tasks. Little consideration was given to real-life activities or life participation issues, and aphasia treatment remained focused on stimulus-response linguistic tasks. Therapy was typically provided in a nondescript therapy room within a medical setting. Given the office setting, individuals with aphasia rarely had the opportunity

to meet others who were dealing with similar challenges, and important psychosocial issues related to coping with aphasia were unlikely to be addressed'.

7. Like functional communication, communication effectiveness subsumes a range of pragmatic behaviours: 'to be communicatively effective, of course, requires the appropriate use of several pragmatic skills' (Wright and Newhoff 2005, p. 242).

Chapter 2
Pragmatic Disorders Across the Life Span

2.1 Introduction

Pragmatic disorders display no preference for the individuals they afflict. People of different ethnicities, socioeconomic classes, and ages can develop pragmatic disorders. Men and women appear to be equally predisposed to pragmatic disorders.[1] Pragmatic disorders are not confined to people living in certain geographical regions, and are no more commonly found in urban over rural dwellers (or vice versa). No lifestyle, culture or type of education places an individual at an increased risk of developing a pragmatic disorder. In view of this lack of discrimination, pragmatic disorders are best examined within a life span perspective. This perspective adopts a chronological approach in which pragmatic disorders are examined in their order of occurrence throughout the life span.

The chapter begins by examining pragmatic disorders which have their onset in the developmental period. These disorders are found in children and adults with autism spectrum disorder and a range of genetic syndromes, amongst other conditions. Beyond the developmental period, older children and adolescents can sustain injuries and develop illnesses that compromise their pragmatic language skills. This age group is challenging for clinicians in that while many pragmatic skills have been acquired, these children do not have adult-like pragmatic competence. In adulthood, events such as cerebrovascular accidents (strokes) and head injuries can disrupt previously intact pragmatic skills. In later life, neurodegenerative diseases such as the dementias can cause significant, progressive loss of pragmatic skills. Each of these life stages raises a unique set of issues that affect the characterization, assessment and treatment of pragmatic disorders. This chapter and book will address many of these issues in its discussion of pragmatic disorders.

Before embarking on this life span survey of pragmatic disorders, it is important to be clear on the structure and extent of this survey. Pragmatic disorders will be examined according to the life stage in which they have their onset. These stages are (1) the developmental period (0 7 years), (2) older childhood

L. Cummings, *Pragmatic Disorders*, Perspectives in Pragmatics, Philosophy & Psychology 3, DOI: 10.1007/978-94-007-7954-9_2, © Springer Science+Business Media Dordrecht 2014

and adolescence (8–17 years), (3) early to late adulthood (18–65 years) and (4) advanced adulthood (66–85 years).

The age range for each life stage is, of course, controversial. Any demarcation of the developmental period is particularly difficult as language and cognitive skills develop and mature at different times in the same individual and also across individuals. Children do not master complex grammar such as raising until 8 or 9 years of age (Perovic and Wexler 2007). Many pragmatic aspects of language are even later to develop than complex grammatical constructions. Levorato and Cacciari (2002) examined the development of figurative language across four age groups: children aged 9.6 and 11.3 years, adolescents aged 18.5 years and adults. These investigators found that the ability to use figurative language required 'a long developmental time span'. In fact, the metalinguistic ability that was needed to make innovative figurative expressions communicatively appropriate and conceptually sensible was found to continue developing up to adulthood. An extended developmental period is the basis of definitions of developmental disabilities, many of which cause significant pragmatic disorders. In the US, the Centers for Disease Control and Prevention (2012a) state that a developmental disability can have its onset at any time during development up to 22 years of age. One developmental disability—intellectual developmental disorder (formerly 'mental retardation')—can have its onset at any point up to the age of 18 years (American Psychiatric Association 2013).

Aside from the developmental period, the distinctions instituted in adulthood are also likely to be problematic. Although 18 years of age is the beginning of adulthood, this is a legal definition which has no bearing on the language and cognitive skills that an individual may be presumed to have at this point in his or her life. As people live to increasingly advanced ages, it is doubtful that 65 years should be viewed as late adulthood or that 66 years should be viewed as the beginning of advanced adulthood. Typically, this transition in adulthood has been taken to reflect the standard (male) retirement age in most Organization for Economic Co-operation and Development (OECD) countries. It is also the age at which many diseases associated with older age become more common. These diseases, which include dementia and cerebrovascular accidents or strokes, often have significant detrimental effects on the pragmatic language skills of those who experience them.

However, in the same way that retirement ages are an administrative convenience that could be otherwise (the retirement age in a number of OECD countries is *not* 65 years, for example), it is important to note that the distinction between adults younger and older than 65 years is not intended to reveal any significant distinction in the pragmatic language skills of these individuals. So, although most people who acquire pragmatic disorders as a result of dementia or a stroke are over 65 years (and will be discussed in this age category for this reason), there are still significant numbers of younger people who also develop pragmatic disorders as a result of these conditions. The demarcation in adulthood used in this chapter is also a matter of convenience, and should be recognised by the reader as such. Notwithstanding these various difficulties, the life stages outlined above provide a convenient chronological framework in which to discuss pragmatic disorders.

2.2 Pragmatic Disorders in the Developmental Period

For a significant number of children and adults, pragmatic language skills are not normally acquired in the developmental period. For children with specific language impairment (SLI), who experience marked difficulties with structural language (e.g. syntax and semantics), pragmatic language skills may also not develop along normal lines. For a subset of children with SLI, pragmatic skills may be disproportionately impaired in relation to structural language skills. Autism spectrum disorder (ASD) is a neurodevelopmental disorder which can have particularly severe implications for a child's communication skills. In those cases where language is acquired, pragmatics is often severely compromised with even high-functioning children and adults with ASD experiencing significant, life-long problems with the pragmatics of language. Although they have been some-what neglected to date by researchers in communication disorders, the emotional and behavioural disorders (EBDs) are beginning to receive systematic examination of their pragmatic difficulties. A significant number of children are born with genetic syndromes (e.g. Down's syndrome) or are exposed during their prenatal development to various teratogens (e.g. alcohol, cocaine, lead) which have an adverse effect on their intellectual and pragmatic development. The pragmatic impairments which attend these various conditions will be examined in the following section.

2.2.1 Specific Language Impairment

For a significant number of children, language acquisition does not proceed along normal lines. These children form a clinically heterogeneous group with developmental language disorder (DLD). In most cases of DLD, problems with language development can be related to organic and cognitive factors. For example, the child who has hearing loss, a craniofacial anomaly or intellectual disability may be slow to acquire language or, in severe cases, not acquire language at all. However, for a significant subset of children with DLD, language fails to develop normally in the absence of a clear underlying aetiology.[2] The diagnostic label 'specific language impairment' (SLI) is applied to these children. This label reflects the fact that the developmental disorder is *specific* to language, with performance in other domains (e.g. motor development) falling within the normal range. (Contrast SLI with pervasive developmental disorder in which development is compromised across a number of domains.) The term 'specific language impairment' replaces a large number of earlier diagnostic labels including 'childhood aphasia' and 'developmental dysphasia'. SLI is now in widespread use among clinical language researchers.

The true extent of SLI has been difficult to establish with epidemiological studies obtaining quite different prevalence rates for the disorder. Tomblin et al. (1997) obtained an estimated overall prevalence rate of SLI in monolingual English-speaking kindergarten children of 7.4 %. On the basis of this prevalence rate, and using information from the 1990 US Census, it was estimated that 273,025 of the 3,689,533 five-year-old children in the US present with SLI. This disorder, Tomblin et al. (1997, p. 1258) concluded, is a 'common condition among kindergarten-age children when compared with the prevalence of many developmental disorders'. More recently, Hannus et al. (2009) obtained a prevalence rate for SLI of 0.6 % for children aged 0–15 years in the Finnish town of Vantaa. This rate is equal to the lowest prevalence rates of other international studies. Where epidemiological studies do not differ is on the greater prevalence of SLI in boys than in girls. Hannus et al. (2009) obtained boy: girl ratios between 2.3 and 3.5:1 in the Finnish town of Vantaa over an 11-year period between 1989 and 1999. These sex ratios are consistent with those obtained in other epidemiological investigations.

Expressive and receptive subtypes of SLI are recognised in the tenth edition of the International Classification of Diseases (ICD-10; World Health Organization 1993). In the expressive subtype (F80.1, ICD-10), expressive language is markedly below the appropriate level for a child's mental age, but language comprehension is within normal limits. In the receptive subtype (F80.2, ICD-10), understanding of language is below the appropriate level for the child's mental age with expressive language markedly affected in nearly all cases also. The structural language impairments of children with SLI have been extensively documented and are increasingly being linked to cognitive deficits (see Sect. 4.4 in Cummings (2008) for a detailed discussion). In a study of 97 Dutch preschool children with SLI, Van Daal et al. (2009) identified four stable language factors that contributed to the language development problems of these children over a 2-year period. These factors were phonology, lexical-semantics, syntax and speech production. Short-term auditory memory showed strong relations with syntax and medium relations with the other language factors, while intellectual capacity showed weak to medium relations with phonology, lexical-semantics and syntax. Language problems in SLI are associated with literacy difficulties and persist well into adulthood (Whitehouse et al. 2009a).

When we turn to pragmatic disorders in SLI, a somewhat complicated clinical picture emerges. The SLI population does contain children who have significant pragmatic disorders. Moreover, not all these disorders can be accounted for by deficits in structural language. These children are diagnosed as having pragmatic language impairment (PLI), which is a successor to the earlier term 'semantic-pragmatic disorder'. Ketelaars et al. (2010, p. 205) state that 'the term 'pragmatic language impairment' is used to describe children who have relatively intact phonology, syntax and verbal fluency, but who do exhibit communicative problems related to understanding and conveying intentions, the ability to adhere to the needs of a conversational partner, and discourse management skills'.

Because these pragmatic deficits are similar to those found in individuals with autism spectrum disorder, there has been considerable debate about whether the PLI label reflects a distinct clinical entity or is more appropriately construed as being part of the autism spectrum (Bishop 2000). There is evidence that while some children with PLI do meet criteria for autism disorder, other children with PLI do not warrant a diagnosis of either autism or pervasive developmental disorder, not otherwise specified (Bishop and Norbury 2002). These latter children tend to use stereotyped language with abnormal intonation/prosody, but yet they are sociable and communicative and have normal non-verbal communication skills. The term 'social communication disorder' in DSM-5 includes children with PLI (American Psychiatric Association 2013). Social communication disorder specifically excludes ASD. It can occur as a primary impairment or can co-exist with other disorders (e.g. intellectual disorders).

Questions of nosology aside, there is now a well-developed literature on the pragmatic impairments of children and adults with PLI and SLI. These impairments are not only found in conversation but also in other forms of discourse (e.g. narrative). Laws and Bishop (2004) found evidence of pragmatic impairments in a significant subgroup of children with SLI examined in their study. Some 41 % of these children scored below the cut-off point for pragmatic impairment on the pragmatic composite of the Children's Communication Checklist (Bishop 1998). Stereotyped conversation was particularly evident in these children compared to controls. In a study of the conversational responsiveness of children with SLI, Bishop et al. (2000) found that a subset of children with PLI were more likely than control children to give no response to adult soliciting utterances. They also made very little use of non-verbal responses such as nodding. Non-verbal responding was not only closely related to the quality of children's responses, but its absence indicated a relatively high level of pragmatically inappropriate responses that could not be accounted for in terms of limited grammar and vocabulary. Ketelaars et al. (2012) examined the narrative competence of 77 children with PLI. Compared to typically developing children, children with PLI demonstrated poorer narrative competence, as indicated on measures of narrative productivity, organization of content and cohesion. Only some narrative problems in these children could be attributed to language impairments. The rest were pragmatic deficits.

Clinical studies of SLI and PLI have also examined the use and understanding of pragmatic features such as implicatures and maxims. Katsos et al. (2011) assessed the comprehension of statements containing quantifiers such as 'some' in Spanish-speaking children with SLI. These expressions have both a logical meaning and a pragmatic meaning, the latter derived by means of the maxim of informativeness.[3] Katsos et al. found that children with SLI performed more poorly than a group of age-matched typically developing peers, but similarly to younger language-matched children. Children with SLI were disproportionately challenged compared to age-matched peers by the pragmatic meaning of the quantified statements. Ryder et al. (2008) posed questions of increasing pragmatic complexity in different contexts to children with SLI and PLI. Children with PLI performed significantly more poorly than children with SLI on questions targeting implicature. Scores on implicature questions accurately identified children with PLI from those with SLI with sensitivity of 89 %. Children with SLI were only able to infer referents and semantic meaning and generate implicatures when they had the support of pictorial (not verbal) context. Several clinical pragmatic studies have examined the use of discourse features such as referential cohesion by children with SLI. Relative to typically developing children, Polite et al. (2011) found that children with SLI made less use of definite articles to refer to a previously established referent in discourse.

All utterance interpretation proceeds on the basis of inferences that are drawn by speakers and hearers. Several studies have shown that the ability to draw inferences is compromised in children with PLI. In a study of 11-year-olds with SLI and primary pragmatic difficulties, Botting and Adams (2005) reported significant problems during an inferential comprehension task that required participants to make logical (text connecting) inferences, bridging (gap filling) inferences and elaborative inferences. The performance of both clinical groups of children was similar to that of younger children aged 7 and 9 years. Moreover, the clinical groups performed similarly to each other on this inferential task.

Holck et al. (2010) examined inferential ability in children with PLI, cerebral palsy and spina bifida with hydrocephalus. Children with PLI performed significantly worse than children with cerebral palsy on questions that required inferential comprehension. Moreover, the PLI group was the only one in which problems with inferential questions exceeded problems with literal questions. Adams et al. (2009) found that children with PLI scored significantly less on an inference comprehension task than control subjects matched for age and sentence comprehension ability. Although there was no evidence for a unique pattern of inference errors in children with PLI, there was a trend for these children to perform more poorly on developmentally more complex inference items. There is also evidence that the ability to produce and comprehend pragmatic inferences about given or presupposed knowledge in mental state verbs is impaired in children with PLI (Spanoudis et al. 2007).

2.2.2 Autism Spectrum Disorder

For a significant number of children, problems with language development occur alongside deficits in other areas of development. To the extent that development in several domains is compromised, these children are described as having a pervasive developmental disorder (as opposed to a *specific* developmental disorder such as SLI, in which only language development is compromised). The construct of a spectrum has clinical utility in representing the wide range of impairments in this heterogeneous population and is the basis of the diagnostic label 'autism spectrum disorder' (ASD).

In DSM-5 (American Psychiatric Association 2013), ASD is diagnosed on the basis of persistent deficits in social communication and social interaction across multiple contexts and by restricted, repetitive patterns of behaviour, interests or activities. Impairments in the social communication domain include deficits in social-emotional reciprocity, non-verbal communicative behaviours and in developing and maintaining relationships. Stereotyped or repetitive behaviours, excessive adherence to routines, highly restricted, fixated interests and hyper- or hypo-reactivity to sensory input are also core symptoms of ASD. These symptoms must be present in the early developmental period, although they may not be fully manifest until social demands exceed limited capacities. They must also impair everyday functioning.

The epidemiology of ASD continues to be extensively investigated. Findings of large-scale epidemiological studies reveal that ASD is a common neurodevelopmental disorder. Moreover, the prevalence of this disorder is increasing over time. The Autism and Developmental Disabilities Monitoring Network (ADDMN) investigates the epidemiology of ASD in 14 sites in the United States. For the 2008 surveillance year, the ADDMN reported that the overall estimated prevalence of ASD was 11.3 per 1,000 (1 in 88) children aged 8 years (Centers for Disease Control and Prevention 2012b). This figure represents an increase in estimated ASD prevalence of 23 % on 2006 surveillance data and 78 % on 2002 data. A consistent finding of epidemiological studies is the greater prevalence of ASD in boys than in girls. According to the ADDMN, one in 54 boys and one in 252 girls were identified as having ASD in 2008. There is now widespread medical consensus that ASD has a strong genetic basis. Genetic research in recent years has identified several vulnerability loci and cytogenetic abnormalities or single-base mutations which are implicated in the causation of autism (Caglayan 2010).

Approximately 50 % of individuals with autistic disorder do not develop functional speech (O'Brien and Pearson 2004). For those individuals who do become verbal communicators, early vocal anomalies as well as prosodic impairments have been identified. Toddlers with ASD have been shown to produce significantly more atypical nonspeech vocalizations than age- and language-matched controls (Schoen et al. 2011). Peppé et al. (2007) reported that children with high-functioning autism performed significantly less well than typically developing children and normal adult controls on receptive and expressive prosody tasks. Deficits in phonology have been noted in several clinical studies. For example, Cleland et al. (2010) identified developmental phonological processes (e.g. cluster reduction) and non-developmental errors (e.g. phoneme specific nasal emission) in the speech of 69 children with ASD. Non-developmental distortions occurred relatively frequently in the speech of these children.

Studies of syntax in ASD reveal a complicated clinical picture. Certainly, there is evidence of syntactic impairments in individuals with ASD. Riches et al. (2010) found that overall error rates on a sentence repetition task did not vary significantly between adolescents with SLI and adolescents with ASD plus language impairment. The repetition task examined relative clauses that varied in syntactic complexity. However, children with ASD have also been found to align their use of syntactic structure (e.g. passive) to that of a conversational partner (Allen et al. 2011) and to map verbs onto causative actions (i.e. engage in syntactic bootstrapping) (Naigles et al. 2011). In terms of lexical semantics,

Norbury et al. (2010) found that word learning in children with ASD was compromised on account of their reduced sensitivity to the social informativeness of gaze cues. Studies have revealed interactions between the lexicon and syntax in ASD. McGregor et al. (2012) found that only children with ASD who were free of syntactic deficits demonstrated age-appropriate word knowledge. Also, the conceptual salience of entities (specifically, their salience) has been found to influence word order choices in individuals with ASD (Lake et al. 2010). For a review of structural language impairments in ASD, the reader is referred to Boucher (2012).

In clinical studies, structural language impairments have been somewhat eclipsed by often severe deficits in the pragmatics of language in ASD. These deficits are typically in excess of those found in other developmental disorders. Philofsky et al. (2007) reported that children with ASD have poorer pragmatic skills, as measured on the Children's Communication Checklist (Bishop 2003), than children with Williams syndrome. MacKay and Shaw (2004) found that children with ASD performed more poorly than controls with no ASD on a test of the understanding, and intentionality behind, figurative utterances. Lewis et al. (2008) found that adults with a diagnosis of ASD performed significantly less well than adults with no disability on two pragmatic subtests of the Right Hemisphere Language battery (RHLB; Bryan 1989). These tests examined the comprehension of inferred meaning and the appreciation of humour. Dennis et al. (2001a) examined a range of inferences in high-functioning children with autism. These children failed to make inferences about what mental state verbs implied in context. They also failed to make inferences about social scripts and to draw the inferences needed to understand metaphor and produce speech acts. For a recent review of the literature on pragmatic inferences in ASD, the reader is referred to Loukusa and Moilanen (2009).

Discourse deficits have also been identified in children and adults with ASD. Asberg (2010) reported significantly lower abilities in narrative discourse comprehension in school-aged children with ASD compared to younger, typically developing children. Structural language impairments could not account for this finding, as there were no significant differences between the groups in either oral receptive vocabulary or reception of grammar. Colle et al. (2008) found that adults with Asperger's syndrome used fewer personal pronouns, temporal expressions and referential expressions than matched controls and adults with high-functioning autism during a story-telling task. Solomon (2004) reported that high-functioning children with ASD were able to engage in introduction sequences during fictional narratives. However, their problems lay in narrative co-telling, which was often not globally organized over an extended course of propositions. In a study of 57 children with autism, Hale and Tager-Flusberg (2005) found a significant relationship between the tendency to respond in conversation in a noncontingent (off-topic) manner and autistic symptomatology. Children with autism or Asperger's syndrome have also been found to have impairments in inferring and building causal relationships within and across story episodes in narrative contexts (Losh and Capps 2003).

Not all aspects of pragmatics are impaired in ASD. Scalar inferences appear to be intact in individuals with ASD, at least on the basis of a small number of studies conducted to date. Chevallier et al. (2010) found that participants with ASD produced as many pragmatic enrichments of 'or' as matched controls (e.g. *John or Mary will come* generates a scalar implicature that not both of them will come). Pijnacker et al. (2009) found that subjects with ASD were as likely as controls to derive scalar implicatures from utterances such as *Some sparrows are birds* (i.e. not all sparrows are birds). Other studies have identified intact pragmatic skills alongside pragmatic impairments in individuals with ASD. As well as problems with the comprehension of inferred meaning and the appreciation of humour, Lewis et al. (2008) found no significant difference between adults with ASD and adults with no disability on the written and pictorial metaphor subtests of the RHLB. The presence of intact pragmatic skills alongside impairments is similar to the pattern observed at other language levels (e.g. syntax) and most likely reflects the broad range of competencies which underlie the pragmatics of language.

2.2.3 Emotional and Behavioural Disorders

In some children and adults, language and communication impairments occur in the presence of significant emotional problems and behavioural disturbances which have their onset in the early years. Although this clinical population is variously defined by educational bodies and health agencies, emotional and behavioural disorders (EBDs) will be taken in this chapter to include the following conditions: attention deficit hyperactivity disorder (ADHD), conduct disorder, and selective mutism.[4] While children with each of these disorders can present with significant communication problems, these problems are most prominently acknowledged in the diagnostic criteria for ADHD. In this way, DSM-5 states that the individual with ADHD who has symptoms of inattention 'often does not seem to listen when spoken to directly' (American Psychiatric Association 2013). A child or adult with symptoms of hyperactivity and impulsivity 'often talks excessively', 'often blurts out an answer before a question has been completed (e.g. completes people's sentences; cannot wait for turn in conversation)' and 'butts into conversations'. With these various conversational anomalies on display, it is not surprising that this population of individuals is beginning to attract the attention of clinical pragmatists.

The prevalence of emotional and behavioural disorders has tended to vary with each epidemiological study. However, one reasonably consistent finding is that ADHD is the most common of these disorders. Using data from the 2010 National Health Interview Survey in the US, Bloom et al. (2011) reported that an estimated 8 % of children under 18 years of age had ADHD. In a study of all 4-year-olds born in 2003 or 2004 in the Norwegian city of Trondheim, Wichstrøm et al. (2012) reported estimated population rates for the following disorders: ADHD (1.9 %), oppositional defiant disorder (1.8 %), conduct disorder (0.7 %) and anxiety disorders (1.5 %). The authors acknowledged a lower prevalence of these disorders among pre-schoolers than has been found in previous studies from the US. Research into the aetiology of emotional and behavioural disorders continues apace. In a review of literature on the aetiology of ADHD, Millichap (2008, p. e363) states that '[a] genetic cause linked to dopamine deficit is frequent and primary, but various environmental factors, including viral infection, maternal smoking during pregnancy, prematurity, cerebral hypoxic ischemia, alcohol exposure, and nutritional and endocrine disorders may contribute as secondary causes'.

Expressive and receptive language disorders are increasingly being identified in children with emotional and behavioural disorders. In a study of 84 public school children with EBDs, Benner (2005) obtained prevalence rates of total, expressive and receptive language disorders of 54, 55 and 42 %, respectively. Mackie and Law (2010) found that 7- to 11-year-old children with emotional/behavioural difficulties were significantly more likely to have structural language and word decoding difficulties than age- and sex-matched controls. Manassis et al. (2007) examined the language skills of 6- to 11-year-old children with selective mutism. These children scored significantly lower on standardized language measures than children with anxiety and normal controls. Kim and Kaiser (2000) reported that children with ADHD performed worse than typically developing children on the sentence imitation (grammar) and word articulation (phonology) subtests of the Test of Language development—Primary (Newcomer and Hammill 1991). Boys and girls with ADHD are at an increased risk of written language disorder and reading disability (Yoshimasu et al. 2010, 2011). For a review of literature on language impairments in ADHD, conduct disorder and other emotional and behavioural disorders, the reader is referred to Sundheim and Voeller (2004) and Bellani et al. (2011).

Pragmatic deficits have been commonly reported in children with EBDs. Donno et al. (2010) reported significantly poorer pragmatic language skills in a group of persistently disruptive school children than in a comparison group. Gilmour et al. (2004) found that two thirds of their sample of 55 children with conduct disorder had pragmatic language impairments as measured on the Children's Communication Checklist (Bishop 1998). The pragmatic impairments of these children were similar in nature and degree to those of children with autism. Kim and Kaiser (2000) found that children with ADHD produced more inappropriate pragmatic behaviours in conversational interactions than typically developing children, despite having similar pragmatic knowledge, as measured by the Test of Pragmatic Language (Phelps-Terasaki and Phelps-Gunn 1992). Mathers (2006) reported that children with ADHD used more tangential and unrelated information during spoken texts than control children. In a study of 76 children diagnosed with ADHD, Bruce et al. (2006) found that almost half displayed moderate to severe language comprehension problems, most often occurring together with communication problems. The comprehension and communication subdomains of language were assessed in this study by means of pragmatic items in a parent-completed questionnaire (e.g. 'tends to misinterpret what is said', 'difficulty carrying on a conversation').

Discourse deficits are also widely reported in children with EBDs, particularly during narrative production and comprehension. Rumpf et al. (2012) examined the organization of narratives in children with ADHD. Only one of 9 children with ADHD (11 %) was able to verbalize the core aspects of the story adequately. This contrasted with 27 % of children with Asperger's syndrome and 82 % of healthy controls. This difference in frequencies was significant and pointed to limited coherence in the narratives of children with ADHD (and Asperger's syndrome also). Berthiaume et al. (2010) found that boys with ADHD were less able than comparison peers to draw inferences, particularly explanatory inferences, which link events in a story. They were also less able than peers to monitor their ongoing comprehension of texts. McInnes et al. (2004) found that children with selective mutism used fewer story elements (viz., settings, initiating events, internal responses) during their production of narratives than children with social phobia. In terms of narrative comprehension, McInnes et al. (2003) reported that children with ADHD, who did not have co-occurring language impairment, comprehended factual information in spoken passages, but were poorer at comprehending inferences. Not all studies have found a relationship between emotional and behavioural disorders and pragmatic and discourse deficits. Cohen et al. (2000) found no support for their hypothesis that ADHD would be associated with narrative discourse and pragmatics.

2.2.4 Intellectual Disability

Language development is often severely delayed and deviant in the presence of cognitive or intellectual disability. Pragmatic language skills are no exception in this regard with many experiencing the same developmental disruption as language in general. In DSM-5, the term 'intellectual developmental disorder' replaces the earlier (and now unacceptable) diagnostic label of mental retardation. Intellectual developmental disorder (IDD) is defined as a disorder that includes both a current intellectual deficit (e.g. in reasoning and problem-solving) and a deficit in adaptive functioning with onset during the developmental period. Adaptive functioning captures how well an individual meets standards of personal independence and social responsibility in daily life activities such as social participation or functioning at school or at work. A diagnosis of IDD is equivalent to performance on standardized tests of intellectual function which is approximately 2 standard deviations below the population mean. This level of performance equates to an Intelligence Quotient (IQ) score of 70 or below. In recent years, diagnosing clinicians have attempted to supplement IQ test scores with performance on a range of social and adaptive criteria. This can be seen in the definitions of severity levels of IDD in DSM-5, which focus on adaptive functioning rather than on IQ test scores.

Recent epidemiological investigations have reported the prevalence of intellectual disability to be less than 1 %. The prevalence of intellectual disability in

China in 2006 was 0.75 % (Kwok et al. 2011). Boyle et al. (2011) estimated the prevalence of intellectual disability between 1997 and 2008 in US children aged 3–17 years to be 0.71 %. The prevalence was higher in boys than in girls (0.78 and 0.63 %, respectively). Prevalence rates were higher in children aged 11–17 years than 3–10 years (0.84 and 0.59 %, respectively), and varied with the race and ethnicity of children—intellectual disability was most prevalent in non-Hispanic Black children (1.06 %) and least prevalent in non-Hispanic white children (0.62 %). In terms of aetiology, a large range of organic conditions is associated with intellectual disability. These conditions include genetic syndromes (e.g. Down's syndrome, fragile X syndrome), prenatal exposure to teratogens (e.g. alcohol, cocaine), cerebral and other infections (e.g. meningitis, rubella), metabolic disorders (e.g. phenylketonuria, congenital hypothyroidism) and birth anoxia. Despite extensive evaluation, the aetiology of intellectual disability cannot be determined in 30–50 % of cases (Daily et al. 2000).

Given the clinical and aetiological heterogeneity of children and adults with intellectual disability, investigators have tended to describe the speech, and expressive and receptive language problems of this population in relation to specific syndromes. Down's syndrome is the most common genetic cause of mild to moderate intellectual disability (National Institutes of Health 2008). In 2002, the prevalence of this syndrome in 10 regions in the US among children and adolescents aged 0–19 years was 10.3 per 10,000 (Shin et al. 2009). Articulation skills in children and adults with Down's syndrome are often poor on account of the presence of flaccid dysarthria. Receptive language is typically superior to expressive language with difficulties particularly evident in phonology and syntax (Martin et al. 2009). Children with Down's syndrome are slow to acquire the phonological system of language and a productive vocabulary (Stoel-Gammon 2001). Vocabulary knowledge and, to a lesser extent, phoneme awareness are strong predictors of reading skills in children with Down's syndrome (Hulme et al. 2012). Syntactic deficits are common in children and adults with this syndrome. During conversation, children with Down's syndrome have been found to produce shorter, less complex utterances overall and less complex noun phrases, verb phrases, questions and negations than typically developing children (Price et al. 2008).

The language features of other, less common syndromes have also been examined. In a study of 32 individuals with Prader-Willi syndrome, Van Borsel et al. (2007) identified problems with expressive language, morphosyntax and vocabulary, while phonology is relatively intact. In verbal individuals with cri du chat syndrome, there are receptive and expressive language delays, although receptive language is generally superior to expressive language (Kristoffersen 2008). Phonological problems are present and include frequent substitutions, omissions and distortions. Consonant inventories are small, syllable shapes are restricted and vowels are variable. In terms of morphosyntax, individuals with cri du chat syndrome can inflect words from all the major word classes. Little is still known about syntactic skills in this syndrome (Kristoffersen 2008). Syndrome-specific characterisations of language enable investigators to address theoretically significant questions. For example, there is little evidence that syntax, morphology, phonology or pragmatics in children and adults with Williams syndrome exceed non-verbal abilities (Brock 2007). This lack of dissociation between verbal and non-verbal abilities provides support for neuroconstructivist accounts of language development. For further discussion of this issue, the reader is referred to Stojanovik (2014).

Pragmatic language skills in individuals with intellectual disability have attracted considerable attention from investigators. This is particularly the case in Williams syndrome, where significant weaknesses in pragmatic language skills and relational/conceptual language occur alongside relative strengths in concrete vocabulary and verbal short-term memory and grammatical abilities which are consistent with general intellectual ability (Mervis and John 2010). Philofsky et al. (2007) reported that school-age children with Williams syndrome have pragmatic language difficulties, as measured on the Children's Communication Checklist-2 (CCC-2; Bishop 2003). The performance of these children on most subscales of the CCC-2 was similar to that of children with ASD. These findings reinforce earlier results obtained by Laws and Bishop (2004). During a referential communication task, children with Williams syndrome have been found to verbalize the inadequacy of messages on less than half the occasions when this was necessary (John et al. 2009).

Several studies have examined figurative language in Williams syndrome. These studies have revealed the contribution of lexical semantic knowledge to the production and comprehension of figurative language. Thomas et al. (2010) reported that individuals with Williams syndrome may access different, less abstract knowledge during the completion of figurative utterances than typically developing individuals. Naylor and van Herwegen (2012) found that synonymy knowledge was the best predictor of figurative language production scores in Williams syndrome. Preschoolers with Williams syndrome can use gestures, particularly pointing, to infer the communicative intent of a speaker. However, significantly more preschoolers with Down's syndrome than with Williams syndrome were able to use communicative gestures for this purpose (John and Mervis 2010). Other pragmatic findings in Williams syndrome include problems with idiom comprehension and failure to interpret ironic jokes (the latter interpreted as lies) (Sullivan et al. 2003; Lacroix et al. 2010).

Pragmatic and discourse deficits have also been documented in a number of other syndromes associated with intellectual disability. A subject with Down's syndrome investigated by Papagno and Vallar (2001) exhibited impaired comprehension of metaphors and idioms in the presence of largely preserved phonological, syntactic and lexical-semantic skills. Adolescents with Prader-Willi syndrome and nonspecific mental retardation have been found to classify ironic jokes incorrectly as lies, because they do not correspond to reality (Sullivan et al. 2003). Estigarribia et al. (2011) obtained evidence of narrative impairment affecting macrostructural story grammar elements in boys with fragile X syndrome. During conversations, individuals with fragile X syndrome have been found to produce more tangential language than clinical control groups, especially within unsolicited comments (Sudhalter and Belser 2001). Comblain and Elbouz (2002) reported that boys with fragile X syndrome were less efficient than typically developing children matched for lexical age in organizing new and old information during referential communication tasks. Thorne et al. (2007) found that the rate of ambiguous nominal reference during picture-elicited narratives was highly accurate in classifying children with a foetal alcohol spectrum disorder. These findings indicate that pragmatic deficits must be considered by clinicians who are working with clients with intellectual disability regardless of aetiology.

2.3 Pragmatic Disorders in Older Childhood and Adolescence

The acquisition of language and pragmatic skills may be developmentally appropriate up to a certain stage. However, even as certain language skills are in place, and other language skills are yet to be acquired, a child may sustain injury or develop disease. For example, the 8-year-old child may develop one of a range of different brain tumours. The growth of these tumours may damage brain tissue and not simply in the areas immediately next to the tumours. The treatment of brain tumours involves a combination of neurosurgery, cranial irradiation and chemotherapy. Each of these interventions can compromise language and cognitive skills, in some cases for many years after the point of treatment. Although there has been little systematic examination of pragmatic skills in children with brain tumours, the neuropsychological profile of these children provides grounds for believing that pragmatics may not emerge unscathed in this group of clients.

Also, children who have already undergone substantial language acquisition may sustain a traumatic brain injury (TBI). So-called childhood TBI is now known to result in marked difficulties with pragmatics and discourse. These children present with a complex clinical picture in that some previously acquired language skills are impaired and the acquisition of later language skills is compromised. Additionally, the neural plasticity of the maturing brain enables it to respond in remarkable and unpredictable ways to traumatic injuries. This range of factors means that the pragmatic and discourse skills of these children are likely to be subject to considerable change in the weeks and months following a traumatic brain injury. This section will examine what is known about the pragmatic disorders of these two clinical populations.

2.3.1 Childhood Brain Tumours

As used in this section, the term 'brain tumour' refers to a mixed group of neoplasms which originate from intracranial tissues and the meninges with degrees of malignancy that range from benign to aggressive. The term specifically does *not* include spinal cord tumours, metastatic tumours (these arise outside the central nervous system) and primary brain lymphomas, which are essentially haematological malignancies (McKinney 2004). Brain tumours are the most common category of solid tumours in childhood (Pollack 2011). In an annual report to the nation on the status of cancer, Kohler et al. (2011) reported astrocytomas to be the most common childhood (0–19 years) brain tumour in the US. Depending on type, the median age of astrocytomas in children is 9.0 and 10.0 years. After astrocytomas, two other significant brain tumours in childhood are malignant gliomas (median age 6.0 years) and medulloblastomas (median age 5.0 years). Kohler et al. also reported that one third of all childhood brain tumours are non-malignant. This is a much lower rate of non-malignancy than in adulthood, where two thirds of brain tumours are non-malignant.

In the 1970s and 1980s, management of malignant brain tumours in children involved a combination of surgery, radiation therapy and chemotherapy, while benign tumours were treated almost exclusively by surgery with radiation treatment as a salvage modality (Pollack 2011). It is now widely acknowledged that these treatments are associated with long-term neurocognitive and other sequelae in a large proportion of treated patients (Aarsen et al. 2004; Maddrey et al. 2005). In a study of 61 long-term survivors of childhood brain tumours, Macedoni-Lukšič et al. (2003) found that 38 patients (62 %) experienced at least one impairment as a result of treatment. Some 16 patients (30 %) had an IQ score of less than 80. Among the risk factors and clinical variables associated with IQ decline in children treated for brain tumours are younger age at time of treatment, longer time since treatment, use of radiotherapy and radiotherapy dose, hydrocephalus,[5] and the volume of brain that received treatment (Kieffer-Renaux et al. 2000; Mulhern et al. 2004). Current treatment strategies focus on reducing treatment-related sequelae for children with therapy-responsive tumours and on improving outcome for children with tumours that have historically been resistant to therapy (Pollack 2011).

There is a high incidence of speech, language and hearing symptoms in children and adolescents with brain tumours. Gonçalves et al. (2008) found speech, language and hearing symptoms in 42 % of a sample of 190 children and adolescents with brain tumours. Dysarthria and dysphagia are widely recognised and studied sequelae in children with brain tumours (Cornwell et al. 2003; Morgan et al. 2008). The incidence of dysarthria and dysphagia following surgery for posterior fossa tumour in children is known to be relatively high, affecting around one in three cases (Mei and Morgan 2011). However, alongside speech and swallowing problems there are often long-term language deficits in children with brain tumours. Ribi et al. (2005) reported language deficits in 56 % of their sample of 26 survivors of paediatric medulloblastoma. Some of these language deficits have been documented in patients prior to surgery.[6] However, many more language problems have been reported in children who have undergone surgical interventions for brain tumours.

In a study of five children who received surgical resection of left thalamic tumours, Nass et al. (2000) reported Broca's aphasia in three children, and mixed transcortical aphasia and conduction aphasia in one child each. De Smet et al. (2009) found language deficits, including agrammatism, anomia, impaired verbal fluency and comprehension deficits, in five children following posterior fossa tumour resection. Riva and Giorgi (2000) reported that children with right cerebellar hemisphere astrocytomas showed a slight but non-significant decline in verbal performance following surgery which was most pronounced in relation to receptive syntax and the formulation of sentences (as measured by MLU). Only lexical components of language (naming and comprehension) were impaired in children after surgery for left cerebellar hemisphere astrocytomas. Two children with cerebellar vermis medulloblastomas developed a post-surgical mutism which evolved into a severe language disturbance with similar features to agrammatic aphasia. These children displayed a lack of language spontaneity and spoke very little even when encouraged to do so. Frank et al. (2008) found mild signs of language disturbance in subjects with right-sided lesions following tumour surgery in the cerebellum.[7]

There has been little systematic investigation of pragmatic and discourse skills in children with brain tumours. One of the few studies to assess these skills has revealed significant disruption of pragmatics in the context of intact structural language. Lewis and Murdoch (2010) examined a female patient aged 14.1 years who had received risk-adapted cranial radiation therapy for medulloblastoma 4 years prior to testing. Although this subject's performance on tests of general language skill was within normal limits (one exception was recalling sentences), her high-level language skills were impaired. Several of these skills were pragmatic in nature, e.g. resolving ambiguity, understanding inferential, metaphoric and figurative language, and producing language within the pragmatic constraints of a given situation.

Docking et al. (2005) reported the case of a boy of 6.7 years who received radiotherapy and chemotherapy for treatment of a brainstem glioma diagnosed at 1.8 years. Although this boy performed within normal limits on measures of receptive language, expressive language and phonological awareness skills, his high-level language skills displayed some weaknesses. These weaknesses were evident on subtests which examined the expression of intents and the interpretation of ambiguous sentences. In a later study, Docking et al. (2007) recorded deficits in linguistic problem solving in two patients with ependymoma and juvenile pilocytic astrocytoma of the right and left cerebellar hemispheres, respectively. Both patients displayed intact general language abilities according to normative data.

Hydrocephalus is commonly associated with childhood brain tumours such as gliomas (Roujeau et al. 2011), astrocytomas and medulloblastomas (Di Rocco et al. 2010). Several clinical studies have revealed significant pragmatic and discourse deficits in children with hydrocephalus of diverse aetiologies. Children aged 6 15 years with early-onset hydrocephalus have been found to perform more poorly than normally developing controls on oral discourse tasks that required them to establish alternate meanings for ambiguous sentences, understand figurative expressions, make bridging inferences and produce speech acts (Dennis and Barnes 1993). Barnes and Dennis (1998) reported that children with early-onset hydrocephalus had difficulty using context to derive meaning. Specifically, these children had difficulty drawing inferences during a narrative comprehension task. Their problems interpreting novel figurative expressions contrasted with their ability to understand idiomatic figurative expressions. Moreover, although they produced the same quantity of story content as controls during retellings of fairy tales, children with hydrocephalus produced less of the core semantic content than controls. Difficulties suppressing contextually irrelevant meanings have also been reported in children with hydrocephalus (Barnes et al. 2004). Pragmatic impairments have been identified in young children with myelomeningocele and shunted hydrocephalus (Vachha and Adams 2003).

2.3.2   Childhood Traumatic Brain Injury

Many children successfully acquire language skills only to have them disrupted by a traumatic brain injury (TBI) in older childhood and adolescence. These injuries can be sustained through falls, road traffic accidents (RTAs), sports injuries and assaults, the latter as a result of child abuse or violence between (particularly male) adolescents. There are two main types of TBI. In an open head injury, the brain is damaged by an external missile which also fractures the skull. In a closed head injury, the skull remains intact while the brain is damaged within it. This may be as a result of shearing forces which are sustained during a RTA and which drive the brain against bony protuberances on the inside of the skull. Both focal pathologies (contusion, haematoma formation) and diffuse pathologies (diffuse axonal injury, diffuse microvascular damage) occur in TBI along with more generalized abnormalities involving widespread neuroexcitation and metabolic changes (Povlishock and Katz 2005). Most TBIs—as many 97 % on some estimates (Koepsell et al. 2011)—are mild in severity. TBI can result in adverse neurocognitive and neurobehavioural outcomes including problems with memory, psychomotor processing speed and language in children with mild TBI (Babikian et al. 2011) and executive functions and social competence in children with severe TBI (Ganesalingam et al. 2011). There is also a high incidence of dysarthria and dysphagia in children with severe TBI (Morgan et al. 2010).

Language deficits are commonly found in the paediatric TBI population. As one might expect, these deficits have been found to vary in nature and severity with the child's developmental level at the time of injury. Ewing-Cobbs and Barnes (2002) reported that linguistic deficits at lexical and discourse levels are more often found in young children who sustain severe TBI, while higher-order discourse functions are more commonly disrupted in older children with TBI. Hanten et al. (2009) found that children who were younger when they sustained a TBI achieved poorer overall performance on measures of oral reading and expressive language skills than children who were older when injured. Anderson et al. (2004) obtained reduced expressive and receptive language scores in children with severe TBI. Moreover, while improvements in expressive language skills occurred in the 30 months post-injury, minimal improvements in receptive language were evident during the same time. Moran and Gillon (2004) found that adolescents who had sustained a TBI before 11 years of age performed more poorly than age-matched peers on measures of receptive vocabulary and grammar. At discourse level, literal text comprehension deficits have been reported in children with severe closed head injury (Dennis and Barnes 2001).

While significant structural language skills are often found in paediatric clients with TBI, by far the most pronounced deficits occur in pragmatic and discourse skills. The adolescents with TBI studied by Moran and Gillon (2004) performed more poorly than age-matched peers on tasks requiring the understanding of metaphors and idioms and the comprehension of (causal) inferences. Adolescents also performed more poorly than peers during discourse comprehension, where questions targeted the understanding of details, main idea, prediction, inference and sequence in spoken texts. The inferential comprehension difficulties of these adolescent subjects were greatest when the working memory demands of tasks were high (Moran and Gillon 2005).[8] The comprehension of inferential language was also significantly impaired in the children with severe closed head injury studied by Dennis and Barnes (2001). Furthermore, these children displayed significant problems understanding the mental states and intentions that are the basis of pragmatic processes such as irony appreciation. Related to these children's difficulties with intentionality, Dennis et al. (2001b) found that 6- to 15-year old children with severe closed head injury displayed poor mastery of a task in which they were required to interpret scenarios involving literal truth, ironic criticism and deceptive praise.

Studies of narrative discourse have revealed high-level difficulties with the thematic organization, event sequencing and informational content of narratives produced by children with TBI. Many of these narrative discourse problems are related to executive function deficits in these children. Chapman et al. (2004) examined the ability of children with severe TBI to interpret and summarize information presented in narratives. Compared to typically developing peers, children with TBI—particularly those who sustained early injuries—produced significantly less transformed information during their summaries. Summarization ability was shown to be related to problem solving skills in these children, but not to their lexical or sentence-level language skills. Similar results were obtained by Chapman et al. (2006). These investigators found that the quality of narratives (measured by means of cohesion and coherence) and quantity of narratives (measured by means of the number of words used) were poorer in children with severe TBI than in typically developing children. The ability to recall explicit and implicit discourse content was also poorer in children with TBI than in control children. Once again, discourse performance was poorer in young children with TBI than in older children. Working memory was shown to be significantly correlated with summarization ability in children with TBI.

Brookshire et al. (2000) examined narrative retelling by children who sustained severe or mild closed head injuries. Narratives were assessed on the basis of information and language variables. Children with severe TBI were found to produce narratives which had reduced content and information, impaired organization, and used fewer words and less complex sentences than narratives produced by children with mild TBI. Discourse production was shown to correlate with general verbal ability as well as executive function measures of problem solving and working memory. Other forms of discourse (e.g. expository discourse) are also problematic for children with TBI. Hay and Moran (2005) investigated narrative and expository discourse retelling abilities in nine children with closed head injury. Discourses were examined according to language variables (number of words and T-units, sentential complexity) and information variables (number of propositions, episodic structure elements and global structure elements). In narrative and expository retellings, children with closed head injury performed significantly more poorly than age-matched peers, with performance on narrative tasks superior to performance on expository tasks. In both types of discourse, children with closed head injury differed significantly from age-matched peers in their ability to formulate a moral or aim of the discourse. Many deficits observed in the spoken discourse of children with TBI have also been reported to occur in the written discourse of these children (Wilson and Proctor 2002).

2.4   Pragmatic Disorders in Early to Late Adulthood

Even when language and pragmatic skills are fully acquired, illness, injury and disease in adulthood can result in their breakdown. The onset of mental illnesses in adulthood can have severe, detrimental effects on the pragmatics of language. The most extensively investigated mental illness by clinical language researchers is schizophrenia, although the communication features of other mental illnesses (e.g. bipolar disorder) are increasingly being examined (see chap. 6 in Cummings (2014a) for discussion). Often, pragmatic impairments are more pronounced in individuals with mental illnesses than any deficits in structural language. Like children, adults can sustain traumatic brain injuries. However, unlike children, these injuries occur against a backdrop of much reduced neural plasticity and fully acquired pragmatic skills. The effects of these injuries on language and pragmatic skills are thus likely to differ from those seen in children. Also, recovery of pragmatic skills is also likely to differ from that witnessed in children. It is for these reasons that adults with traumatic brain injury will be discussed as a distinct clinical population in this section.

In middle to late adulthood, several neurodegenerative conditions are beginning to be diagnosed with increasing frequency. These conditions include multiple sclerosis, motor neurone disease and Parkinson's disease (and the less frequently occurring Huntington's disease). Adults with these conditions are at risk of pragmatic disorders often as a result of the significant cognitive deficits that attend these neurodegenerative diseases. However, only in one of these conditions—Parkinson's disease—has there been any systematic examination of pragmatic language skills. This section will examine what is known about pragmatics in these neurodegenerative disorders alongside other disorders which have their onset in early to late adulthood.

2.4.1   Schizophrenia

Schizophrenia is a serious mental illness which has adverse implications for an individual's social, occupational and academic functioning. According to DSM-5, the disorder is diagnosed when two or more of the following symptoms are present: (1) delusions, (2) hallucinations, (3) disorganized speech, (4) grossly abnormal psychomotor behaviour (including catatonia), and (5) negative symptoms (e.g. diminished emotional expression or avolition). The incidence and prevalence of schizophrenia vary with different epidemiological studies. In an overview of three related systematic reviews, McGrath et al. (2008) calculated the median incidence of schizophrenia to be 15.2/100,000 persons, while the median lifetime prevalence was 4.0 per 1,000 persons. The disorder was found to occur more commonly in males than in females in a ratio of 1.4:1. The onset of symptoms in schizophrenia occurs earlier in males than in females. Schürhoff et al. (2004) identified two subgroups of schizophrenic patients according to age of onset. The group with a mean age of onset of 19.91 years consisted predominantly of males, while the group with a mean age of onset of 33.48 years consisted predominantly of females. Antipsychotic medications are the mainstay in the pharmacological treatment of schizophrenia. Notwithstanding these medications and other interventions, the prognosis in schizophrenia is generally poorer than in other types of psychotic and nonpsychotic disorders (Harrow et al. 2005).

Language impairments in clients with schizophrenia affect the phonology, syntax and semantics of language. Deficits in phonological processing (e.g. phonological awareness) have been identified in adults with schizophrenia and are related to reading impairments in these clients (Arnott et al. 2011; Birkett et al. 2011). Receptive and expressive syntax or grammar is impaired in clients with schizophrenia. Semkovska (2010) reported the case of a schizophrenic patient with formal thought disorder in whom syntactic and morphological components of expressive grammar were equally impaired. Condray et al. (2002) reported deficits in receptive syntax, as measured by accuracy of responses to 'who' questions, in male subjects with schizophrenia. Semantic deficits have been reported extensively in this clinical population. Adults with schizophrenia have been found to make significantly more semantic errors on naming tasks, to produce fewer meanings for homophones and to produce fewer items in semantic fluency tasks than healthy control subjects (Vogel et al. 2009). While some authors attribute semantic deficits in this population to problems in lexical-semantic retrieval (Vogel et al. 2009), other authors point to a storage deficit of semantic memory as the cause of semantic impairments (Rossell and David 2006). For a review of language impairments in schizophrenia, the reader is referred to Covington et al. (2005).

By far the most marked linguistic deficits in schizophrenia occur in pragmatics and discourse. Pragmatic impairments are known to compromise the comprehension and recognition of speech acts, maxims and implicatures (Tényi et al. 2002; Mazza et al. 2008). The understanding of non-literal language, including metaphors, irony, proverbs, idioms and humour, is also impaired in adults with schizophrenia (Langdon et al. 2002; Tavano et al. 2008; Thoma et al. 2009; Polimeni et al. 2010). Alongside these receptive pragmatic deficits are a number of expressive deficits in the pragmatics of language. Typically, these are characterized in story-telling contexts. Perlini et al. (2012) reported deficits in local and global coherence during a story-telling task in 30 Italian-speaking patients with schizophrenia. During story retellings, patients with schizophrenia have been found to produce irrelevant information and engage in derailments (Marini et al. 2008). Consistent with this finding of derailments in expressive language, Meilijson et al. (2004) reported that topic was a pragmatic parameter on which their subjects with schizophrenia exhibited a high degree of inappropriate abilities. Clients with schizophrenia also display reduced context processing (Schenkel et al. 2005), are impaired in recognizing and repairing communicative failures (Bosco et al. 2012a) and have problems with referential communication (Champagne-Lavau et al. 2009).

A range of cognitive problems, including theory of mind impairments and executive function deficits, are believed to underlie the pragmatic and discourse impairments of adults with schizophrenia (see Sect. 3.4 in Cummings (2009) and Chap. 3 in this volume for further discussion). One cognitive problem in particular, an impairment of inference and reasoning in schizophrenia (Kruck et al. 2011), is likely to compromise pragmatics more than other cognitive deficits. This is because utterance interpretation is an inferential activity through and through.[9] There is much empirical evidence in support of the claim that inference and reasoning is compromised in schizophrenia. Clients with schizophrenia display impaired probabilistic inference (Averback et al. 2011), transitive inference (Titone et al. 2004), associative inference (Armstrong 2012), analogical reasoning (Simpson and Done 2004), inductive reasoning (Corcoran 2003) and deductive reasoning (Mirian et al. 2011). Moreover, some types of inference and reasoning have been shown to be linked to pragmatic language skills in individuals with schizophrenia. For example, Corcoran (2003) found a substantial correlation between the performance of clients with schizophrenia on an inductive reasoning task and a hinting task. The latter task is a measure of pragmatic language which requires subjects to infer a speaker's intention.

2.4.2 Adult Traumatic Brain Injury

It is important to consider the pragmatic impairments of children and adults who sustain TBI separately. This is because children and adults who sustain TBI have different states of learning and knowledge in place at the time of injury. Disruption of full, adult linguistic competence has a very different clinical manifestation from disruption of the partial linguistic competence of the developing child. This is a point that is frequently attested to in the literature, but is then overlooked as investigators proceed to base interventions for and clinical models of language impairment in childhood TBI on the language impairments of adult clients with TBI. Also, the mature, adult brain which is damaged by a traumatic event is likely to mount a different neural response from that which occurs in the developing brain of a child. Certainly, differences in the neural plasticity of the child and adult brain are commonly acknowledged. This neural response will have implications for the recovery of language in general, and pragmatics in particular, alongside a number of other cognitive functions. It is with these considerations in mind that we discuss adult TBI apart from childhood TBI, notwithstanding certain similarities that will be apparent to the reader between these discussions.

Depending on the clinical criteria used to diagnose TBI, the incidence of TBI in adults has been found to vary substantially. Based on a population in South East Finland, Numminen (2011) reported an annual incidence rate of 221 per 100,000. The majority of patients (71 %) had mild TBI. When cases were excluded which did not exhibit a lack of consciousness or post-traumatic amnesia, the incidence rate was reduced to 137 per 100,000. The incidence of severe TBI is lower still with a rate of 4.1 per 100,000 reported by Andelic et al. (2012) for the adult population of Norway in 2010. Typically, more adult males than females sustain a TBI. In 2010, Andelic et al. (2012) reported the annual incidence of severe TBI for males to be 5.6 per 100,000 while for females the incidence was 2.0 per 100,000. The mean age of adults with severe TBI was 46.7 years. The most common cause of injury was falls (50 %) followed by transport accidents (40 %), assaults (5 %) and other causes (5 %). The median age of patients with TBI hospitalizations caused by transport accidents and assaults was 29 years and 35 years, respectively.

Structural language impairments are relatively common in adults who sustain TBI. The frequency of aphasia following TBI is reported to vary between 11 % and 30 % (Demir et al. 2006). The most common form of aphasia among the 51 subjects studied by Demir et al. was Broca's aphasia (26.5 %) followed by anomic aphasia (19.6 %) and transcortical motor aphasia (15.7 %). Deficits can be found in the reception and production of language across different modalities (e.g. spoken and written language) and language levels (e.g. syntax and semantics). Ellis and Peach (2009) found evidence of language production problems in individuals with TBI during a task that required subjects to produce sentences which varied in syntactic complexity. Subjects with TBI have been found to produce less semantic information during verbal definitions of objects (living and non-living), a deficit which is attributed to difficulty accessing semantic information despite intact organization of semantic knowledge (McWilliams and Schmitter-Edgecombe 2008). Adults with severe TBI also exhibit impaired reading performance (Mathias et al. 2007). In the acute care setting, impairments of language comprehension and expression in patients with TBI are predicted by education and TBI severity as measured on the Glasgow Coma Scale (Leblanc et al. 2006).

Adults with TBI form one of the few clinical populations in which pragmatic and discourse deficits have been more extensively investigated than impairments of structural language. In terms of pragmatics, adults with TBI have been found to exhibit difficulties in the Gricean domains of quantity, relation and manner (Douglas 2010a). During casual conversations with friends, adults with severe TBI have been observed to produce tangential language (Bogart et al. 2012). (Tangential language violates the Gricean maxim of relation.) Moreover, these adults were also found to have difficulty identifying communication breakdown, asking questions (a type of speech act) and engaging in conversational joking (jokes and humour in general make extensive use of non-literal language). Rousseaux et al. (2010a) examined pragmatic skills in dyadic interaction in 18 patients with severe TBI during rehabilitation (2–12 months post-injury) and at the chronic phase in recovery (2 years post-injury). Patients displayed impaired greeting behaviour. They also exhibited difficulty in responding to open questions, presenting new information and introducing new themes, organizing discourse and adapting to interlocutor knowledge.

Dardier et al. (2011) reported pragmatic strengths and weaknesses in 11 French-speaking adults with severe TBI. Adults with TBI were able to comprehend a range of requests (direct, conventional indirect, unconventional indirect) as well as controls. Moreover, no single request type was more difficult than any other for these adults (but see Angeleri et al. below). However, adults with TBI displayed poorer metapragmatic knowledge than controls in that they were less able to give a relevant explanation of their comprehension of requests. They also produced fewer topic-maintaining speaking turns and more speaking turns containing a digression than controls. In fact, compared to controls, adults with TBI adhered to the topic of conversation four times less often and digressed more than 10 times more often. Problems with topic management in TBI—specifically topic repetitiveness—have also been reported by Body and Parker (2005). Angeleri et al. (2008) demonstrated a trend of increasing difficulty in understanding and producing different pragmatic phenomena in patients with TBI. Standard communication acts were easier for these patients than deceits which, in turn, were easier than ironies. This trend was observed in both linguistic and extralinguistic modalities.

A range of discourse deficits has been reported in the adult TBI population. More often than not, narrative discourse is the context in which these deficits are investigated. Carlomagno et al. (2011) examined narrative discourse in 10 non-aphasic adults with TBI. Although the information content of narratives produced by these adults did not differ from those produced by healthy controls (but see below), adults with TBI were found to produce more errors of cohesion, local coherence and global coherence in their narratives than control subjects. Narrative discourse deficits have also been found to occur in adults with TBI who have intact language skills. Marini et al. (2011) examined the narratives of 14 non-aphasic adults with severe TBI. Although the lexical and grammatical skills of these adults were normal, their narratives contained errors of cohesion and coherence. These errors were on account of frequent (self-) interruption of ongoing utterances, derailments and extraneous utterances. The narratives of these adults contained a normal amount of thematic units, but this information was not correctly organized. Investigators have used a range of propositional measures (e.g. propositional complexity index) to account for the reduced informativeness of discourse in adults with TBI. These measures typically indicate that adults with TBI produce significantly fewer propositions per T-unit than controls (Coelho et al. 2005a).

2.4.3 Neurodegenerative Disorders

Several neurodegenerative disorders become increasingly common as people proceed through adulthood. These disorders include, but are by no means limited to, Parkinson's disease (PD), Huntington's disease (HD), multiple sclerosis (MS) and motor neurone disease (MND; also known as amyotrophic lateral sclerosis or ALS). Until recently, it was thought that these disorders only had implications for speech production (and swallowing) with interventions by speech and language therapists aimed almost exclusively at the management of dysarthria (and dysphagia). However, it is becoming increasingly clear that language skills in general, and pragmatic skills in particular, are disrupted in clients with neurodegenerative disorders. These linguistic impairments are often related to the significant cognitive problems that attend these disorders, particularly in relation to executive function skills (see Chap. 3, this volume). Clinical speech and language literature is beginning to reflect this growing appreciation of the pragmatic impairments of clients with neurodegenerative disorders. However, published studies to date are still quite limited in number and have mostly been undertaken in clients with Parkinson's disease. This section will examine what is currently known about the pragmatic skills of these clients and individuals with other neurodegenerative disorders.

Before embarking on an examination of pragmatic deficits in this population, something must be said about the epidemiology and neuropathology of the neurodegenerative diseases which will be examined in this section. Parkinson's disease results from a depletion of dopamine-producing cells in the substantia nigra of the brain. The disease has an incidence rate of 13.4 per 100,000 person-years (Van Den Eeden et al. 2003). This increases rapidly over the age of 60 years, with only 4 % of cases in people under the age of 50 years. In multiple sclerosis, the protective myelin sheath, which covers the axons of neurones in the central nervous system, is degraded in a neuropathological process called demyelination. MS has a lower incidence than Parkinson's disease—7.5 per 100,000 person-years on one estimate (Mayr et al. 2003). The median age at onset varies with different forms of MS. In relapsing-remitting MS, the most common form, the median age at onset is 28.7 years (Confavreux and Vukusic 2006).

In motor neurone disease, a progressive deterioration of upper and lower motor neurones results in reduced innervation to, and consequent atrophy of, muscles that are responsible for a range of motor functions (speech, walking, breathing, etc.). MND is a low incident disorder. Hoppitt et al. (2011) calculated the incidence to be 1.06–2.4 per 100,000 person-years. The peak age of onset of MND for both sexes is 60–64 years (Fong et al. 2005). Huntington's disease is an autosomal dominant neurodegenerative disorder that affects the basal ganglia, leading to affective, cognitive, behavioural and motor decline (Reiner et al. 2011). The disease has an incidence of 0.44–0.78 per 100,000 person-years (Hoppitt et al. 2010). In one study of 680 patients with Huntington's disease, the mean age at onset (as determined by neurologists) was 44.0 years (Tsai et al. 2012).

In addition to significant difficulties with speech, voice and swallowing, clients with neurodegenerative disorders also exhibit language problems. This is the case even when there is no cognitive impairment or dementia in these clients. Adults with Parkinson's disease have been found to have problems with intonational marking of syntactic boundaries (MacPherson et al. 2011), lexical-semantic processing (Arnott et al. 2010) and receptive syntax (Walsh and Smith 2011). Klugman and Ross (2002) found that 63.3 % of their sample of 30 patients with MS reported language difficulties. Aphasia, alexia and agraphia have been reported rarely in MS individuals (Lacour et al. 2004; Mao-Draayer and Panitch 2004; Varley et al. 2005). Other language impairments in MS include lexical access problems, as indicated by naming deficits (Sepulcre et al. 2011), and difficulties with linguistic expression (Mackenzie and Green 2009). Language impairments, which are not a consequence of dementia or aphasia, have been reported in adults with MND. These impairments include syntactic comprehension problems and agraphic writing errors (Bak and Hodges 2004; Ichikawa et al. 2008). Language impairments are found in early and late Huntington's disease. Teichmann et al. (2005) found that patients in the early stage of HD were impaired in rule application in the domains of morphology and syntax. Saldert and Hartelius (2011) described a woman with advanced HD who had word retrieval problems, reduced comprehension and whose speech was characterized by echolalia.

Pragmatic disorders have been most extensively investigated in adults with Parkinson's disease. These adults present with marked pragmatic impairments, even in the absence of dementia. These impairments include problems with the comprehension of speech acts (Holtgraves and McNamara 2010a), irony (Monetta et al. 2009) and metaphor (Monetta and Pell 2007; McKinlay et al. 2009). McNamara et al. (2010) reported that patients with PD are less likely than control subjects to automatically activate indirect meanings of implicatures. They are also overly confident in their interpretations and unaware of errors of interpretation. McNamara and Durso (2003) reported significant impairments of pragmatic communication abilities in 22 patients with PD, particularly in the areas of conversational appropriateness, turn-taking, prosodics and proxemics. Less research has been conducted into expressive aspects of pragmatics in adults with PD. Holtgraves and McNamara (2010b) found that patients with PD used less polite strategies than control subjects and had difficulty varying the politeness of requests in relation to features of social context such as the power of the recipient. Pragmatic impairments have been shown to correlate with the duration and severity of Parkinson's disease (Hall et al. 2011). They also appear to be linked to cognitive deficits (particularly of working memory) related to frontostriatal dysfunction (Monetta and Pell 2007).

Pragmatic and discourse deficits in adults with other neurodegenerative disorders are increasingly being investigated. Saldert et al. (2010) studied pragmatic and discourse skills in a group of 18 patients with Huntington's disease. These subjects were significantly less able than pair-matched controls to comprehend metaphors, explain lexical ambiguities in sentences and respond to questions about the (explicit and implicit) content of narrative discourse. Notwithstanding similar performance on primary language tasks, patients with HD have been found to be significantly impaired relative to controls on tasks that require the interpretation of ambiguous, figurative and inferential meaning (Chenery et al. 2002). Murray (2000) reported that patients with HD produced the same amount of verbal output as control subjects during a picture description task. However, this output was less informative than that produced by controls. In a study of picture description abilities in six patients with HD, Jensen et al. (2006) reported that patients used significantly fewer action information units than a non-neurologically impaired control group.

Patients with multiple sclerosis have also been found to produce the same quantity of information as controls during narrative discourse (Arnott et al. 1997). However, the narratives of these patients contained less essential story information, and more incorrect and ambiguous information, than the narratives produced by controls. Laakso et al. (2000) reported that a group of patients with MS and self-reported language problems had lower mean scores than healthy control subjects and patients with MS and no reported language problems on tests that required them to comprehend ambiguous sentences and sentences with metaphorical expressions, as well as make inferences and understand implied relationships in the script of a text. None of the language difficulties of these patients were detected by a standard aphasia test. Roberts-South et al. (2012) also found language difficulties in patients with ALS which were not apparent on standardized language tests. Sixteen patients with ALS without dementia, who did not differ from control subjects on any standardized language test, displayed discourse production difficulties during a picture description task. These difficulties were most apparent in discourse content which was more impaired than discourse productivity.

2.5 Pragmatic Disorders in Advanced Adulthood

The post-retirement years are coincident with an increase in cerebrovascular disease and a number of neurodegenerative pathologies. Cerebrovascular accidents or strokes can compromise neuroanatomical areas in the left and right cerebral hemispheres as well as sub-cortical structures. When the language centres in the brain's left hemisphere are damaged, aphasias of various types are the result. Traditionally, clinicians have subscribed to the view that while structural language is impaired in the aphasias, pragmatics is relatively intact. It has become increasingly apparent that this is not the case with many studies of clients with aphasia revealing significant pragmatic problems, not all of which can be accounted for in terms of structural language deficits. The brain's right hemisphere is even more closely associated with pragmatic disorder. Since Penelope Myers' first formal study of right-hemisphere language disorder in 1979, clinical studies have consistently revealed marked pragmatic and discourse deficits in clients with right-hemisphere lesions.

Although cerebrovascular disease is a common cause of pragmatic disorder in the latter years, it is by no means the only organic problem to affect the brain which has implications for language and communication. Dementias of various types are becoming increasingly common in people of advanced years. Although pragmatic skills in clients with Alzheimer's disease, the most common cause of dementia, have been extensively investigated by clinical researchers, relatively little is known about these skills in individuals with one of the non-Alzheimer's dementias. These dementias will be introduced in this chapter in preparation for a more detailed examination of their pragmatic deficits in Chap. 6.

2.5.1 Left-Hemisphere Damage

The language centres in the brain's left hemisphere can be compromised by injury and disease. Among the organic conditions and other events which can damage these centres are traumatic brain injury, cerebrovascular accidents, infections (e.g. meningitis) and benign and malignant neoplasms. The language and pragmatic impairments that result from adult TBI have already been examined and will not be considered further in this section. Among the remaining organic causes listed above, cerebrovascular accidents (CVAs) or strokes are the most significant cause of left-hemisphere damage (LHD) in adults. The World Health Organization states that stroke is the second leading cause of death above the age of 60 years (Mackay and Mensah 2004). It is also the single biggest cause of major disability in the UK. Aphasia is one of the sequelae of stroke, occurring in 35 % of adult stroke patients—an incidence rate of 60 per 100,000 persons per year (Dickey et al. 2010). Less commonly, aphasia is caused by cerebral infections and neoplasms (Mukand et al. 2001; Kastenbauer and Pfister 2003). While aphasia often attends LHD, it is important to acknowledge that LHD can also occur without any resulting aphasia. This section will examine the pragmatic and discourse deficits that are found in adults with aphasia and in adults with left-hemisphere damage in the absence of aphasia.

Language impairment in aphasia can affect the production and reception of language at all levels (e.g. phonology, syntax, semantics[10]) and across all modalities (i.e. speech, writing and signing). Linguistic symptoms tend to coalesce around a number of aphasia syndromes which can be broadly classified as fluent and nonfluent. A comprehensive discussion of these symptoms and aphasia syndromes is beyond the scope of this chapter (see Bastiaanse and Prins (2014) for a detailed account). Not all symptoms have equal implications for pragmatics and discourse. Through their disruption of the linguistic processes of encoding and decoding upon which utterance production and interpretation depend, syntactic and semantic deficits often have adverse consequences for pragmatics and discourse. But even in the presence of these deficits, adults with aphasia can still display pragmatic competence. For example, the adult with agrammatic (non-fluent) aphasia produces utterances in which there is reduced syntactic complexity and omission of grammatical morphemes. These utterances lack the syntactic structure needed to produce conventional indirect speech acts (e.g. the subject pronoun-auxiliary verb inversion present in *Can you open the window?*). However, the relative preservation of content words means that the adult with agrammatic aphasia is often still able to produce informative discourse.

An extensive literature exists on pragmatic and discourse deficits in adults with aphasia. Among these adults, studies have found evidence of impaired comprehension of idioms with understanding taking the form of literal interpretation

(Papagno et al. 2004; Papagno and Caporali 2007), problems with the processing of metaphoric meaning (Giora et al. 2000; Gagnon et al. 2003) and speech acts (Soroker et al. 2005) and impaired comprehension of proverbs (Chapman et al. 1997) and sarcasm (Giora et al. 2000). Rousseaux et al. (2010b) found severe verbal pragmatic disorders during conversation in stroke patients with cortico-sub-cortical lesions and sub-cortical lesions. Narrative and procedural discourse deficits have also been reported in adults with aphasia (Weinrich et al. 2002). Andreetta et al. (2012) examined the narrative discourse skills of 10 subjects with chronic anomic aphasia. These subjects produced more errors of cohesion and global coherence and fewer lexical information units than healthy control individuals. Moreover, these discourse problems were related to the lexical retrieval difficulties of the subjects with anomic aphasia (but see below). The written narratives of eight adults with aphasia were examined by Behrns et al. (2010). Alongside linguistic deficits, these adults were found to produce narratives in which there was reduced productivity and coherence. All but two adults with aphasia produced narratives with relatively well crafted initiating events and last episodes.

The traditional view of pragmatic and discourse deficits in adults with LHD is that these deficits are the consequence of structural language impairments in aphasia. However, there is clear evidence that this is not always the case. Firstly, pragmatic language impairments have been shown to persist despite improvements in structural language in adults with aphasia. Coelho and Flewellyn (2003) examined coherence in the story narratives of a subject with anomic aphasia over a 12-month period. These researchers found that although microlinguistic skills improved over this period, local and global coherence failed to improve appreciably.

Secondly, pragmatic and discourse impairments have been found in adults with LHD who have no aphasia. Ellis et al. (2005) examined cohesion in the narrative discourse of 12 subjects who sustained left-hemisphere strokes. None of these subjects were diagnosed with aphasia or were generally language impaired. Notwithstanding this fact, 8 % of all cohesive ties used by these subjects were incomplete or erroneous, with errors involving ties of reference type (82 %) and lexical type (18 %). Thirdly, pragmatic impairments have been found in extra-linguistic communication where they cannot be related to the presence of linguistic deficits. Cutica et al. (2006) found that subjects with LHD were unable to use videotaped fictions in which actors performed gestures to establish an actor's communicative intention. Studies such as these indicate that researchers must look beyond aphasia-related structural language impairments to explain the pragmatic and discourse deficits of adults with LHD.

2.5.2 Right-Hemisphere Damage

The brain's right hemisphere is at risk of injury and disease from the same illnesses and events which cause lesions in the left hemisphere. Focal lesions of the right hemisphere are most often caused by a CVA but may also result from a brain tumour. Beyond the different functions of the left and right hemispheres, there are reasons for viewing stroke-induced lesions of the right hemisphere differently from those of the left hemisphere. Compared to patients with left-hemisphere stroke, adults with right-hemisphere stroke present later to emergency departments, are less likely to receive thrombolysis, and have worse clinical outcomes (Di Legge et al. 2006; Palmerini and Bogousslavsky 2012). Delays in, and lack of, medical treatment are related to poorer awareness of neurological deficits in right-hemisphere stroke among patients (Ito et al. 2008) as well as insensitivity of stroke severity scales to these deficits (Yoo et al. 2010).

Even as right-hemisphere strokes are underreported and not fully diagnosed, so too are the language deficits caused by these strokes. The high-level language deficits associated with right-hemisphere damage (RHD) are quite unlike the structural language impairments associated with aphasia. Moreover, standardized language batteries are known not to be sensitive to these deficits (Joanette et al. 2014). With these considerations in mind, it can be seen that right-hemisphere language disorder following a stroke is likely to be a somewhat neglected consequence of a cerebral event that is itself not fully recognised and diagnosed.

Clinical researchers have come to the study of right-hemisphere language disorder much later than that of aphasia. However, there is now widespread awareness among investigators of the part played in communication by the brain's right hemisphere and of the substantial number of people who experience communication disorders when this hemisphere is damaged. The incidence of (nondysphasic) language and communication problems in RHD has been estimated to be 50 %, with marked difficulties for 20 % (Benton and Bryan 1996). More recently, Côté et al. (2007) estimated the incidence of these problems to be higher than 50 % in a rehabilitation centre setting. Pragmatic and discourse impairments in the RHD population have been extensively investigated since the late 1970s when Penelope Myers' study of patients with RHD first brought this client group to the attention of clinicians (Myers 1979). Some of the results of this research are considered below.

Findings of pragmatic impairments in adults with RHD are commonplace in the clinical literature. Most often, they describe impaired comprehension of non-literal language. This impairment affects the interpretation of implicatures (Kasher et al. 1999), metaphors (Rinaldi et al. 2004), idioms (Papagno et al. 2006), humour (Heath and Blonder 2005), sarcasm (Giora et al. 2000; Shamay-Tsoory et al. 2005) and indirect speech acts (Hatta et al. 2004). Typically, comprehension problems in RHD are characterized by a tendency towards literal interpretation of utterances. Adults with RHD have been found to have difficulty establishing a speaker's communicative intention in producing non-literal utterances (Cheang and Pell 2006) and contributing to the development of the intentional structure of conversation (Hird and Kirsner 2003). Problems with the interpretation of non-literal language in RHD have been attributed to theory of mind deficits (Winner et al. 1998), visuo-perceptual and visuo-spatial deficits (Papagno et al. 2006) and impaired processing of affective (emotional) prosody and language (Lehman Blake 2003).

Discourse deficits were the focus of Myers' early work[11] and have been extensively documented in adults with RHD. Non-aphasic adults with RHD have been found to produce narratives which contain tangential errors and conceptually incongruent utterances (Marini 2012). Compared to normal controls, adults with RHD have been shown to produce picture descriptions which have poorer information content, cohesion and coherence (Marini et al. 2005). Lehman Blake (2006) reported that discourse produced by adults with RHD during a thinking-out-loud task was rated as more tangential and egocentric than the discourse of healthy older adults. RHD discourse also contained extremes of quantity (i.e. extreme verbosity or paucity of speech). Adults with RHD are less able than non-brain-damaged individuals to use discourse context to resolve lexically ambiguous words (Grindrod and Baum 2005).

In a series of studies by Tompkins and colleagues, discourse deficits in RHD have been related to difficulties in generating and suppressing inferences. Adults with RHD have been found to have difficulty drawing high-level inferences about the motives of characters in narratives (Tompkins et al. 2009). Although adults with RHD are able to generate predictive inferences during the presentation of narratives, they are less able to maintain those inferences than non-brain-damaged adults (Lehman-Blake and Tompkins 2001). The suppression of inappropriate inferences is a significant predictor of narrative discourse comprehension in adults with RHD (Tompkins et al. 2000, 2001). Conversely, greater activation for contextually inappropriate interpretations is associated with poorer discourse comprehension performance in adults with RHD (Tompkins et al. 2004). Tompkins et al. (2008) found that adults with RHD who had difficulty sustaining activation for the peripheral semantic features of nouns—a phenomenon known as coarse coding—were also relatively poor comprehenders of implied information from narratives. For further discussion of this research, the reader is referred to Joanette et al. (2014).

2.5.3 Dementias

The dementias are a large and varied group of neuropathologies that lead eventually to the loss of cognitive and physical functions in affected individuals. People with dementia may experience mild cognitive impairment initially which develops over time into mutism, incontinence, immobility and dependence on others for all aspects of care. Dementias can be caused by infections (e.g. HIV infection), excessive alcohol consumption over an extended period of time (e.g. Korsakoff's syndrome), cerebrovascular disease (e.g. vascular dementia) and age-related degenerative changes in the brain (e.g. Alzheimer's disease).

Many people who develop dementia do so outside of the period we are describing as advanced adulthood (i.e. 66–85 years). These cases of early-onset dementia are often associated with certain types of dementia. In a sample of 948 patients meeting established clinical criteria for a dementing illness,

McMurtray et al. (2006) found that 278 patients (about 30 %) had an age of onset less than 65 years. These patients had significantly more dementia which was attributed to TBI, alcohol, HIV and frontotemporal lobar degeneration. Nevertheless, the age of onset for the large majority of people (about 70 %) who develop dementia is greater than 65 years. These cases of late-onset dementia are typically associated with Alzheimer's disease (McMurtray et al. 2006). It is these latter cases which we will examine in this chapter. The non-Alzheimer's dementias will be discussed in Chap. 6.

Alzheimer's disease (AD) is a common condition which places a large economic and health burden on developed countries with aging populations. Currently, it is estimated that approximately 5.4 million Americans have AD, a figure which is expected to nearly triple to 14.5 million people over the next 40 years (Lopez 2011). The prevalence of AD is 4.9 % while the incidence is 2.3 per 100 person-years (Katz et al. 2012). Although AD rates increase with age, they do not differ by sex (Katz et al. 2012). The neuropathological processes of AD are relatively well understood even if what triggers these pathological changes to occur has still to be established. Brain tissue is characterized by the presence of amyloid plaques, neurofibrillary tangles, neuronal loss (and synapses) and cerebral amyloid angiopathy, which is the build-up of proteins called amyloid on the walls of the arteries in the brain (Lopez 2011). Once symptoms appear, the disease has a relentless progression. On one estimate, the median survival from initial diagnosis is 4.2 years for men and 5.7 years for women (Larson et al. 2004).

Along with other cognitive functions, language deteriorates with the onset and progression of Alzheimer's disease. However, there is evidence that this deterioration does not affect all language levels to the same extent or at the same time. The language hierarchy, which proceeds from simple to more complex units of language along the ranks of phonology, morphology, syntax and semantics, was the focus of a review of studies of language impairment in AD by Emery (2000). It was concluded that the decline of language in AD is hierarchical in nature, with late-acquired aspects of language deteriorating before aspects of language which are acquired early in development. Semantic and lexical aspects of language are thus more vulnerable to early deterioration in AD than phonological and syntactic aspects. Even within language levels there is an age of acquisition effect. This effect has been demonstrated for word production and recognition, for example. On a semantic fluency task, Sailor et al. (2011) found that patients with AD produced words which have an earlier age of acquisition. Cuetos et al. (2010) observed a similar age of acquisition effect during a word recognition task, with AD patients recognizing fewer late than early acquired words correctly.

Pragmatic and discourse aspects of language are still being acquired long after phonology and syntax are well established components of a child's linguistic competence (Levorato and Cacciari 2002; Nippold et al. 2005). To this extent, one might reasonably expect pragmatic and discourse skills to be particularly vulnerable to early deterioration in AD. There is evidence to indicate that this is the case. In one of the few studies to document longitudinal deterioration of language skills in patients with Alzheimer's disease, Bayles et al. (1992) found significant discourse impairments at stages of the disease when structural language skills were still relatively intact. Two discourse tasks examined the ability of patients with AD to produce relevant information units about the setting, events and main idea of a picture (picture description task) and to provide relevant, non-redundant and truthful information about an object (object description task). The Global Deterioration Scale (GDS; Reisberg et al. 1982) was used to determine the stage of dementia in patients. Of the seven stages of dementia recognized by the GDS, three will be examined here.

Patients at GDS = 3 exhibit the earliest, clear-cut clinical deficits of dementia. While these patients scored at the 90 % or better level of the normal mean on oral reading, superordinate identification, auditory comprehension and writing to dictation, they performed at only 55 % of the normal mean on both discourse tasks. Patients at GDS = 4 are in the late confusional stage. These patients still approximate normal performance on oral reading, reading comprehension and auditory comprehension. However, their performance on picture description is 50 % of the normal mean and is even less than that on object description. Patients at GDS = 5 have moderately severe cognitive decline and exhibit early dementia. These patients' performance on auditory and reading comprehension is still greater than 50 % of the normal mean, while their performance on object and picture description is less than 50 % of the normal mean. The pattern of linguistic impairments is consistent across these stages—the performance of patients with AD on structural language tasks surpasses that on discourse tasks. In a later study, Papagno (2001) reported that decline of figurative language was not an early symptom of dementia in 39 patients with probable AD. Clearly, more research needs to be undertaken into the stage at which language skills in general, and pragmatic skills in particular, deteriorate in AD.

Stage of deterioration aside, pragmatic language skills have been repeatedly found to be impaired in adults with AD. In some studies, impairment of these skills is associated with cognitive decline but not aphasia (Hays et al. 2004). Comprehension of non-literal language is particularly affected. Amanzio et al. (2008) reported that patients with probable AD displayed impaired comprehension of non-conventional or novel metaphors, although their comprehension of conventional metaphors and idioms was intact. Papagno (2001) found that metaphor comprehension in patients with probable AD decreased significantly over time, a pattern not observed for the comprehension of idioms. Idiom comprehension was found to be poor in the patients with AD examined by Rassiga et al. (2009), with comprehension performance correlating with executive tests. Even when literal comprehension in patients with AD is normal or only mildly impaired, idiom comprehension has been found to be very poor (Papagno et al. 2003). Comprehension errors typically take the form of literal interpretation. Of 350 idiom comprehension errors committed by the patients with AD examined by Papagno (2001), 149 (47.3 %) were 'literal or concrete' interpretations.

Studies of the comprehension of sarcasm or irony in patients with AD have produced mixed results. The patients with AD examined by Kipps et al. (2009) had no difficulty appreciating sarcastic statements. Shany-Ur et al. (2012) found that patients with AD did not demonstrate impaired comprehension of sarcasm when overall cognitive deficits were accounted for. However, Bara et al. (2000) reported a significant difference in the percentage of correct responses of 14 patients with AD (19 %) and controls (59 %) on a pragmatic task examining recognition of non-verbal ironies. Leyhe et al. (2011) found that the performance of patients with early AD on a proverb interpretation test was significantly worse than that of healthy controls. Errors produced by the these patients included concrete answers and senseless answers. The completion of proverbs has also been shown to be compromised in patients with AD (Lindholm and Wray 2011). Chapman et al. (1998) found that patients with AD exhibited significant difficulty formulating correct non-literal explanations for proverbs and selecting the correct abstract interpretation of proverbs during a multiple choice proverb interpretation task. Often, patients chose the abstract foil which took the form of another proverb (e.g. selecting *There's more than one way to skin a cat* as the meaning of 'One swallow doesn't make a summer').

Discourse deficits in patients with AD have been examined in conversational and narrative contexts and during referential communication and picture description tasks. Mentis et al. (1995) identified problems with topic management during casual conversational interaction. Patients with AD exhibited reduced ability to change topics, difficulty contributing to the propositional development of topics, and a failure to maintain topics in a clear and coherent manner. Carlomagno et al. (2005) examined the discourse skills of patients with AD during a referential communication task and a picture description task. These patients displayed reduced lexical encoding of information during both tasks, and reduced efficiency in establishing reference during the referential communication task. They also produced confounding and irrelevant information during the referential communication task. As well as expressive discourse deficits, patients with AD have significant difficulty with the comprehension of discourse. Welland et al. (2002) reported poorer overall comprehension of narratives in subjects with early-stage and middle-stage AD than in subjects with no brain damage. The comprehension of subjects with AD was better for main ideas than for details, and for stated information than for implied information.

2.6   Summary

This chapter has examined pragmatic disorders from a life span perspective. This perspective takes a chronological approach to pragmatic disorders, from problems with the development of pragmatic language skills in childhood to the disruption of those skills by injury and disease in adulthood. The organic and other conditions which cause pragmatic disorders have been examined throughout the chapter in a wide-ranging discussion of the aetiology of pragmatic impairment. The chapter has also addressed the prevalence and incidence of pragmatic disorders, most often through an examination of the epidemiology of the conditions that cause these disorders.[12] Pragmatic findings have included the results of experimental studies, analyses of conversation and investigations of non-dialogical discourse (e.g. narrative). These studies have revealed a broad spectrum of pragmatic disorder in children and adults which will be examined further in subsequent chapters.

Notes

1. Several clinical conditions which have marked pragmatic disorders (e.g. autism spectrum disorder, or ADS) are more commonly found in males than in females (see Sect. 3.3.1 in Cummings (2008) for a discussion of sex ratios in ASD). To this extent, more males than females do have pragmatic disorders. However, apart from these specific populations, there is no evidence to suggest that being male per se places one at greater risk of having a pragmatic disorder.
2. It should be noted that substantial investigation of the genetic basis of SLI has been undertaken in recent years. For reviews, the reader is referred to Bishop (2009) and Newbury and Monaco (2010).
3. Katsos et al. are testing these children's understanding of scalar implicatures. A scalar implicature is a type of generalized conversational implicature. In the utterance 'Mike attended some of the classes' there is a scalar implicature to the effect that he did not attend all the classes. The terms <all, most, many, some> differ in informational strength, with 'all' the semantically strongest and 'some' the semantically weakest terms in the set. By asserting the weakest term 'some', a speaker may be taken to implicate 'not all/most/many'.
4. In DSM-5, ADHD is included in the category Neurodevelopmental disorder while selective mutism is a specifier in the category Social anxiety disorder (Social phobia). Conduct disorder occurs alongside a number of other conditions (e.g. oppositional defiant disorder) in the category Disruptive, Impulse Control, and Conduct disorders.
5. The presence of hydrocephaly has been identified as a factor in reduced language outcomes (Lewis and Murdoch 2011a).
6. Di Rocco et al. (2011) identified pre-surgical language impairment in children with posterior fossa tumours. Moreover, pre-surgical language impairment was found to be a risk factor for the development of cerebellar mutism syndrome following surgery.
7. It is important to note that the treatment of childhood brain tumours does not always result in language impairments. Docking et al. (2005) found that six children treated for brainstem tumour demonstrated intact language and phonological awareness abilities. In a later study, Docking et al. (2007) reported intact abilities in receptive language (including vocabulary), expressive language and naming in four children treated with surgery and/or radiotherapy for cerebellar tumour. Richter et al. (2005) found no signs of aphasia in 12

children and adolescents who underwent surgery for cerebellar astrocytoma. Frank et al. (2007) found preserved naming and verb generation accuracy in nine children and adolescents following surgery for cerebellar tumours. Lewis and Murdoch (2011b) reported intact language skills and semantic processing in a 14-year-old female who received fractionated cranial radiation dosages for treatment of medulloblastoma at 10 years and 3 months. In other cases, treatment has actually resulted in improvements in language function. Mabbott et al. (2007) found improvement in receptive language in a preschool child who received surgery, chemotherapy, stem cell transplant and radiation for the treatment of medulloblastoma.

8. Many higher-level pragmatic and discourse impairments in childhood TBI are related to memory deficits and other executive function disorders in this population (see Chap. 3, this volume). The relationship of pragmatic and discourse impairments to executive function deficits, often in the absence of structural language problems, is the basis for the use of the term 'cognitive communication disorder' in relation to the communication difficulties of both children and adults with TBI.

9. It should be noted, however, that the exact nature of the inferences involved in utterance interpretation is still unknown. The reader is referred to chap. 3 in Cummings (2005) for further discussion.

10. Not all language levels are impaired in individuals with aphasia. El Hachioui et al. (2012) examined phonology, syntax and semantics in 141 subjects with acute stroke-induced aphasia. In 22.4 % of subjects, deficits were found in only one of three linguistic levels. Phonology was the language level most likely to be disrupted (16.3 %) followed by syntax (3.4 %) and semantics (2.7 %). Also, the recovery of language levels does not follow a parallel course, with evidence of earlier recovery (up to 7 weeks post-stroke) for syntax and semantics and somewhat later recovery (up to 4 months) for phonology.

11. Myers (1979) had her subjects with RHD describe the cookie theft picture from the Boston Diagnostic Aphasia Examination (Goodglass and Kaplan 1972).

12. This 'indirect' approach to the epidemiology of pragmatic disorders is necessitated by the lack of epidemiological work on communication disorders. Some indication of the extent to which epidemiology has been neglected in the study of communication disorders is apparent from a workshop held in March 2005 by the National Institute on Deafness and Other Communication Disorders (NIDCD). At this workshop, it was reported that only 1.1 % of all NIDCD funded grants are associated with epidemiology.

Chapter 3
Disorders of the Pragmatics-Cognition Interface

3.1 Introduction

The interpretation of any utterance involves a complex interplay of cognitive processes. These processes resolve into two types. Firstly, a hearer must use a range of general cognitive skills such as attention and memory in order to attend to a linguistic stimulus (an utterance) and retain this stimulus in memory while other cognitive operations can be performed upon it. These general cognitive skills are not unique to utterance interpretation and, indeed, are also used in the cognitive processing of non-linguistic stimuli (e.g. visual perception). Theorists have standardly characterized them as executive function skills. Secondly, a hearer must also deploy cognitive skills which, although they are not unique to utterance interpretation, assume a form that is nevertheless specific to this linguistic process. Within this category is included a set of metarepresentational skills of the type identified by theorists and researchers as a theory of mind. Both types of cognitive process are integral to utterance interpretation. It is to be expected, therefore, that deficits of these processes will have adverse consequences for a range of pragmatic phenomena in language.

In this chapter, we examine the cognitive skills involved in utterance interpretation and the different ways in which utterance interpretation may be disrupted by impairments of those skills. This examination will include a range of clinical populations in which cognitive deficits are believed to play a central role in disorders of the pragmatics of language. The chapter will also consider theories of these cognitive processes, and assess if these theories can explain the types of communicative problems encountered by children and adults with pragmatic disorders. To begin with, however, the role of cognition in utterance interpretation will be examined by considering how cognitive skills contribute to a range of pragmatic phenomena in language.

L. Cummings, *Pragmatic Disorders*, Perspectives in Pragmatics,
Philosophy & Psychology 3, DOI: 10.1007/978-94-007-7954-9_3,
© Springer Science+Business Media Dordrecht 2014

3.2 Pragmatics and Cognition

While enlightening on some occasions, standard ways of talking about cognition in relation to utterance interpretation can also lead to misconceptions. One such misconception is the idea that cognitive processes as wide-ranging as linguistic decoding, perception and reasoning are essentially separable from the processes of pragmatic interpretation. This is particularly clearly demonstrated in the case of linguistic decoding where syntactic and semantic rules are assumed to arrive at the decoded content of an utterance to which inferential processes of pragmatic interpretation are then applied. (It will be shown below that this overlooks the important role of inferential processes in arriving at decoded content.) The problem with this view of the relationship between pragmatics and other aspects of cognition is that it assumes that there is a clear boundary between these domains when, in fact, every aspect of utterance interpretation is cognitive through and through. To demonstrate this, consider the following exchange between Bob and Sue:

> Bob: Did Sally come home late last night?
> Sue: Her car is not in the driveway.

This short exchange between Bob and Sue contains examples of the following central pragmatic phenomena: implicature, presupposition, speech acts and deixis. It is a *presupposition* of Bob's question that Sally did come home. Sue clearly recognises Bob's utterance as a particular type of *speech act*—a question—to which she must offer a response. Sue's response is intended to address the presupposition of Bob's utterance—not only did Sally not come home late, but she did not come home at all. However, Sue does not directly override this presupposition. Rather, she does so indirectly by way of *implicature*. Moreover, two aspects of *deixis* in Bob's utterance—the verb 'come' and the noun phrase 'last night'—tell us something about Bob's spatial location (he is at home) and the time period to which he refers (Bob is talking about the hours which elapsed overnight and are immediately prior to his utterance). Even apart from these core pragmatic concepts, Bob and Sue have employed other linguistic features in their utterances which are also pragmatic in nature. Bob is able to include the name 'Sally' in his utterance because he knows Sue will know the referent of this proper noun. It is this same shared knowledge between the participants in the exchange that allows Sue to use 'her car' without fear of ambiguity—Sue will expect Bob to readily identify Sally as the owner of the car.

This apparently simple exchange between Bob and Sue belies a complex array of cognitive processes in the absence of which this interaction would not be possible. Specifically, both participants must attend to the linguistic utterances of the other. However, Bob and Sue's *attention* must extend beyond the purely linguistic stimulus of the utterance to include attention to facial expressions, aspects of the physical context of the exchange, and much else besides. Having directed attention to linguistic and non-linguistic stimuli, Bob and Sue must engage in *perception* of those stimuli. It is their capacity for perception that allows Bob and Sue to distinguish their utterances from a range of other ambient sounds and as something distinctly linguistic in nature. As well as perception, Bob and Sue must hold the utterances in the above exchange in working or short-term memory while linguistic decoding takes place. The fleeting representation of the utterance that is held in short-term memory is of sufficient duration to allow a range of specialised phonological, syntactic and semantic processes to determine the propositional content of what each has said. These processes are still cognitive operations, albeit ones which are adapted to linguistic input alone. Information stored in long-term memory such as semantic knowledge also comes into play during linguistic decoding.

To this point, we have described a range of cognitive processes that are integral to the interpretation of the utterances in the above exchange. Yet, we have still not described how a cognitive capacity for mental state attribution (i.e. theory of mind) also plays a key role in the interpretive processes by means of which Bob and Sue understand the utterances in this exchange. It is now widely acknowledged by theorists that there is substantial intrusion of pragmatics into the propositional content of utterances.[1] For example, Bob and Sue must use pragmatic skills to establish the referents of 'Sally' and 'her car' in the utterances in the above exchange in order to arrive at the propositional content of these utterances. But these pragmatic skills are at all possible because Bob and Sue are able to attribute certain *knowledge* states to each other's minds, specifically, knowledge of who Sally is and that she owns a car.

This same ability to attribute mental states to the minds of others is also evident in how Bob and Sue manage the implicature, speech act and presupposition in the above exchange. Bob must attribute a certain *belief* to Sue—Sue believes that Sally did not come home at all—if he is to understand the relevance of Sue's utterance as a response to his question. Sue communicates this belief indirectly to Bob by way of implicature, and Bob recovers this implicature when he establishes the *communicative intention* that motivated Sue's utterance. By the same token, Sue must be able to establish that Bob is asking a question because he *wants* to be given certain information. Finally, Bob can only presuppose that Sally came home because he believes this information is part of Sue's knowledge (as it turns out, he is mistaken). In short, each of these mental states—knowledge, belief, communicative intention, and desire—speaks to the central role of theory of mind skills in the interpretation of utterances.

As the above discussion demonstrates, it makes little sense to attempt an account of utterance interpretation in the absence of the cognitive processes that make such interpretation possible. In fact, cognitive processes are so deeply interwoven with utterance interpretation that it is misleading to view the cognitive domain as having a discrete or separable relationship to pragmatics. Utterance interpretation is cognitive through and through. A fortiori, the pragmatic processes that speakers and hearers use to generate and interpret utterances must have a cognitive quality that extends beyond that of a mere influence of the cognitive domain on pragmatics. In Sects. 3.3 and 3.4, the two main types of cognitive process discussed above—theory of mind and executive function—will be examined in detail. With this examination complete, it will then be possible to address what is known about the relationship of deficits in these cognitive processes to pragmatic disorders in Sect. 3.5.

3.3 Theory of Mind

Theory of mind (ToM), also known as mentalizing or mind-reading, describes the ability to attribute mental states both to one's own mind and to the minds of others. Mental states so attributed allow us to predict and explain the behaviour of others. The term was originally used by Premack and Woodruff, two primatologists, in a 1978 paper entitled "Does the chimpanzee have a 'theory of mind'?". In that paper, Premack and Woodruff defined this concept as follows:

> In saying that an individual has a theory of mind, we mean that the individual imputes mental states to himself and others [...] A system of inferences of this kind is properly viewed as a theory, first because such states are not directly observable, and second, because the system can be used to make predictions, specifically about the behaviour of other organisms. (1978, p. 515)

Leaving aside questions in primatology, theory of mind has been a hugely influential concept in the study of human psychology. For over 30 years, psychologists have subjected theory of mind to rigorous experimental investigation in children and adults. False belief tests have become the standard means of testing ToM skills. In a false belief test, a story is enacted through the use of two dolls. (These tests have become known as Sally-Anne experiments on account of the names of the dolls first used in these experiments.) Children observe a scenario in which one doll (Sally) switches the location of an object that is subsequently requested by the other doll (Anne). Importantly, Anne is unaware that this switch has been made and believes that the object is still in the original location where she placed it. The child who appreciates that Anne now has a false belief about the location of the object, a false belief that leads her to search for the object in its original location, is said to have passed the test. This child is aware that other agents (represented here by the doll Anne) can have beliefs that differ from his or her own. False belief tests can be used to examine ToM skills of increasing complexity. The simplest of these tests examines first-order ToM skills, i.e. the ability to attribute to another mind a mental state such as *Anne believes that the object is in the cupboard* (the object's original location).

Much is now known about the normal development of theory of mind in children. The mental states which are attributed to other minds include knowledge, ignorance, beliefs, intentions, desires and pretence. Some of these states are more readily acquired by normally developing children than others. For example, there is evidence that infants can appreciate pretence from around 15 or 16 months of age (Bosco et al. 2006a; Onishi et al. 2007). Ruffman et al. (2002) found that children's desire talk preceded their talk about beliefs. Developmental precursors of ToM skills have also been investigated and include most notably joint attention (Charman et al. 2000). Although normally developing children pass false belief tests for the first time at around 4 years of age, younger children can also pass these tests under certain conditions. Wellman and Lagattuta (2000, p. 25) identify these conditions as downplaying the salience of the real state of affairs or making salient the prior mental state of the actor in the scenario (both encourage the child to consider the actor's false belief), the active engagement of the child in the deception of the target person, phrasing the false belief question in certain ways, and overlearning the main features of the false belief narrative. Baillargeon et al. (2010) review results from investigations which suggest that when spontaneous-response tasks are used—false belief tests typically use elicited-response tasks—infants can already attribute false beliefs in the second year of life.

While most ToM research has been conducted in young children, some studies have examined the ToM achievements of older children and adolescents (Dumontheil et al. 2010). Children of 10 and 11 years of age can pass first- and second-order ToM problems, perform slightly above chance on third-order ToM problems and perform at chance on fourth-order ToM problems (Liddle and Nettle 2006). ToM skills have also been found to decline in later years. For example, Maylor et al. (2002) found that performance on ToM stories in an old age group (mean age = 81 years) was significantly worse than that of two other age groups (mean ages = 19 and 67 years) across all conditions in the study.

Theory of mind has also been examined in a range of clinical populations. Chief amongst these populations are children and adults with autism spectrum disorder (ASD). An early study of the ToM skills of autistic children was conducted by Baron-Cohen et al. (1985) who found that while 85 % of normal children and 86 % of children with Down's syndrome passed the belief question in a false belief test, 80 % of autistic children failed this same question. Of significance was the fact that the four autistic children who did pass the belief question had chronological ages from 10.11 to 15.10 years (it is now widely acknowledged that it takes children with autism until around 10 years of age to pass the same false belief tests that normally developing children can pass at 4 years of age).

This early study has been followed by a plethora of investigations into the ToM skills of children and adults with ASD. Some of the findings from these investigations are that subjects with ASD have diminished awareness of their own and others' intentions (Williams and Happé 2010), display impaired visual perspective-taking (i.e. knowledge that different people may see the same thing differently at the same time) (Hamilton et al. 2009), and have impaired understanding of the perception-knowledge relationship (Lind and Bowler 2010). There is also clear evidence that subjects with ASD have difficulty inferring complex emotions and mental states from faces and voices (Golan et al. 2006; Kleinman et al. 2001; Rutherford et al. 2002), and in social contexts and from non-verbal social cues (David et al. 2010; Golan et al. 2008). It is worth remarking that while impaired ToM has been dominant in cognitive accounts of autism, other theorists have viewed the social cognitive deficits of autism as arising from impairments of social motivation (Chevallier et al. 2012). On this view, disruption of social motivational mechanisms, not impairments of ToM, constitute a primary deficit in autism.

ToM impairments in autism spectrum disorder are developmental in nature, i.e. ToM skills do not develop along normal lines in children with ASD. Other clinical populations in which there are significant developmental ToM deficits are children and adults with specific language impairment (SLI), intellectual disability or one of the emotional and behavioural disorders (EBDs). Clinical studies have revealed that children with SLI exhibit delayed development of visual perspective-taking and make less frequent use of cognitive state predicates than their mental-age peers (Farrant et al. 2006; Johnston et al. 2001). Perhaps unsurprisingly given their language deficits, ToM performance in children with SLI has been found to be related to the language skills of these children. When the linguistic complexity of false belief tests is low, children with SLI have been found to perform similarly to same-age peers (Miller 2001). Furthermore, the performance of children with SLI on false belief tests is predicted by their proficiency in processing the syntax of complement structures (Miller 2004). (A complement structure is an integral part of the mental states that are attributed to agents during false belief tests: *Anne believes that the object is in the cupboard.*)

ToM skills in clients with intellectual disability, often in the presence of various syndromes, have also been examined. ToM deficits have been reported in subjects with Williams syndrome, fragile X syndrome, Down's syndrome and foetal alcohol spectrum disorders (Abbeduto et al. 2001; Cornish et al. 2005; Grant et al. 2007; Rasmussen et al. 2009; Santos and Deruelle 2009; Sullivan and Tager-Flusberg 1999; Yirmiya et al. 1996). Finally, there is some evidence that children with emotional and behavioural disorders such as attention deficit hyperactivity disorder (ADHD) display impairments of ToM skills. Children with ADHD display poorer recognition of emotional facial expressions, lower levels of social perspective-taking and worse performance on second-order ToM tasks than normally developing children (Buitelaar et al. 1999; Marton et al. 2009; Pelc et al. 2006).

With the onset of a number of conditions in adulthood, previously intact ToM skills may become impaired. Clients with adult-onset schizophrenia are known to have significant ToM deficits. These clients perform poorly on first- and second-order ToM tasks (Bozikas et al. 2011). Negative symptoms in schizophrenia have been found to be associated with ToM difficulties, while positive symptoms (e.g. delusions) are linked to overmentalizing (Lincoln et al. 2011; Montag et al. 2011). Although studies have revealed ToM and mentalising deficits in clients with right-hemisphere damage (RHD) (Griffin et al. 2006; Happé et al. 1999; Weed et al. 2010), a review of this area by Weed (2008) judged that evidence for a specific ToM deficit in RHD is still inconclusive.

The evidence for ToM impairments in subjects who sustain a traumatic brain injury (TBI) is also not conclusive. While subjects with severe TBI have been found to perform as well as control subjects on first-order false belief tasks (Muller et al. 2010), other studies have reported that the recognition of basic emotions and capacity for mental state attribution in subjects with TBI are both significantly reduced relative to controls (Henry et al. 2006). ToM impairments in clients with TBI have also been found to remain stable between the time of injury and at 1-year follow-up (Milders et al. 2006). Finally, clinical investigators are increasingly examining ToM deficits in neurodegenerative disorders. ToM deficits have been identified in patients with frontal and behavioural variant frontotemporal dementia (Fernandez-Duque et al. 2009; Gregory et al. 2002; Lough et al. 2006; Torralva et al. 2009), Alzheimer's disease (Castelli et al. 2011; Fernandez-Duque et al. 2009; Gregory et al. 2002), Parkinson's disease (Bodden et al.

2010; Saltzman et al. 2000; Santangelo et al. 2012), multiple sclerosis (Henry et al. 2011), Huntington's disease (Brüne et al. 2011) and motor neurone disease (Cavallo et al. 2011; Gibbons et al. 2007; Girardi et al. 2011).

The neural correlates of ToM are increasingly the focus of brain imaging studies. To the extent that neural correlates can contribute to the development of cognitive theories, some mention should be made of the findings of these studies in this section. Brain imaging studies of ToM are of two types. Firstly, there are investigations of the neural underpinnings of ToM in normal, healthy subjects. The neural basis of ToM is generally taken to consist of the medial prefrontal cortex, posterior cingulate/precuneus and bilateral temporal parietal junction (Mar 2011). Although some of the same neural processes are involved in affective and cognitive aspects of ToM, only the medial/ventromedial prefrontal cortex was recruited during affective ToM tasks in adolescents who underwent functional magnetic resonance imaging (fMRI) (Sebastian et al. 2012). In an investigation of the neural correlates of false belief reasoning, Sommer et al. (2010) found that children aged 10–12 years did not selectively recruit the right temporoparietal junction. This was not the case for adults in the same study, a finding which suggested modulation of the cortical network involved in false belief reasoning during development.

Secondly, brain imaging studies have also examined the neural correlates of ToM in subjects with mentalizing impairments. In an fMRI study of patients with schizophrenia, Lee et al. (2011) found reduced neural activation in the temporoparietal junction and medial prefrontal cortex of these patients compared to controls during false belief tasks. Lombardo et al. (2011) reported that the right temporoparietal function was the only neural region to respond atypically during an fMRI investigation into mentalizing judgements in adult males with an autism spectrum disorder. Unlike normal controls, neural activation during an animated social attribution task in adolescents with moderate to severe TBI has been found to exclude the medial prefrontal cortex (Scheibel et al. 2011).

For further discussion of the issues examined in this section, the reader is referred to Cummings (2013a, 2014b).

3.4 Executive Function

The second class of cognitive processes to play a role in utterance interpretation is executive function. Definitions of executive function abound, each with a slightly different emphasis or orientation. Unlike theory of mind, executive function lacks a unitary concept. Accordingly, a typical definition of executive function takes the form of a list of cognitive skills as follows:

> The key elements of executive function include (a) anticipation and deployment of attention; (b) impulse control and self-regulation; (c) initiation of activity; (d) working memory; (e) mental flexibility and utilization of feedback; (f) planning ability and organization; and (g) selection of efficient problem-solving strategies. (Anderson 2008, p. 4)

As this list demonstrates, executive function is integral to the planning, execution and regulation of goal-directed behaviour. It is the ability of executive function to coordinate and direct the brain's cognitive functions that has found it likened to the conductor of an orchestra (Brown 2006, pp. 36–37). In the same way that skilled musicians will produce poor music if their individual contributions are not successfully integrated, significant executive function deficits can occur in the presence of intact cognitive skills if these skills are not properly coordinated.

In this section, we examine what studies have revealed about the development of executive function in children. Of necessity, this large and disparate body of research can only be examined in brief in the present context. We then consider some of the executive function deficits that have been found in clinical populations with significant pragmatic impairments. Some of these executive function deficits are developmental in nature, such as those found in children and adults with autism spectrum disorder. Others are acquired, and include the executive function deficits that occur in individuals who sustain a traumatic brain injury. Finally, much is now known about the neural substrates of executive function. Although this set of cognitive skills is typically linked to the brain's frontal cortex, so much so in fact that the terms 'executive function' and 'frontal lobe function' are often used synonymously, there is now clear evidence that striatal structures also play a role in executive function processes (Elliott 2003, p. 49). We conclude this section with a brief examination of the results of brain imaging studies of executive function in healthy and clinical subjects.

Notwithstanding a large literature on executive function in children, there has been little attempt to generate a developmental account of executive function skills throughout childhood and adolescence. Best and Miller (2010) make a start in this regard by examining the development of three foundational components of executive function: inhibition, working memory and shifting. These three executive functions are separable, but correlated skills in adults (Miyake et al. 2000). However, there is evidence that executive function is a unitary, domain-general process at 3 years of age, when executive function skills are emerging (Wiebe et al. 2011).

Inhibition is defined as 'one's ability to deliberately inhibit dominant, automatic, or prepotent responses when necessary' (Miyake et al. 2000, p. 57). A typical response inhibition task is the day–night task, in which a subject must say 'night' to a picture of the sun and 'day' to a picture of the moon ('day' and 'night' are the prepotent responses, respectively). Young, normally developing children typically fail these tasks. However, under certain conditions (e.g. the presence of a delay between stimulus and response), children of 4 years of age have been found to succeed on these tasks (Diamond et al. 2002). Urben et al. (2011) reported an improvement in the ability of children to inhibit a prepotent response between 5 and 10 years of age. (Although Urben et al. found no role for working memory and processing speed in age-related improvements in inhibition, other investigators (e.g. McAuley et al. 2011) have linked inhibitory improvements to these cognitive skills.) Other cognitive skills which have been shown to be related to inhibition include attention. Reck and Hund (2011) found that sustained attention is a predictor of inhibitory control in 3- to 6-year olds. Friedman et al. (2007) reported that attention problems in children aged 7–14 years predicted response inhibition at 17 years.

Working memory, or rather the updating and monitoring of working memory representations, is a key executive function. This function 'requires monitoring and coding incoming information for relevance to the task at hand and then appropriately revising the items held in working memory by replacing old, no longer relevant information with newer, more relevant information' (Miyake et al. 2000, p. 57). As this description suggests, the updating function has a number of constituent processes. Ecker et al. (2010) found that three components—retrieval, transformation and substitution—make independent contributions to updating performance. Working memory updating can be examined through a range of tasks including the keep track task, the letter memory task and the tone monitoring task (Miyake et al. 2000).

Some investigations of updating have used a time-monitoring task, in which subjects have to indicate the passing of time every 5 min while watching a movie. Forman et al. (2011) reported that adolescents aged 12–16 years displayed reduced clock checking and increased timing error than they had done 4 years earlier at 8–12 years of age. Adolescents with greater relative gains in the development of working memory achieved better calibration than subjects with less developed working memory functions. Mäntylä et al. (2007) found that children needed more clock checks in order to obtain the same level of response accuracy as adults, a finding which was related to the children's difficulties in temporary maintenance and updating of working memory contents. Working memory updating has been shown to be related to reading comprehension ability and scholastic attainment in children (Carretti et al. 2005; St Clair-Thompson and Gathercole 2006).

Shifting—also known as attention switching or task switching—involves shifting back and forth between mental sets, multiple tasks or operations (Miyake et al. 2000, p. 55). A range of tasks may be used to examine shifting. One of the most popular is the Wisconsin Card Sorting Test. This assessment requires subjects to sort cards according to different principles such as form, colour or number. As the task progresses, the subject is required to change his approach as he encounters unannounced shifts in the sorting principle (from colour to number, for example). This task was used by Huizinga and van der Molen (2007) to examine developmental change in set-switching and set-maintenance in children and adults. These investigators found adult levels of performance on set-switching in 11-year-olds and set-maintenance in 15-year-olds.

Kalkut et al. (2009) examined the development of set-shifting ability from childhood to early adulthood. Modest effects of age and gender were observed on set-shifting tasks. Set-shifting abilities continued to improve during adolescence with women displaying better performance in general on set-shifting tasks than men. Crone et al. (2006) examined children's ability to use feedback cues to switch between different sorting rules in a rule change task. The number of perseverative errors was less in 16- to 18-year-olds than in 8- to 10-year-olds. Children aged 12–14 years performed at an intermediate level on this task. Shifting in young children is influenced by language skills. Okanda et al. (2010) found that bilingual children and monolingual children with higher verbal ability performed a set shifting task significantly better than matched monolingual children. Shifting has been found to be related to non-verbal reasoning and reading in children aged 9–12 years (van der Sluis et al. 2007).

Executive function deficits have been characterized in several of the clinical populations examined in Chap. 2. Investigators have examined executive functions in children with autism spectrum disorder (ASD), specific language impairment (SLI), emotional and behavioural disorders, traumatic brain injury (TBI), brain damage related to a cerebrovascular accident and in intellectual disability. Robinson et al. (2009) reported significant impairments in the inhibition of prepotent responses and planning in 54 children with ASD and normal IQ. Tasks examining self-monitoring also resulted in atypical age-related patterns of performance in children with ASD compared to controls. Henry et al. (2012) found that children with SLI had significantly lower performance than typical children on (verbal and non-verbal) working memory and fluency and (non-verbal) inhibition and planning. These executive function deficits remained even when adjustments were made for these children's verbal abilities.

Inhibition deficits have been reported in preschool children aged 3.5–5.5 years with attention deficit hyperactivity disorder (Schoemaker et al. 2012). Utendale et al. (2011) found inhibitory control deficits in preschool and early elementary school children with externalizing problems. Executive function deficits involving goal setting and processing speed have been found to persist in children 10 years after sustaining a severe TBI (Beauchamp et al. 2011). Long et al. (2011) reported deficits in attentional control, cognitive flexibility and information processing in children who sustained a stroke at least 12 months prior to neuropsychological testing.

Increasingly, investigators are examining executive functions in clients with intellectual disability often in the presence of genetic and chromosomal syndromes. Lanfranchi et al. (2010) found that adolescents with Down's syndrome performed at a significantly lower level than mental age-matched typically developing children on tasks assessing set shifting, planning/problem-solving, working memory and inhibition/perseveration. A sustained attention task was also problematic for these adolescents. Menghini et al. (2010) reported deficits of selective and sustained attention, short-term memory and working memory, planning and inhibition in individuals with Williams syndrome whose mean mental age was 6.10 years.

Hooper et al. (2008) examined executive functions in boys with fragile X syndrome (FXS) who were aged 7–13 years. Compared to a group of typically developing boys, boys with FXS displayed significant deficits in inhibition, working memory, cognitive flexibility/set shifting and planning. A set shifting task and memory for word span task were successfully completed by 25.9 and 94.4 % of boys with FXS, respectively. Executive function deficits have also been reported in Kabuki syndrome and in 22q11 deletion syndrome, although in the latter they have been associated with the presence of ASD/ADHD and schizophrenia-prodrome symptoms (Niklasson and Gillberg 2010; Rockers et al. 2009; Sanz et al. 2010). Pei et al. (2011) reported substantial difficulties in organization, accuracy and memory on a test of memory and executive functioning in children aged 6–12 years with foetal alcohol spectrum disorders.

Executive function deficits can arise in adulthood for the first time with the onset of aphasia, schizophrenia or a neurodegenerative disorder such as dementia or motor neurone disease. Similarly, adults may display executive dysfunction subsequent to traumatic brain injury or right brain damage. Purdy (2002) studied three dimensions of performance—accuracy, speed and efficiency—in the context of neuropsychological tests examining cognitive flexibility and goal-directed planning in 15 subjects with aphasia. These subjects displayed significant differences compared to healthy control subjects on all speed and efficiency variables. Hutton et al. (1998) examined executive function in 30 patients with first-episode schizophrenia. These patients performed more poorly than 30 normal volunteers on all tests, with performance non-uniform across areas. Although patients with schizophrenia were able to inhibit prepotent responses and switch attention, they displayed limitations in memory, ability to think ahead and organize responses.

There is also evidence that executive function deficits persist in schizophrenia beyond the onset of the disorder, and that these deficits vary in relation to the symptom profile of patients. Greenwood et al. (2008) found impairments of the same executive functions in 22 patients with first-episode schizophrenia and 35 patients with chronic schizophrenia. Also, executive impairments differed in patients with disorganization symptoms and patients with psychomotor poverty (negative) symptoms. Greenwood et al. concluded that the executive profile in patients with schizophrenia is related to symptom type rather than chronicity.

Executive function deficits have been reported in subjects with right brain damage in a range of neuroanatomical locations and related to different aetiologies. Davidson et al. (2008) described executive function deficits in patients who underwent right frontal lobe tumour resection. Schweizer et al. (2008) studied a patient with persisting executive dysfunction after a right cerebellar haemorrhage. Rainville et al. (2003) identified a severe executive function syndrome in a patient with lesions in the subcortical structures of the right hemisphere. Executive function deficits are commonly amongst the neuropsychological sequelae of traumatic brain injury in adults. Zgaljardic and Temple (2010) examined executive function in 20 patients with moderate-to-severe TBI. These patients performed significantly worse than normal on tests that examined cognitive flexibility, selective and divided attention, psychomotor speed and verbal memory. Executive function problems also occur in mild TBI. Erez et al. (2009) reported deficits in planning and shifting in 13 adults with mild TBI an average of 4.7 months after injury.

Increasingly, investigators are characterizing executive function deficits in clients with a range of neurodegenerative disorders. McGuinness et al. (2010) examined working memory and executive functioning in patients with mild-moderate Alzheimer's disease and patients with vascular dementia. Although both groups of patients were significantly impaired on all working memory and executive functioning measures, there were no significant differences between these groups on any measure. Weintraub et al. (2005) found that planning deficits and diminished inhibitory control accounted for 75 % of the variance in scores on executive function tests in a sample of 46 patients with Parkinson's disease. Arnett et al. (1997) attributed the poor performance of their patients with multiple sclerosis on the Tower of Hanoi test to a combination of poor planning and slowed information processing speed. Raaphorst et al. (2011) recorded executive and memory impairments in 17 % of their patients with progressive spinal muscular atrophy (the lower motor neuron variant of motor neuron disease).

Studies have also examined the neural correlates of executive functions. The findings of these studies have permitted investigators to develop an understanding of the neuroanatomical areas and neural circuits involved in executive functions. Increasingly, this understanding has gone beyond the traditional characterization of executive functions as 'frontal lobe functions'.[2] In healthy subjects, executive functions depend not only on the prefrontal cortex, but also on the intact functioning of corticostriatal circuitry mediated by dopaminergic transmission (Elliott 2003). That striatal processes play a role in this neural mechanism is suggested by the executive function deficits found in patients with Parkinson's disease (Dirnberger et al. 2005).

Other brain-imaging studies of clinical subjects have also helped investigators elucidate the neural mechanisms involved in executive functions. They include Covey et al. (2011), who used magnetic resonance imaging (MRI) to measure structural brain damage in patients with multiple sclerosis during tasks examining information processing speed, neural efficiency and working memory. Slowed processing speed and processing inefficiency were associated with white matter atrophy in these patients, while decreased accuracy during a high working memory load condition was associated with grey and white matter atrophy. Impairments of inhibitory control in patients with schizophrenia are associated with a failure to activate the right striatum, the right inferior frontal cortex, and the left and right temporoparietal junction during fMRI (Zandbelt et al. 2011). Using single-photon emission computed tomography (SPECT), Terada et al. (2011) found that hypoperfusion of the bilateral rectal and orbital gyri was closely associated with the number of perseverative errors on the modified Wisconsin Card Sorting Test in patients with mild Alzheimer's disease. Further studies of this type are needed to confirm these initial research findings.

3.5 Cognitive Substrates of Pragmatic Disorders

Research into theory of mind and executive functions as cognitive substrates of pragmatic disorders is a relative newcomer in clinical pragmatics. Yet, this nascent area of work is beginning to reveal a hitherto neglected role for ToM and executive function in a cognitive explanation of pragmatic impairments. In this section, we examine the small, but growing, clinical literature that now exists on the relationship between pragmatic disorders on the one hand and ToM and executive function deficits on the other hand. The studies that form this literature are limited in several respects. They are often based on small clinical samples. Even when a relationship between ToM impairments, executive function deficits and pragmatic disorders is demonstrated, it is difficult to ascertain the direction and nature of that relationship. So statements to the effect that ToM impairments and executive function deficits *cause* pragmatic disorders cannot often be justified. (It is possible that another variable (e.g. IQ) could be making an independent contribution to impairments in ToM, pragmatics and executive function.)

Nevertheless, I contend that this body of work represents a new, and more robust, type of cognitive explanation of pragmatic disorders than has previously been available and one which warrants serious consideration by all those with an interest in pragmatic disorders. Having considered the results of studies that examine the relationship between pragmatic disorders, and ToM and executive function deficits, the stage will then be set to discuss a number of theoretical proposals regarding ToM and executive function. Although these proposals have currency among cognitive theorists, they are not all equally suited to a cognitive explanation of the processes that are involved in utterance interpretation. Only some of these theories, it will be argued, can demonstrate 'pragmatic adequacy'. But before addressing these cognitive theories, we must consider the empirical evidence in support of the view that ToM and executive function deficits contribute to the pragmatic disorders of children and adults.

A number of clinical studies have examined the relationship between ToM and pragmatic disorders in children and adults with neurodevelopmental disorders. Martin and McDonald (2004) found that second-order ToM reasoning was significantly associated with the ability of subjects with Asperger's syndrome in their study to interpret non-literal utterances (ironic jokes). Hale and Tager-Flusberg (2005) examined discourse skills—specifically, the use of topic-related contingent utterances—and ToM in 57 children with autism. ToM contributed unique variance in the contingent discourse skills of these children beyond the significant contribution made by language skills. Losh et al. (2012) examined ToM and pragmatic language in children with idiopathic autism and children with fragile X syndrome (FXS) with and without autism. Children with FXS and autism performed similarly to children with idiopathic autism, and performed more poorly than typically developing controls, on measures of pragmatic language and ToM. Children with FXS only did not differ from controls on these measures. ToM was related to pragmatic language ability in all groups.

John et al. (2009) examined the referential communication skills of 57 children with Williams syndrome aged 6–12 years. These children were required to verbalize to a speaker when a message was inadequate, and also to communicate effectively the way in which it was inadequate. Three inadequate message conditions were used, all of which were intended to prompt the child to seek clarification from the speaker: impossible condition (the child lacked the relevant picture to complete the task); ambiguous condition (the speaker's request was sufficiently vague that it did not identify the picture to be used); and unknown word (the speaker used a word, which was not in the child's vocabulary, to identify the picture). In the inadequate message conditions, children with Williams syndrome indicated that the message was inadequate less than 50 % of the time. The likelihood that they would effectively communicate the way in which a message was inadequate varied as a function of condition. ToM contributed significantly to the prediction of variance in overall verbalization of message inadequacy. Children with Williams syndrome who had first-order ToM skills were significantly more likely to verbalize message inadequacy effectively in the unknown word condition (26 %) and the ambiguous condition (22 %).

There is also evidence to indicate that acquired ToM impairments in adults contribute to the pragmatic problems of these clients. Monetta et al. (2009) examined ToM performance and irony comprehension in 11 non-demented patients with Parkinson's disease. These investigators found a significant correlation between these patients' ability to interpret an utterance as a lie or an ironic remark and performance on second-order belief questions. Cuerva et al. (2001) reported a significant association between performance on a test of second-order false belief and pragmatic deficits in the interpretation of conversational implications and indirect requests in 34 patients with probable Alzheimer's disease. The population of adults with schizophrenia has been the focus of several investigations. Brüne and Bodenstein (2005) found that approximately 39 % of the variance of proverb comprehension in patients with schizophrenia was predicted by their ToM performance.

Mo et al. (2008) studied 29 patients with schizophrenia who were in remission. Although these patients had a ToM deficit and were impaired in their comprehension of metaphor and irony, only metaphor comprehension was significantly correlated with second-order false belief understanding. In a study of patients with schizophrenia and formal thought disorder, Langdon et al. (2002) reported that poor ToM performance was associated with impaired understanding of irony, but not with impaired metaphor comprehension. Mazza et al. (2008) examined ToM and pragmatic language skills in 38 patients with schizophrenia. These patients performed significantly worse than healthy controls on ToM tasks and a pragmatics task examining appreciation of Gricean maxims, even after controlling for IQ and executive function scores. Moreover, a significant correlation was found between the number of errors on the Gricean maxim task and ToM performance in these patients.

Although most studies have accounted for poor pragmatic skills in clinical subjects in terms of ToM impairments, some studies have attributed ToM deficits in subjects to impairments of pragmatics. Muller et al. (2010) found that patients with traumatic brain injury performed significantly worse than controls on a task examining the interpretation of direct and indirect speech acts and on a faux pas test (a test of ToM). The interpretation of indirect speech acts was shown to be significantly correlated with performance on the faux pas-related questions of the faux pas test as well as performance on second-order false belief stories. Muller et al. suggested that impairment in these patients' language skills, specifically pragmatic abilities, may at least partially explain their problems with ToM.

Surian and Siegal (2001) reported difficulties on verbally presented ToM tasks in patients with right-hemisphere damage. These patients also displayed reduced sensitivity to violations of Gricean maxims in conversation. Surian and Siegal attributed these patients' difficulties with ToM tasks to their problems with utterance interpretation. This view of the direction of the relationship between ToM impairments and pragmatic disorders is the opposite of that proposed by the studies above. Finally, it should not be overlooked that some investigations have failed to establish a relationship between ToM impairments and pragmatic disorders in clients. Losh and Capps (2003) examined the narrative discourse abilities of 28 high-functioning children with autism or Asperger's syndrome. These investigators found that the narrative abilities of these subjects were associated with performance on measures of emotional understanding, but not with ToM or verbal IQ.

Executive function deficits have also been found to be correlated with pragmatic disorders in children and adults (but see below). Eddy et al. (2010) examined the understanding of sarcasm, metaphor and indirect requests in patients with Tourette's syndrome, a chronic neurodevelopmental disorder that is characterized by motor and phonic tics. The ToM skills of these patients were also examined using a faux pas task. These subjects displayed significant impairments in the comprehension of all three non-literal forms and in the ToM task compared to healthy controls. There was a significant relationship between errors on the Pragmatic Story Comprehension Task (a test of the understanding of sarcasm and metaphor) and the time taken to respond to items during the inhibitory condition of the Black and White Stroop Test (one of two inhibitory measures used in the study). Bishop and Norbury (2005) reported a significant relationship between generativity (as measured on two fluency tasks) and autistic-like communicative abnormalities in children with pragmatic language impairment.

Several studies have examined the relationship between pragmatic impairments and executive dysfunction in traumatic brain injury (TBI). In a study of 43 adults who sustained a severe TBI, Douglas (2010b) found pragmatic difficulties involving violations of the Gricean maxims of quantity, relation and manner on the La Trobe Communication Questionnaire (LCQ; Douglas et al. 2000). Executive function measures predicted 37 % of the variability in LCQ scores. Channon and Watts (2003) found less discrimination between direct, literal interpretations and correct, indirect interpretations of brief vignettes in a group of subjects with closed head injury (CHI) than in a control group. In subjects with CHI, pragmatic performance was found to be associated with an executive measure of inhibition.

Although a relationship between ToM deficits and pragmatic impairments is a relatively consistent finding across clinical studies, investigators have not infrequently failed to establish a correlation between pragmatic impairments and executive function deficits. Donno et al. (2010) found that significantly more persistently disruptive primary school children than children in a comparison group obtained scores in the clinical range on the pragmatic composite scale of the Children's Communication Checklist. It appears unlikely that executive function deficits played any role in the pragmatic impairments of these children, as no significant difference was found between disruptive and comparison groups on any executive function tested.

In a study of 18 patients with right-hemisphere damage, McDonald (2000) found that pragmatic performance was correlated to right hemisphere (visuospatial) function and not to executive function. Dardier et al. (2011) examined pragmatic and executive function skills in 11 subjects with frontal lesions following TBI. These investigators found areas of strength and weakness in the pragmatic skills of these subjects. Interindividual differences in pragmatic skills were not systematically linked to performance on executive function tests. Among four subjects who showed no executive impairment, only one attained good scores on all pragmatic and metapragmatic tasks. In the four patients with the best pragmatic and metapragmatic performance, only one had no executive deficit. This pattern of results, Dardier et al. argue, confirms earlier findings of a lack of a clear link between pragmatic deficits and executive dysfunction.

3.6 A Cognitive Explanation of Pragmatic Disorders

As the discussion of the above section demonstrates, there are clear empirical grounds for pursuing a cognitive explanation of pragmatic disorders in terms of ToM impairments and executive function deficits. Although these cognitive deficits were characterized as relative newcomers to a cognitive explanation of pragmatic disorders, they are preceded by and contemporaneous with other cognitive accounts that have arisen within pragmatics itself. These accounts are relevance theory (Sperber and Wilson [1986] 1995), modular pragmatics theory (Kasher 1991a, b) and cognitive pragmatics theory (Bara 2010). The contribution of these cognitive pragmatic accounts to an explanation of utterance interpretation in general, and pragmatic disorders in particular, will be examined in Chap. 4. Instead, the focus of this section will be on theoretical proposals concerning theory of mind and executive function.

These proposals have not been systematically examined by pragmatists, let alone studied with a view to accounting for the cognitive basis of pragmatic disorders.[3] In the absence of this discussion, it is not possible to say which, if any, of these theoretical proposals displays 'pragmatic adequacy', i.e. the capacity to capture certain hallmark features of utterance interpretation. The aim of this section will be, first, to establish what these hallmark features are and, second, to assess the pragmatic adequacy of each theoretical proposal in turn. Even if it is concluded that these cognitive theories are poorly suited to an explanation of the pragmatic processes involved in utterance interpretation, the exercise of stating why this is the case will bring us closer to formulating a cognitive theory that will explain pragmatic disorders.

3.6.1 Defining Pragmatic Adequacy

Although pragmatists are divided along well established theoretical lines concerning the pragmatic processes involved in utterance interpretation, there is at least general consensus on the features of utterance interpretation that a pragmatic theory should attempt to explain. These features are that (1) utterance interpretation has an *open texture* which is not seen in language decoding; (2) utterance interpretation involves *reasoning* or the use of inferences in addition to other cognitive processes that are present in language decoding; (3) utterance interpretation requires engagement with *mental states* in a way that language decoding does not; and (4) utterance interpretation displays *defeasibility* that is not present in language decoding. To demonstrate each of these features, consider the following exchange between Fred and Sue:

Fred: Will you join us in Spain this summer?
Sue: Bill's contract doesn't expire until the autumn.

Clearly, Sue is implicating by way of her utterance that she will not join Fred in Spain in the summer. The cognitive and linguistic processes by means of which Sue produces this implicature, and Fred interprets it, provide demonstration of the four points described above. In relation to (1), Fred must draw on both linguistic and world knowledge in order to recover the implicature of Sue's utterance. He must know what a contract is and what it means for it to expire (semantic knowledge). Fred must also know who Bill is, that a contract involves employment which normally requires a person to be present at a place of work (and thus not in Spain), and that the autumn season follows the summer (world knowledge). Also, Fred must be able to assess the relevance of Sue's utterance to his question which has the function of an invitation in this context (pragmatic knowledge).

The knowledge that Fred uses in his interpretation of Sue's utterance is not just of different types, but is indefinably large. In fact, when we begin to examine the knowledge that Fred must possess in order to interpret Sue's utterance, there is no point at which we can stop. Beyond knowledge of the meanings of individual words and rules of conversation, Fred must also have knowledge of Sue's interests, lifestyle and other commitments in order for him to believe that she might seriously entertain an invitation of this type. Each of these aspects of knowledge presupposes, in turn, further knowledge—one's lifestyle, for example, presupposes certain values and beliefs. Put quite simply, knowledge—and utterance interpretation which draws on it—has an open texture in which interconnectedness between its component parts precludes any attempt to circumscribe it. Fred is not bringing a limited amount or type of knowledge to his interpretation of Sue's utterance so much as his full knowledge of life itself.

In order to draw an implicature from Sue's utterance, Fred must use a range of cognitive skills. He must attend to, and perceive or recognise auditory stimuli. He must hold information in memory as phonological, syntactic and semantic operations are performed on it. The linguistic processes which are involved in the decoding of an utterance are of a particular type. They are fixed, rule-based processes which take certain information as input and return the same, pre-determined information as output on every occasion that they are activated. These processes are not subject to contextual influences in the way that utterance interpretation is and they do not involve higher-level cognitive processes of reasoning or inference. For example, the semantic rule which returns a meaning of FEMALE PARENT for the word 'mother' does so automatically in the absence of any reasoning about what this word means.

The situation is quite different, however, when Fred is confronted with an utterance of the type Sue has produced. Of course, Fred must use all the cognitive processes (e.g. auditory perception) and linguistic operations just described in his decoding of this utterance. But he must also go beyond these processes and operations and employ a rational competence that does not come into play during language decoding. It is the fact that Fred is not just activating an algorithm in his interpretation of Sue's utterance, but exercising a rational competence, that sets the cognitive processes involved in language decoding apart from those which are central to utterance interpretation. Specifically, Fred is employing high-level processes of reasoning and inference in order to establish the implicature of Sue's utterance. These high-level cognitive processes are in addition to those he must use to establish the encoded meaning of Sue's utterance in this exchange.

Point (3) above describes a feature of utterance interpretation which has been apparent to pragmatists since Grice first gave prominence to the role of intentions in communication. Merely decoding Sue's utterance will not lead Fred to the particular communicative intention that motivated the production of that utterance. Yet, that intention is exactly what must be recovered if Fred is to establish the implicature of Sue's utterance. En route to establishing this intention, Fred must also attribute other mental states to Sue. He must attribute *knowledge* to her, for example, knowledge that Spain is a European country and that the summer spans several months in the year. He must also attribute certain *desires* to Sue. For example, Fred must have reason to believe that Sue wants to travel to Spain in order to issue her with an invitation to visit the country. Fred must also attribute *beliefs* to Sue, such as the belief that Bill's contract prevents him from leaving the country.

For her part, Sue must also attribute mental states to Fred, such as knowledge that Bill is Sue's husband, and the belief that employment can limit opportunities for foreign travel. Beyond the attribution of first-order mental states about the world to each other's minds (e.g. Sue knows that Spain is a European country), Fred and Sue must also attribute second-order mental states to each other's minds. These second-order mental states are not about the world, but about the content of another mind (e.g. Sue believes that Fred believes that Bill is Sue's husband). The attribution of mental states is at the very heart of all utterance interpretation and must be accounted for by any cognitive account of the pragmatic processes by means of which interpretation proceeds.

Point (4) captures the feature of defeasibility in utterance interpretation. An interpretation of an utterance may need to be revised or rejected altogether if certain circumstances arise that demand it. For example, imagine a situation in which Sue extends her turn in the above exchange in the following way: 'Bill's contract doesn't expire until the autumn. But I'll join you in Spain anyway'. In this case, the implicature to the effect that Sue will not join Fred in Spain is overturned. This feature of defeasibility or cancellability is a general characteristic of all utterance interpretation and reflects the wider sensitivity of interpretative processes to features of context. In this way, Fred may also have to revise his understanding of the implicature of Sue's utterance if he suddenly recalls an earlier conversation with Sue in which she described marital problems and expressed an interest in spending some time away from Bill. In this case, Sue may be taken to implicate that she would like to travel to Spain to spend time with Fred.

Quite simply, no interpretation of any utterance is beyond revision if features of context suggest that such revision is necessary. The defeasibility of utterance interpretation places certain requirements on the cognitive processes by means of which interpretation proceeds. Specifically, these processes must be dynamic and responsive to changes in context. At a minimum, they must include defeasible forms of reasoning in which a conclusion (an interpretation) can be overridden when a feature of context requires it. In general, these forms of reasoning will be non-deductive in nature and exhibit non-monotonicity (as opposed to deductive or monotonic modes of reasoning, in which inferences are not overturned by the emergence of new information). It remains to be seen if cognitive theories can address this feature of utterance interpretation.

3.6.2 The Pragmatic Adequacy of Theory of Mind Theories

It emerges that a pragmatically adequate cognitive theory is one which can draw on any item of knowledge or information (feature 1), explain the type of reasoning or inferences that are involved in utterance interpretation (feature 2), accommodate mental state attribution and, specifically, the attribution of communicative intentions (feature 3), and capture the defeasibility of interpretation (feature 4). The success or otherwise of cognitive theories of ToM and executive function within an explanation of pragmatic disorders will be judged in terms of how well these theories satisfy these four criteria of pragmatic adequacy.

In this section, we assess the pragmatic adequacy of theory of mind theories. Although there is a bewildering array of theoretical possibilities, ToM theories are basically of two types. First, there are theorists who argue that we understand, and can make predictions about, the minds of others by constructing a folk psychological theory of those minds (so-called theory-theorists). Second, there are theorists who claim that the ability to understand, and make predictions about, other minds does not involve any type of theory construction, but rather the ability to project ourselves imaginatively into another person's mind, thus simulating their mental activity with our own (so-called simulation theorists). Within these two basic types of theory, there are a number of other theoretical possibilities. For example, theory-theorists differ on the extent to which the constructed theory is accessible to consciousness and oral report, and involves a tightly structured and interrelated set of principles.

Theory-theorists also differ on the mechanism by means of which this folk psychological theory is acquired, whether this is through the biological growth of an innate, genetically endowed module, or learning by means of theorising, or teaching and enculturation. Simulation theorists are further sub-divided according to whether the simulation involves first-person awareness of one's own mental states with an argument from analogy the basis of the inference from self to other, or a type of imaginative identification which proceeds without introspective self-awareness. Simulation theorists believe that the ability to simulate is an innate genetic endowment, but differ on whether simulation is an ability to imagine, to think counterfactually, to entertain suppositions or to take one's reasoning 'off-line' (Carruthers and Smith 1996, pp. 4–5).

Obviously, limitations of space preclude an examination of the pragmatic adequacy of each of these theoretical possibilities. Nevertheless, certain of them will be examined with a view to assessing their contribution to an explanation of pragmatic disorders. The idea of a ToM module has been particularly dominant in recent years. There is reason to believe that the open texture of utterance interpretation (feature 1) may prove to be a difficult aspect of pragmatic adequacy for a modular account of ToM to satisfy. A cognitive module is a specialized sub-system of the mind which is designed to process certain types of information to the exclusion of other information. A visual perception module, for example, is only equipped to handle visual data.

In the same way, a theory of mind module can only process intentional data relating to mental states. Because they are adapted to process a particular type of data, the specialized internal processes of the ToM module can only receive a certain type of input. More specifically, these processes do not have access to information contained in the mind's central system, or to information that is processed by other cognitive modules (e.g. the language faculty). This restriction on the information that is available to the inner workings of a module is known as informational encapsulation and is one of the defining features of cognitive modules, as originally envisaged by Jerry Fodor. This is how Fodor (1983) captures the notion of informational encapsulation and how Segal (1996) applies this notion to a ToM (intentional) module:

> In a nutshell: one way that a system can be autonomous is by being encapsulated, by not having access to facts that other systems know about. I am claiming that [...] they [input systems] are, to an interesting degree, autonomous in this informational sense. (Fodor 1983, p. 73).

> In Jerry Fodor's (1983) terminology, intentional modules may be 'informationally encapsulated': some of the information in the subject's mind outside a given module may be unavailable to it. For example, information in the conscious mind is often not available to the Freudian unconscious [...] I suggest that if a set of appropriately related psychological states exhibits [...] informational encapsulation [...] then they constitute an intentional module. (Segal 1996, p. 143).

The informational encapsulation of cognitive modules confers an important efficiency on the operation of modules. To the extent that modules are processing data of a particular type, their internal processes are fast.[4] But the same informational encapsulation that makes this significant cognitive efficiency possible in certain domains can also have limitations in other domains. One such domain is utterance interpretation. As a cognitive model of the pragmatic processes—or even the ToM skills—involved in utterance interpretation, it is difficult to see how a ToM module can succeed in capturing the open texture of these processes. In Sect. 3.6.1, we described how Fred could draw on an indefinable range of knowledge in order to establish the implicature of Sue's utterance. In the same way, Fred must be able to draw on diverse sources and types of information in order to attribute any particular mental state to Sue.

In Sect. 3.6.1, one of the mental states that Fred was credited with attributing to Sue was the desire that Sue *wants* to travel to Spain. The attribution of this mental state to Sue involves a range of information that is no more easily circumscribed than was the information Fred used to derive the implicature of Sue's utterance. For example, Fred may recall an earlier conversation with Sue in which she described her love of Spanish food and culture at the point when he attributes this particular desire to Sue. But Fred may also attach salience to Sue's animated facial expression when he mentions Spain, or the fact that Sue is studying Spanish at evening class as the basis of his attribution of this particular desire to Sue. It is difficult to see how Fred's ToM module can have access to this information located, as it is, within the mind's central system (prior beliefs about Sue's interests) and visual perception module (Sue's facial expression). There is, thus, strong reason to doubt that a modular view of ToM can satisfy feature (1) of the criterion of pragmatic adequacy.

For similar reasons, it is also doubtful that a ToM module can satisfy feature 2 (reasoning and inference) and feature 3 (mental state attribution) of the criterion of pragmatic adequacy. To the extent that mental state attribution proceeds by means of ToM reasoning, and ToM reasoning is integral to utterance interpretation, features 2 and 3 are related. Utterance interpretation is achieved at the point at which a hearer attributes a communicative intention to the mind of the speaker. Certainly, this is ToM reasoning *par excellence*. But this is not a type of ToM reasoning that can be captured by an informationally encapsulated cognitive module. In attributing a communicative intention to Sue, Fred is drawing on knowledge and beliefs which are located in the mind's central system. Yet, the contents of this system are unavailable to a ToM module.

Of course, the proponent of a modular view of ToM will contend that the output of a ToM module interacts with knowledge and beliefs in the mind's central system. To this extent, it is argued, there is the interaction between ToM information and other knowledge and beliefs deemed necessary to utterance interpretation. But this vital involvement of knowledge and beliefs in the mind's central system only takes place *after* the ToM module has executed its internal procedures and arrived at a particular mental state for attribution to a speaker's mind. Prior knowledge and beliefs along with visual perception data, as we saw above, must be able to influence the workings of a ToM module, and are not merely added to the output of this module.[5] To the extent that a cognitive module has no access to the type of central system information that plays a role in ToM reasoning, it is doubtful that a modular view of ToM adequately captures the reasoning and inference processes at work in utterance interpretation.

The same feature of informational encapsulation creates further difficulties for a ToM module when we turn to the defeasibility of utterance interpretation (feature 4). The defeasibility of utterance interpretation is only possible to the extent that any cognitive mechanism involved in interpretation is able to revise its output in response to contrary information. To the extent that a ToM module forms at least part of this mechanism, it too must be capable of revising its output should conditions require it. A problem for cognitive modules is that they are fully demarcated from the information that might suggest some revision of their contents is required. So Fred may be about to attribute to Sue's mind the desire that Sue wants to travel to Spain. However, he may then use Sue's sullen expression on hearing Fred's invitation as grounds to revise his initial attribution of this mental state to Sue's mind. However, to the extent that the visual data Fred needs to revise his attribution of this mental state is contained within his visual perception module, it is difficult to see how Fred's attribution of this mental state to Sue can be overridden. This is because from its location in the visual perception module, this information has no access to Fred's ToM module.

Furthermore, another feature of modules is that once the input conditions of their internal algorithms are satisfied, an invariant output is automatically returned. It is not possible for information that might override mental state attribution of the type between Fred and Sue to influence the workings of these algorithms. On both counts—the informational encapsulation of cognitive modules and the invariant operation of algorithms—there is little prospect of a ToM module being able to accommodate the type of defeasibility that is a hallmark feature of utterance interpretation.

So far, we have only discussed the pragmatic adequacy of a modular account of ToM. Simulation theories of ToM may be able to circumvent some of the difficulties of a modular account. Although there are several theoretical possibilities, according to one prominent simulation account, that of Gordon (1986), simulation proceeds as follows:

> Our decision-making or practical reasoning system gets partially disengaged from its "natural" inputs and fed instead with suppositions and images (or their "subpersonal" or "sub-doxastic" counterparts). Given these artificial pretend inputs the system then "makes up its mind" what to do. Since the system is being run off-line, as it were, disengaged also from its natural output systems, its "decision" isn't actually executed but rather ends up as an anticipation…of the other's behaviour. (1986, p. 170).

To appreciate how simulation works, let's consider how it might be applied to the case of mental state attribution between Fred and Sue above. To the extent that Fred is attempting to establish what Sue's communicative intention is in producing her utterance, the simulation theorist who subscribes to Gordon's view would argue that Fred proceeds by taking his practical reasoning system 'off-line'. This system is then 'fed' with 'suppositions and images'. In the case of Fred, these suppositions and images will be information of the following type: Sue's facial expression when Fred extends his invitation to her; Fred's recall of an earlier conversation with Sue in which she described her love of Spanish food and culture; Fred's knowledge of who Bill is, and so on. Fred's practical reasoning system then 'makes up its mind' and produces a 'decision'. This decision is an 'anticipation' of the communicative intention that Sue must hold in order for her to have produced the particular utterance she did.

Although a somewhat sketchy account, this description of how simulation might proceed in the case of the type of mental state attribution required for utterance interpretation reveals what is problematic with the simulation approach. One can see how Fred's practical reasoning system may arrive at the particular communicative intention that motivated Sue's utterance when it is presented with certain inputs. This much can be explained in terms of a non-deductive process of reasoning leading from certain premises ('inputs') to a conclusion (a 'decision'). But the task of a pragmatic theory of utterance interpretation is much more than simply accounting for this process of non-deductive reasoning (not that this has been definitively established by pragmatists either). Rather, it is to explain how the inputs which are fed into Fred's practical reasoning system are selected or chosen. The issue for a pragmatic theory is what gives these particular inputs salience over a vast range of other inputs which could undergo processing in the practical reasoning system. To the extent that simulation theory—at least on the account of it given by Gordon (1986)—simply assumes that these inputs can be identified, rather than offers an account of how this identification proceeds, it is unlikely to succeed as an account of the type of mental state attribution that is involved in utterance interpretation. A fortiori, simulation theory cannot satisfy a criterion of pragmatic adequacy when the type of ToM reasoning it captures leaves unexplained the key feature of utterance interpretation for a pragmatic theory, namely, how in Sperber and Wilson's terminology a context is 'chosen' for the interpretation of an utterance rather than determined in advance.[6]

3.6.3 The Pragmatic Adequacy of Executive Function Theories

With an increasing number of clinical studies revealing a role for executive function deficits in pragmatic disorders, it is now relevant to ask if executive function theories display pragmatic adequacy.[7] Mateer (1999) proposes a clinical model of executive functions in which impairment of one or more of the following six functions is found in clients with dysexecutive syndrome: (1) initiation and drive; (2) response inhibition; (3) task persistence; (4) organization; (5) generative thinking; and (6) awareness. Communicative impairments, which are largely pragmatic in nature, are linked to deficits of specific executive functions.

In this way, the client who has an impairment of initiation and drive does not initiate conversation and exhibits flat affect with limited expression. The client with deficits of response inhibition makes inappropriate comments and does not wait for a turn in conversation. The client who loses interest in conversation and cannot maintain a topic has an impairment of task persistence. Problems of organization are manifested in poor verbal organization with an affected individual jumping from topic to topic, talking around a subject and not getting to the main idea. Generative thinking is compromised in the subject who is unable to generate conversation, seems to have little to say, and has difficulty responding to open-ended questions. Finally, the client with a lack of awareness appears to be unaware of his or her communicative deficits and does not appear to notice if others are not interested in a topic.

To the extent that this clinical model of executive functions provides an explanation of pragmatic disorders in clients, there is a mundane sense in which it displays 'pragmatic adequacy'. But pragmatic adequacy in this sense does not take us beyond the isolated operation of each of these executive functions, when the question of real theoretical significance is the extent to which the relationships between these components are able to capture the features of utterance interpretation. When ToM theories were examined, especially those in which ToM is conceived of as a cognitive module, it became apparent that the informational encapsulation of modules is the feature which limited their pragmatic adequacy. Specifically, a ToM module needed to have access to beliefs in the mind's central system in order for a listener to be able to attribute mental states such as communicative intentions to the speaker of an utterance. However, to the extent that there is a restriction on the flow of information between the central system and input modules such as a ToM module, this access to central system beliefs is effectively denied.

If we keep to a Fodorian conception of the mind's cognitive systems and examine the distribution of the various operations we have been calling 'executive functions' within it, it emerges that executive function theories may be better placed that ToM theories to satisfy a requirement of pragmatic adequacy. Specifically, the mind's central system contains a range of general-purpose cognitive skills. These skills, which Fodor (1983) calls horizontal processes, include memory, attention and problem-solving. The extent and nature of the interaction of these cognitive skills with domain-general beliefs in the mind's central system is critical to an assessment of the pragmatic adequacy of executive function theories.

The working memory model of executive functions, first proposed by Baddeley and Hitch (1974), provides fertile ground for an examination of the notion of pragmatic adequacy. A ToM module is not suited to the type of mental state attribution involved in utterance interpretation, it was argued, because background knowledge and beliefs are not accessible to the cognitive processes which are internal to this module. It is interesting to ask if Baddeley's working memory model is any better equipped to integrate information with the cognitive processes which must act upon it. Working memory stands at the crossroads between attention, memory and perception (Baddeley 1992, p. 559). As originally conceived by Baddeley and Hitch, the model consists of three sub-components. (A fourth sub-component, the episodic buffer, was later added to address deficiencies in the model.)

The three sub-components of the original working memory model are a central executive and two 'slave' systems, a visuospatial sketch pad and a phonological loop. The sketch pad and phonological loop manipulate visual images, and store and rehearse speech-based information, respectively. As the more tractable components of the model, the visuospatial sketch pad and phonological loop have received most experimental investigation. The central executive was originally characterized as an attentional control system which was 'capable of integrating the two slave systems, of linking them with information from long-term memory, and of manipulating the resulting representation' (Baddeley 2002, p. 246). This characterization of the central executive remained until Baddeley (1986) began in earnest to address this theoretical void in the model. As details of the central executive have started to be filled in, it has become clear that this system is fractionating in the same way that the slave systems have done so (Baddeley 2002).

Based on extensive experimentation in healthy subjects and subjects with Alzheimer's disease, the functions of the central executive have been found to include dual task performance and the switching of attention from one task to another. At the same time, the absence of a separate storage capacity in the central executive necessitated the introduction of an episodic buffer into the working memory model. The buffer allows information from the two slave systems to be integrated and the central executive to interface with long-term memory (LTM). Baddeley (2002, p. 256) describes the function of the episodic buffer as follows:

> The *episodic buffer* is assumed to be a limited capacity storage system, capable of temporarily holding and manipulating information registered in terms of a multi-dimensional code [...]. It is termed *episodic* to reflect its capacity to hold integrated episodes that extend both spatially and temporally. It is a buffer in the sense that it offers a multidimensional code that allows information from different subsystems to be integrated with and linked to long-term memory. (Italics in original).

Representations in long-term memory are in semantic and linguistic form, and include individual words, phrases, general concepts and higher level schemata (Baddeley 2002). The background beliefs and knowledge that are so integral to utterance interpretation may also be assumed to be represented in propositional or linguistic form in LTM. But unlike in a modular approach to mental architecture, these beliefs and knowledge are fully integrated with all other components in the working memory model. Baddeley (2002, p. 256) states that '[w]hereas our initial approach to working memory emphasized the importance of fractionation, developing methods of establishing separate subsystems, the principal function of the episodic buffer involves integration'.

It is this level of integration in Baddeley's working memory model which better equips it to address the informational requirements of utterance interpretation than an approach based on cognitive modules. These modules are truly 'separate subsystems'. And restrictions on the flow of information both between modules and between modules and the central system further guarantee their separateness. Through the integration afforded by the episodic buffer, representations in long term memory have a synergistic relationship with other components of the model: '[T]here appears to be a synergistic relationship between material held in the phonological store and that held in semantic and linguistic form, presumably in long-term memory' (Baddeley 2002, p. 255). Such a relationship is not possible within a modular framework. The enhanced integration of the working memory model, at least as conceived by Baddeley and colleagues, suggests that this model has the potential to be a pragmatically adequate theory of the cognitive processes involved in utterance interpretation.

3.7 Summary

There is still much that we do not know about the cognitive basis of utterance interpretation in language intact subjects. Even less do we understand how cognitive deficits contribute to a range of pragmatic disorders in clinical subjects. Despite a burgeoning literature on ToM deficits and executive function deficits, most clinical studies have not sought to relate these cognitive impairments to pragmatic aspects of language. The somewhat undeveloped state of empirical research in this area is compounded by a lack of theory construction that might be usefully applied to utterance interpretation. Where ToM and executive function theories do exist, they are often difficult to assess in pragmatic terms. It is hoped that the discussion of this chapter will place new emphasis on the need to consider the role of cognitive deficits in pragmatic disorders, and suggest ways in which disorders of the pragmatics-cognition interface can be further examined.

Notes

1. For an excellent discussion of the different theoretical proposals concerning the nature and extent of this pragmatic intrusion, the reader is referred to Jaszczolt (2012).
2. In fact, it is now recognised that to label executive functions as frontal functions is inaccurate. Leh et al. (2010, p. 70) state that '[t]raditionally, the frontal cortex has been considered the major brain structure involved in executive functions. More recently, however, several studies in subjects with frontal lesions have shown a large variety of behavioral disturbances other than executive dysfunctions that include, for example, apathy, poor motivation, irritability, euphoric state, etc., highlighting the importance of not using the term executive functions interchangeably with frontal functions'.
3. Two exceptions are: Sperber and Wilson (2002), who have examined theoretical proposals relating to ToM in the context of normal utterance interpretation; and Martin and McDonald (2003), who have assessed ToM impairments and executive dysfunction as theoretical contenders in an explanation of pragmatic disorders.
4. Fodor (1983, p. 70) captures this feature of modules as follows: 'to the extent that input systems are informationally encapsulated, of all the information that might *in principle* bear upon a problem of perceptual analysis only a portion (perhaps only quite a small and stereotyped portion) is actually admitted for consideration. This is to say that speed is purchased for input systems by permitting them to ignore lots of the facts'.
5. This point addresses an issue raised by Fodor (1983). Fodor claims that background knowledge must be shown to influence an input system prior to its production of an output in order for this top–down influence to represent a proper challenge to modularity. He expresses this point as follows: 'We sometimes know that the world can't really be the way that it looks, and such cases may legitimately be described as the correction of input analyses by top–down information flow [...] However, to demonstrate *that* sort of interaction between input analyses and background knowledge is not, in and of itself, tantamount to demonstrating the cognitive penetrability of the former; you need also to show that the locus of the top–down effect is

internal to the input system. That is, you need to show that the information fed back interacts with interlevels of input-processing and not merely with the final results of such processing. The penetrability of a system is, by definition, its susceptibility to top–down effects at stages *prior* to its production of output' (Fodor 1983, pp. 73–74). The discussion of the main text demonstrates that a ToM module is penetrable in exactly this sense.

6. Sperber and Wilson (1995, p. 137) state that '…assuming that context is uniquely determined leads to absurdities. However, there is nothing in the nature of a context or of comprehension, which excludes the possibility that context formation is open to choices and revisions throughout the comprehension process.'

7. It is also worth pointing out that several studies have demonstrated an association between executive function and ToM. They include developmental investigations, studies of the relationship between executive function and ToM throughout adulthood and in subjects with a range of clinical disorders. In a study of 82 preschoolers, Müller et al. (2012) found that executive function at ages 2 and 3 significantly predicted ToM at ages 3 and 4, respectively. However, ToM at ages 2 and 3 failed to explain a significant amount of variance in executive function at age 4. Phillips et al. (2011) found that difficulties in updating information in working memory partially mediated age differences in false belief (ToM) reasoning in 129 adults between the ages of 18 and 86 years. In a review of studies of ToM and executive function in patients with acquired neurological pathology, Aboulafia-Brakha et al. (2011) found that executive function and ToM are tightly associated. However, no executive sub-process was specifically associated with ToM performance.

Chapter 4
Theoretical Models and Pragmatic Disorders

4.1 Introduction

For approximately 40 years, investigators have attempted to characterize impairments of pragmatics in children and adults. During this time, certain trends have been evident in how investigators have pursued this work. One of the most noteworthy trends has been the relentless drive to demonstrate skills and behaviours which are disrupted in children and adults with pragmatic disorders. The result has been an abundance of empirical findings, many of which have considerable interest for clinical researchers and practitioners. For example, it is a fact worth knowing if children and adults with autism spectrum disorder cannot recover the sarcastic intent of certain utterances, or if the adult with schizophrenia fails to observe the relation maxim in his contribution of turns to a conversation. However, at the same time as there has been a proliferation of empirical findings, many of these findings can appear poorly interconnected and of limited significance. They can also often lack proper explanatory value. It is important to interrogate why this is the case. As I will argue in this chapter, the answer lies in the lack of theoretical models in clinical pragmatic research. In the absence of these models, clinical pragmatic studies have produced copious findings. However, only some of these findings have the type of theoretical significance that can advance our understanding of pragmatic disorders.

This chapter will examine the contribution of theory to clinical pragmatics. As the above discussion indicates, that contribution has not been as substantial as it might have been over the years. Nonetheless, there is theoretical input into clinical pragmatics which warrants detailed, critical examination. That examination will develop as follows. In the next section, the source of the lack of theory in clinical pragmatics will be traced to the disciplines which have shaped this field of study. Principally, these disciplines are pragmatics and language pathology. It will be argued that there are features of these disciplines which have poorly equipped them to deliver the type of theory which would be most suitable for clinical pragmatics. A distinction is made between strong and weak cognitively-oriented

L. Cummings, *Pragmatic Disorders*, Perspectives in Pragmatics,
Philosophy & Psychology 3, DOI: 10.1007/978-94-007-7954-9_4,
© Springer Science+Business Media Dordrecht 2014

pragmatic theories. In Sect. 4.3, the content of theories which have been influential in clinical pragmatics will be examined. Also in that section, several studies which have employed these theoretical frameworks to examine pragmatic skills in subjects with clinical disorders will be discussed. In Sect. 4.4, theoretical frameworks will be critically evaluated from a clinical pragmatic perspective. Finally, the implications of this evaluation for future theory construction in clinical pragmatics will be considered.

4.2 The Status of Theory in Clinical Pragmatics

To the extent that there is a lack of theoretical models guiding clinical pragmatic research, the question naturally arises of how this situation has come about. Clinical pragmatics reflects the disciplinary influences of the various fields which have shaped its development. Most notably, these fields include pragmatics and language pathology. Pragmatics is a linguistic discipline which is steeped in philosophical tradition as is evident from the formative influences of philosophers of language such as Grice, Austin and Searle. This tradition has contributed many of the core concepts and ideas that pragmatists are still working with today. Notions such as implicature, for example, are at the forefront of pragmatic theorising as recent controversies at the semantics-pragmatics interface demonstrate (see Jaszczolt (2012) for discussion). This theorising has undoubtedly resulted in profound insights into the nature of utterance interpretation. But its inherently abstract nature means that it is often poorly equipped to deal with the more cognitively-oriented issues that are of interest to clinical pragmatists. Body et al. (1999, p. 89) have expressed this same concern in relation to TBI as follows:

> The studies of TBI that take an aspect of pragmatics as a starting point have provided valuable insights into the complex communication patterns of this group. However, we would suggest that there is a need to re-examine the background to pragmatics and to inform the clinical application of pragmatic theories from the perspective of cognition.

A cognitive orientation to pragmatic theorising is necessary for a number of reasons. Firstly, more than any other aspect of language, pragmatics lies at an intersection between language and cognition. In Chap. 3, this intersection was described as the pragmatics-cognition interface. From its position at this interface, pragmatics is uniquely sensitive to, and dependent on, a range of cognitive operations (e.g. reasoning) in a way that structural levels of language (e.g. syntax) are not. Pragmatic theories can only truly reflect this interrelationship between pragmatics and cognition if they are cognitively oriented. Secondly, a pragmatic theory of utterance interpretation must do more than simply explain utterance interpretation in normal subjects. To have validity, a pragmatic theory must also be able to account for aspects of disordered performance. Many pragmatic disorders are related to cognitive deficits—the so-called cognitive-communication disorders seen in TBI and dementia are cases in point. In order to account for disordered interpretation, and the contribution of cognitive factors to such interpretation, pragmatic theory must be cognitively oriented. Thirdly, a pragmatic theory that is not cognitively oriented cannot make predictions about mental processes during utterance interpretation. In the absence of such predictions, the theory cannot be tested and falsified or disconfirmed. A pragmatic theory that is not testable falls short of epistemic standards that we expect of theory construction in general. This final reason why pragmatic theories should be cognitively oriented is possibly the most important of all.

Although cognitively-oriented pragmatic theories are limited in number, they do exist in both strong and weak forms. In strong form, these theories have cognition as their overarching structure so that every aspect of theorising is guided by what is cognitively plausible in terms of mental processes. The entire framework within which utterance interpretation sits is cognitive in orientation. In this chapter, three 'strong' theories will be examined: Sperber and Wilson's relevance theory, Bara's cognitive pragmatics theory, and Kasher's modular pragmatics theory. In the 30 years since it was first proposed, relevance theory has achieved considerable prominence. Its success is due in large part to its capacity to explain many different aspects of utterance interpretation in both normal and impaired subjects. Several relevance-theoretic constructs have been usefully applied to the study of utterance interpretation in children and adults with pragmatic disorders.

Cognitive pragmatics theory is a relative newcomer to clinical pragmatics. Unlike relevance theory, which continues in the tradition of Grice, cognitive pragmatics theory takes the language games of Wittgenstein to be a model of cooperative communication between agents. Also unlike relevance theory, the performance of clinical subjects during utterance interpretation has shaped cognitive pragmatics theory since its inception, i.e. clinical studies are not a later application of the theory as they are in relevance theory. Finally, Kasher's modular pragmatics theory is an attempt to develop a theory of utterance interpretation within the explicitly cognitive framework of modularity. Cognitive modularity makes certain assumptions about the structure of the human mind, assumptions which have held considerable sway in cognitive science over many years. These will be examined as part of a wider discussion of modular pragmatics theory in Sect. 4.3.

Unlike strong theories, 'weak' theories do not set out to frame utterance interpretation in cognitive terms. These theories are concerned with conceptual and logical considerations as they relate to utterance interpretation. For example, one such theory proposes the notion of an impliciture and argues for its role as an intermediate level of meaning between what is said and an implicature (Bach 1994). Several of these theories address the extent to which pragmatic processes contribute to the development of the logical form of an utterance (see Jaszczolt (2012) for discussion). But in saying that these theories do not set out to frame utterance interpretation in cognitive terms, it is important to emphasize that they do not operate with disregard for human cognition. For example, the notion of defaults appears in various guises in theoretical work on the semantics-pragmatics interface including Jaszczolt's default semantics (Jaszczolt 2005) and Levinson's presumptive meanings or default interpretations (Levinson 2000). From the form that these defaults take (usually subconscious, automatic inferences) to the need for such defaults (default interpretations are cognitively 'cheap' and avoid a costly consultation of context), the cognitive character of defaults is unmistakeable. Moreover, 'weak' theories are also guided by the results of psychological experiments such as the finding that Levinson's strong notion of defaults is not supported by experimental evidence (Jaszczolt 2012). These theories are thus not divorced from features of the cognitive sphere.

So, to be of service to clinical pragmatics, theories originating within pragmatics must be cognitively oriented. But even when this requirement is met, as it is in the case of the strong theories and (to a lesser degree) weak theories described above, these theories are only infrequently used in clinical pragmatic research. To understand the reason for this lack of use, we need to examine the other major discipline that has shaped clinical pragmatics, the field of language pathology. Like clinical pragmatics, language pathology is a hybrid discipline with influences ranging from linguistics and neurology to psychology and child development. These fields equip language pathologists well to understand the nature and causes of language disorder. However, what is often neglected in the clinical education of students in language pathology is a sense of how theoretical developments in disciplines such as linguistics can contribute to an understanding of language disorder. It is important to understand the reasons for this neglect.

Some of this neglect can be accounted for quite simply by different priorities. For the clinician who must assess and treat clients with language disorder, theoretical debates in linguistics, many of which are abstract in nature, can appear to be of limited clinical relevance. Understandably, clinicians may view theory construction in linguistics and elsewhere as an indulgence which they can ill-afford when faced with the more pressing demands of busy clinics and targets for patient management. But an even more significant cause of this neglect is that theorists in pragmatics have tended to view clinical applications of their work as a rather low priority (or, indeed, as no priority at all). If clinical application is considered, it is usually as a type of afterthought and when theory construction is complete. When clinical application is treated in this way, it is unable to influence the key constructs of a theory. The result is a type of theory development which has limited clinical utility and which is perceived as such by clinicians.

In summary, theoretical models have not been particularly prominent in clinical pragmatics. The reasons for this lack of prominence are complex and include aspects of the clinical education of students, the lack of priority afforded to clinical application in theory construction, and the development of theories which are not cognitively oriented. In the next section, theories which have guided clinical pragmatic research to greater or lesser extents will be examined in detail. These theories include Sperber and Wilson's relevance theory, Bara's cognitive pragmatics theory and Kasher's modular pragmatics theory. As well as describing the key constructs and proposals of these theories, the findings of clinical studies which have been guided by these theories will also be considered. The stage will then be set for the critical evaluation of theoretical models in Sect. 4.4.

4.3 Theoretical Models in Clinical Pragmatics

The decision to restrict the discussion of this section to only cognitively 'strong' pragmatic theories is justified on the following grounds. Strong theories have been used in studies of language-intact subjects as well as subjects with a range of pragmatic disorders. Theories based on implicitures and defaults have been the subject of experimental pragmatic investigations in normal subjects for some time.[1] However, these cognitively 'weak' pragmatic theories are only just beginning to be examined in clinical subjects.[2] As such, they do not warrant discussion on the grounds that they are not yet significant theoretical frameworks in clinical pragmatic research. Even when weak theories are the focus of experimental investigations, more often than not this is with a view to testing the key claims and constructs of those theories. In this way, Garrett and Harnish (2007) report finding experimental evidence for the existence of implicitures, a meaning construct proposed by Bach (1994). The theories which will be examined in this section assume a quite different role in experimental studies. They are used to explain the pragmatic language skills of clinical subjects and to make predictions about those skills. If these theories perform this role badly, then some revision of their content would be in order. But theory testing and revision is not the primary role of the theories which will be considered in this section.

4.3.1 Relevance Theory

In relevance theory, Sperber and Wilson (1986, 1995) build on Gricean insights about meaning by developing a theory of utterance interpretation from within a cognitive psychological framework. In a landmark paper entitled 'Meaning' published in 1957, Grice delineated a notion called non-natural meaning (meaning$_{NN}$). The meaning$_{NN}$ of an utterance is to be understood in terms of the expression and recognition of (communicative) intentions. This is how Grice (1989, p. 219) captures this notion in *Studies in the Way of Words*:

> 'A meant something by x' is roughly equivalent to 'A uttered x with the intention of inducing a belief by means of the recognition of this intention'.

These intentions cannot be arrived at by the linguistic decoding of utterances. Indeed, the linguistic content of utterances (called 'what is said' by Grice) is often very different from the meaning which speakers intend to communicate by way of their use of utterances (in the case of irony, for example, linguistic content is the opposite meaning to that intended by the speaker). Rather, communicative intentions are recovered by an inferential process which is guided by certain rational expectations. Grice characterizes those expectations by means of his cooperative principle and maxims of quality, quantity, relation and manner. In relevance theory, a principle of relevance is advanced to perform the same role:

> [A]ll of Grice's maxims can be replaced by a single principle of relevance—that the speaker tries to be as relevant as possible in the circumstances—which, when suitably elaborated, can handle the full range of data that Grice's maxims were designed to explain (Wilson and Sperber 1991, p. 381).

A hearer is warranted in believing that a speaker's utterance is relevant to the conversational exchange, even when it seems that it is not, because of a presumption of optimal relevance. This presumption provides the hearer with a guarantee of sorts that the speaker's utterance is worth the cognitive effort of processing it—the hearer's expenditure of cognitive effort will be rewarded by the eventual recovery of the speaker's communicative intention in producing the utterance. In relevance theory, the hearer arrives at this intention by means of the relevance processing of factual assumptions in a deductive device. The assumption which produces the greatest number of contextual implications[3] for the least processing effort is the one which the hearer may take to represent the speaker's communicative intention. An example can be used to demonstrate how this relevance-theoretic procedure unfolds.[4] Consider the following exchange between Sally and Peter:

Sally: Was Jenny's presentation informative and interesting?
Peter: It was informative.

On the basis of this exchange, Sally may be expected to derive a certain implicature from Peter's response, an implicature to the effect that Jenny's presentation was *not* interesting. How does relevance theory account for Sally's seemingly effortless act of utterance interpretation in this exchange? Peter's utterance comes with a presumption of optimal relevance. To this extent, Sally knows that she will not be wasting cognitive effort if she processes this utterance and that there will be some reward for her expenditure of cognitive resources such as memory and reasoning. This reward may be the increased accuracy of her mental representation of the world by the inclusion of a new fact, namely, that Jenny's presentation was not interesting. And so Sally begins her quest to establish the relevance of Peter's response. In establishing a context in which to process the relevance of Peter's utterance, Sally will draw on perceptual data from her senses, on information stored in memory, on her knowledge of Peter's mental states, on preceding utterances in the conversational exchange and on her knowledge of conversational rules. Collectively, these various sources might make the following context available to Sally:

(1) Jenny is a friend of Sally's who has applied for a job at Peter's company (memory)
(2) Peter is the director of human resources at his company (memory)
(3) Presentations are typically required of candidates at interview (memory)
(4) Peter has frowned while producing his utterance (visual perception)
(5) Peter's intonation suggests disagreement with Sally's description (auditory perception)
(6) Peter knows Jenny and Sally are close friends (mental state attribution)

(7) Peter has been describing to Sally the day's events at work (preceding utterances)

(8) Sally has knowledge of conversational rules (metalinguistic knowledge).

Against this context, one can see how Sally might derive a certain implicature from Peter's utterance. Specifically, Sally will know that Peter is attempting to be cooperative in the exchange and, to this end, is presenting only truthful and relevant information to her (conversational knowledge). Sally also knows that she has asked about two attributes of Jenny's presentation and that Peter has only remarked on one attribute (linguistic decoding of Peter's utterance). Further, Sally knows that Peter knows that Sally and Jenny are close friends (mental state attribution). Therefore, it is likely that Peter will wish to avoid producing any statement that is directly critical of Jenny's presentation (politeness constraints). With these various considerations all brought together in Sally's deductive device, it is easy to see how Sally might go on to interpret Peter's under-informative response as implicating that Jenny's presentation was not interesting. With the relevance of Peter's utterance established, further processing of his utterance for its contextual implications ceases. The recovery of any other implicature from Peter's utterance would considerably extend the context that would have to be activated and, with it, the cost of processing this utterance.

Much of the success of relevance theory can be accounted for by the fact that the theory's claims about the relevance processing of utterances are sufficiently specific in nature that they can be used to make predictions about cognitive performance in a number of areas (Van der Henst and Sperber 2004). In the 30 years since relevance theory was first proposed, it has been used to explain results of spatial reasoning experiments (Van der Henst 1999) and the Wason selection task (Sperber et al. 1995; Fiddick et al. 2000; Girotto et al. 2001; Sperber and Girotto 2002), to account for features of child language development (Foster-Cohen 1994; Ryder and Leinonen 2003; Loukusa et al. 2007b), and to address theoretical questions in pragmatics such as whether the generation of implicatures is automatic (the neo-Gricean view of Levinson) or not automatic and effortful (the view of relevance theory) (Noveck and Posada 2003; De Neys and Schaeken 2007) (see Wilson (2010) for discussion of these different strands of relevance-theoretic research). Relevance theory has also been applied to the study of pragmatic disorders in children and adults with a range of clinical conditions. In the rest of this section, these studies will be examined with a view to demonstrating how theoretical models can make a significant contribution to clinical pragmatic research.

One of the earliest studies to apply relevance theory to the study of individuals with pragmatic disorder was Happé (1993). Drawing on relevance theory and the well-known theory of mind (ToM) deficits of children and adults with autism, Happé made predictions about how subjects with autism would process different types of figurative language. Specifically, similes can be comprehended on the basis of literal meaning alone and so should be understood by subjects with autism who have no ToM ability. However, metaphors and irony[5] can only be understood by the hearer who is able to attribute communicative intentions to the speaker's mind. On the basis of relevance theory, Happé predicted that metaphors and irony would be understood by subjects with autism who had first-order and second-order ToM ability, respectively. These relevance-theoretic predictions were borne out by experiments in which 18 subjects with autism listened to verbally-presented sentences and short passages and either selected words to complete the sentences or responded to questions based on the passages. Happé (1993, p. 115) captures the theoretical contribution of relevance theory to an understanding of figurative language in autism in the following terms:

> Relevance theory allows us to reason from the now well-known work showing a deficit in autistic subjects' theory of mind to the well-documented autistic communication handicap. It goes further than this, too, in relating *degree* of metarepresentational ability to *degree* of communicative ability in a quite specific way. The application of relevance theory to autism, therefore, both generates testable predictions about the nature of the autistic communication handicap, and leads to a possible method of testing relevance theory (italics in original).

More recently, Loukusa et al. (2007a) used relevance theory in a study of the responses of children with Asperger syndrome or high-functioning autism (AS/HFA) to contextually demanding questions. According to Sperber and Wilson's principle of relevance, subjects should use a relevant context in generating their responses to questions, but then cease relevance processing when a relevant response is made. The relevancy of responses in this study was defined in relevance-theoretic terms. Three categories of erroneous response were identified. In type 1 errors, children answered the question incorrectly. In type 2 errors, the correct answer was given but in a follow-up question children explained the answer incorrectly. In type 3 errors, children gave a correct answer or explanation. However, they continued answering which eventually led them to give an irrelevant answer.

There were only some significant differences between children with AS/HFA and control children on type 1 errors. This suggested that even when answers were incorrect, they were not totally irrelevant. In terms of type 2 errors, children with AS/HFA had more incorrect explanations than control children particularly in the category of 'incorrect use of world knowledge'. Type 3 errors were common in the children with AS/HFA but were almost non-existent in the control group. The children with AS/HFA were unable to cease relevance processing when they had given the correct response. The resulting topic drifts were explained in relevance-theoretic terms as a failure to achieve optimal relevance. Loukusa et al. (2007a, p. 375) stated that 'we are not suggesting that pragmatic difficulties can be explained by relevance theory alone, but it can help us in locating elements that may cause communication breakdown'.

Leinonen and Kerbel (1999) use the framework of relevance theory to account for the pragmatic difficulties of three children. Relevance theory proposes a level of utterance meaning which is distinct from an implicature. Known as an explicature,[6] this level of meaning is the explicit content of the utterance which is arrived at by means of the pragmatic processes of disambiguation, reference assignment, and loosening (e.g. 'flat' used to mean *relatively flat*). Leinonen and Kerbel demonstrate the different ways in which the children in this study fail to achieve the explicature of an utterance. For example, the pragmatic difficulties of a girl called Sarah (9.8–10.3 years at the time of study) can be traced in part to her problems with enrichment. Specifically, Sarah fails to enrich an instruction to continue telling a story which the researcher has started, and ends up repeating what the researcher has said instead.Having obtained the explicature of the utterance, further relevance processing is required in order for the hearer to derive the implicit meaning (implicature) of an utterance. Here, again, Sarah displays problems when she fails to recover an implicature of remarks made by the researcher during a conversation about holidays. The researcher utters 'It'll be a bit cold in January, after Christmas, won't it?' with the intention of implicating that Sarah's holiday cannot be a beach holiday. This implicature is missed by Sarah altogether. Leinonen and Kerbel (1999, p. 388) summarize the contribution of relevance theory to the analysis of these children's pragmatic difficulties in the following terms:

> [R]elevance theory offers a way of explaining why, in a given context, a particular expression is problematic. The theory thus moves us away from mere description of surface behaviours to an understanding of how the communication difficulty came about.

Relevance theory has also been used to examine pragmatic language difficulties in adults. Dipper et al. (1997) used relevance theory to explain difficulties with bridging inference in adults with right-hemisphere damage (RHD). Three types of bridging inference—textual, textually reinforced and encyclopaedic—were examined in six subjects with RHD and 12 control subjects. A textual bridging inference is based on the linguistic content of the text, e.g. Kathy took the long hose to water the garden. She was wearing her new waterproof suit (inference: she was wearing a waterproof suit because she was watering the garden). A textually reinforced bridging inference is dependent on a discourse connective that directs the way in which a second sentence must be understood in light of the first sentence, e.g. The exam was even harder than Paul had expected. Still he came top of the class (inference: it was not expected that Paul would come top of the class given the difficult nature of the exam).

An encyclopaedic bridging inference draws upon knowledge in encyclopaedic memory, e.g. My sister chopped the onions. Tears were running down her face (inference: tears are caused by the chopping of onions). Subjects with RHD performed worse than control subjects overall and performed differentially on the three types of inference. Inferences based on discourse connectives were harder than other inference types for subjects with RHD and were significantly harder than encyclopaedic inferences. A relevance-theoretic explanation of this difference in performance is that the clinical subjects in this study have difficulty using linguistic information from the text in the deductive system and are over-reliant on encyclopaedic information. Such information is lacking in the case of inferences based on discourse connectives, thus explaining the poor performance of subjects with RHD on this type of inference.

In addition to the above studies, relevance theory has been used to investigate referent specification in children with specific language impairment (SLI) (Schelletter and Leinonen 2003) and the over-interpretation of utterances by individuals with schizophrenia who have paranoid delusions (Cram and Hedley 2005). The theory has also been used to develop an assessment of pragmatic language comprehension in children with SLI (Ryder et al. 2008). In studies where relevance theory has been used to investigate pragmatic language disorders, it is clear that researchers believe it has made a significant contribution to the understanding of these disorders. In Sect. 4.4, we examine that contribution in more detail and assess what merits (and drawbacks) have resulted from the use of relevance theory in clinical pragmatic research. In the meantime, we turn to examine another theoretical model that has been applied to the study of pragmatic disorders in children and adults.

4.3.2 Cognitive Pragmatics Theory

As the name suggests, cognitive pragmatics theory takes a strong cognitive stance to the interpretation of utterances. This cognitive orientation is evident in the preface to Bara's book of the same name: 'I will take a standpoint within the mind of the individual participants, trying to explain how each communicative act is generated mentally—before being realized physically—and then comprehended mentally by the other interlocutors' (Bara 2010, p. ix). While Bara follows Sperber and Wilson in casting the mental processes of communication in terms of an inferential mechanism, he explicitly rejects relevance theory's reliance on deductive rules, claiming that '[h]uman beings reason not by applying innate logical rules, but by constructing and manipulating mental models that subjectively represent states of affairs in the world' (Bara 2010, p. 22). He also doubts that a single principle of relevance is 'sufficient to explain all of the phenomena that make up communication' (2010, p. 22). Given these and other significant differences in theoretical approach, the reader is assured a distinctive cognitive treatment of utterance interpretation in cognitive pragmatics theory. It is to an examination of that distinctive treatment that we now turn.

At the conceptual heart of cognitive pragmatics theory is the notion of a behaviour game. The expression 'behaviour game' is not an accidental coinage. Rather, Bara intends it to hark back to the Wittgensteinian concept of a language game. For Wittgenstein, a range of games may be played out through the use of language. According to Bara (2010, p. 93), Wittgenstein's idea that one should focus on the *use* of language, rather than on language *form*, is 'one that is definitely revolutionary and that still maintains its validity more than 50 years later'. As applied to cognitive pragmatics, a behaviour game is a structure which allows the interpersonal actions of actors to be coordinated, and enables actors to select the intended meaning of an utterance from the many different meanings that an utterance could, in theory, convey. To see how this is achieved, Bara (2010, p. 95) presents the following example in which two actors, *A* and *B*, are discussing exam arrangements:

A: Tomorrow's Thursday. Will you coordinate the exam supervision?
B: Actually, the Vice Chancellor has fixed a meeting for 9 am.

B's response may be taken to be a refusal of *A*'s request to coordinate the exam supervision. The concept of a behaviour game, Bara contends, allows us to explain how the actors in this case arrive at this particular interpretation of the interaction. Specifically, through her request, *A* is proposing that she and *B* play a behaviour game called 'pedagogical duties'. This game stipulates who is responsible for running departmental activities on certain days of the week. It is mutual knowledge of this game that allows the actors in this case to achieve conversational cooperation, even if a particular actor fails to execute a certain move specified by the game, in which case behavioural cooperation is not achieved. Actors need not be fully aware of a behaviour game in order to play it, as a tacit representation of the game suffices to direct their actions. As well as containing actions, behaviour games also have validity conditions which specify the conditions under which games may be played. These conditions are an extension of Austin's (1962) felicity conditions and can apply to any move in a game (and not just performatives à la Austin). Like felicity conditions, validity conditions can describe the mental states of participants, the time and place in which games may take place, etc.

There are many other aspects of cognitive pragmatics theory which we cannot address in the current context. (The reader is referred to Bara (2010, 2011) for a detailed account of the theory.) However, on the basis of the discussion so far, we can describe how Bara applies cognitive pragmatics to the interpretation of a range of different utterances. Regardless of the type of utterance produced by the speaker, the hearer's first task in interpreting an utterance is always identifying the behaviour game to which it refers: 'The key point for the partner is always that of recognizing the opening bid in a behaviour game, in whatever form that move is expressed' (Bara 2010, p. 147). It is the complexity of the inferential chain which connects a speaker's expression act to the opening of a behaviour game which determines the ease or difficulty with which hearers interpret utterances. Certain speech acts are more complex than other speech acts because they require a larger number of inferences to link them to a game. Inferential complexity is thus a key criterion in Bara's categorization of speech acts such as irony and deceit:

> I will speak of *simple irony* when the interlocutor can grasp speaker meaning instantly, moving directly from the utterance to the behaviour game of which the utterance may be considered a move…I define *complex irony* as irony in which the interlocutor must carry out a series of inferences in order to grasp speaker meaning…the difficulty of an act of deception depends on the number of inferences B requires to reach the hidden game, starting from A's untruthful communication act (Bara 2011, p. 469–470; italics in original).

As well as the inferential chain that is needed to link an utterance to a behaviour game, Bara contends that the type of mental representation also plays a role in predicting the ease with which actors comprehend speech acts. Specifically, in standard communication there is no conflict between a speaker's expression act and the speaker's communicative intention. Standard communication acts (e.g. direct and conventional indirect acts) will thus be easier to comprehend than non-standard communication acts (e.g. deceit and irony) where there is a conflict between the expression act and the speaker's communicative intention. The reader can see that

two straightforwardly testable empirical claims lie at the centre of cognitive pragmatics theory: the difficulty of interpreting utterances increases with the number
of inferences that are required to link an utterance to a behaviour game (inferential load) and when there is a conflict between the expression act and a speaker's
mental states (type of mental representation). These empirical claims have been
directly addressed by Bara and colleagues in a series of experimental studies conducted on normal and clinical subjects.[7]

Bara's cognitive pragmatics theory has received much support from studies of developmental pragmatics in normal children. Bara et al. (2000) examined the comprehension of communication acts in an extralinguistic modality
in 80 children across four age groups: 2.6–3 years; 3.6–4 years; 4.6–5.6 years
and 6–7 years. The emergence of acts in these children was expected to follow a trend of difficulty based on cognitive pragmatics theory. It was predicted
that standard communication acts would emerge before non-standard communication acts (the former involve less complex mental representations) and
that deceits would appear before ironies (the former involve a lower inferential load). These predictions were supported. A similar trend of difficulty was
reported in a study by Bucciarelli et al. (2003). As well as examining the comprehension of communicative gestures (extralinguistic modality), these investigators also studied the comprehension of speech acts (linguistic modality).
A total of 160 children were divided equally across the same four age groups
used in Bara et al.'s study. The expected trend of difficulty in the comprehension of these acts, based on the predictions of cognitive pragmatics theory, was
confirmed in both linguistic and extralinguistic modalities. Bosco et al. (2006b)
examined the recognition and repair of communicative failures in children aged
3–8 years. The performance of these children conformed to a trend of difficulty
predicted by cognitive pragmatics theory, based on the representational complexity and inferential load of communicative failures.

The central tenets of cognitive pragmatics theory also accord with pragmatic
performance in a range of clinical subjects. Cutica et al. (2006) examined extralinguistic pragmatic ability in 10 patients with right-hemisphere damage, 9 patients
with left-hemisphere damage and 10 healthy controls. On the basis of cognitive
pragmatics theory, these investigators predicted that non-standard communication would be more difficult than standard communication for patients and controls (only the former type of communication involves a conflict between what is
expressed and what is privately entertained by an actor). They also predicted that
direct and conventional indirect acts would be equally difficult for both patients
and controls, as they require a single-step inferential chain. Finally, because non-
conventional indirect acts involve a longer inferential chain for their comprehension than either direct or conventional indirect acts, they should be more difficult
to comprehend both for patients and controls. In all but one case, these predictions
were confirmed. The exception was the comprehension of conventional indirect
acts by patients with RHD which was more difficult for these subjects than the
comprehension of direct acts. Cutica et al. attribute this aspect of performance of
patients with RHD to a loss of knowledge of conventional social games.

Also using an extralinguistic pragmatic protocol, Bara et al. (2000) demonstrated that impaired comprehension of speech acts in patients with Alzheimer's disease followed the expected trend of difficulty based on cognitive pragmatics theory. Ironies were more impaired than deceits with both of these non-standard communication acts more impaired than standard communication acts. Moreover, the pattern of speech act deterioration in these patients was better explained by cognitive pragmatics theory than by the performance of patients on neuropsychological tests. Angeleri et al. (2008) extended earlier clinical studies by examining the understanding *and* production of communicative acts in 21 subjects with TBI. Subjects were tested on a pragmatic assessment—the Assessment Battery of Communication—which is based on cognitive pragmatics theory. Subjects with TBI not only displayed poorer pragmatic performance than control subjects, but their performance in both linguistic and extralinguistic modalities followed the same trend of difficulty that was evident in other studies: standard communication acts were easier for these subjects than deceits which, in turn, were easier than ironies. Yet again, the predictions of cognitive pragmatics theory were confirmed.

This discussion is by no means exhaustive. It omits a number of clinical studies in which cognitive pragmatics theory has been used to explain patterns of pragmatic impairment, such as in subjects with closed head injury (Bara et al. 1997) and in mute children with autism (Bara et al. 2001) (For further discussion, the reader is referred to Bara et al. (1999) who examine several other clinical conditions in addition to closed head injury and autism). However, what this account does demonstrate is the wide base of experimental evidence which exists in support of cognitive pragmatics theory. It remains to be seen if this theory can withstand the critical evaluation of Sect. 4.4. In the meantime, we turn to the final theoretical model to be examined in this chapter. This model is Kasher's modular pragmatics theory.

4.3.3 Modular Pragmatics Theory

The modular pragmatics theory of Asa Kasher has been outlined in several articles and chapters published over a number of years (e.g. Kasher 1984, 1991a, 1991b, 1994). The theory is of significance to our present discussion for the following reasons. Firstly, modular pragmatics theory takes a strong cognitive orientation to utterance interpretation. It, therefore, satisfies the requirement that a pragmatic theory must be cognitively oriented in order to be plausible. Secondly, the theory is sufficiently specific in its predictions about the processing of different pragmatic phenomena that its central tenets are testable. We will consider some of the experimental evidence which supports the theory. Thirdly, like relevance theory and cognitive pragmatics theory, modular pragmatics theory has been applied to the study of pragmatic language skills in several clinical populations. The findings of these studies have direct relevance to clinical pragmatics and we will examine them below. In this section, we begin the discussion of modular pragmatics theory by outlining its theoretical orientation and claims. We then turn to consider evidence in support of the theory. Finally, we examine how the theory has been used to explain pragmatic impairments in a range of clinical subjects.

As its name suggests, modular pragmatics theory bears more than a superficial resemblance to a cognitive thesis known as modularity of mind. Although there are historical antecedents of the view of mind contained in this thesis, the modularity of mind claim can be said to have originated in the philosophical work of Jerry Fodor. It was in Fodor's 1983 book *The modularity of Mind* that the content of the modularity thesis was first laid bare. In that book, Fodor makes a number of significant claims about mental architecture. Specifically, he believes that certain cognitive functions of the mind (e.g. perception) are mediated by modules which perform these functions by virtue of their possession of particular properties. Chief among these properties is informational encapsulation. An informationally encapsulated cognitive module only has access to information of a certain type or within a circumscribed domain. The visual perception module, for example, only has access to visual perceptual data. It does not have access to linguistic data (only the language module has such access) or to information in the mind's central system (the central system is the locus of belief fixation in the Fodorian view of mind). In addition to informational encapsulation, modular cognitive systems are also domain specific, innately specified, hardwired, autonomous, and not assembled (the reader is referred to Meini (2010) for an accessible account of these features and the modularity of mind thesis). Fodor's work, and particularly his thesis of modularity, has had a profound influence on disciplines in cognitive science. As one of those disciplines, pragmatics has also been influenced by the modularity thesis.

A question of interest to pragmatists has been the extent (if any) to which pragmatic or communicative competence can be modelled in terms of a cognitive module. For cognitive pragmatists like Bara, it is clear that modularity has no place in an account of communicative competence:

> Communicative competence is not a Fodorian module, at least because it is intentional (that is, representational) and because it is not encapsulated (that is, it does not function independently of the rest of what is going on in the agent's mind) (Bara and Tirassa 2000, p. 12).

Relevance theorists such as Sperber and Wilson would concur with Bara that pragmatics cannot be captured by a classical Fodorian module. However, they are not thereby sceptical about the prospects of success of the entire modular project in pragmatics. According to Wilson (2005), pragmatics is a type of mind-reading which is performed by a domain-specific inferential module. And while pragmatic interpretation is not merely the application of general mind-reading abilities to the communicative domain, it is nonetheless a dedicated module which trades on certain regularities within this domain:

> Verbal communication presents special challenges, and exhibits certain regularities, not found in other domains, and these may have led to the development of a dedicated comprehension module with its own special-purpose principles and mechanisms (Wilson 2005, p. 1131).

This relevance-theoretic view supersedes an earlier, and more pessimistic, view about the prospects of arriving at a modular account of pragmatics. This view was captured by Wilson and Sperber (1991, p. 583) in the following terms: 'There are no special-purpose pragmatic principles, maxims, strategies or rules; pragmatics is simply the domain in which grammar, logic and memory interact'. We will see below that Kasher was already advocating a modular approach to pragmatics in 1991, when such an approach was outwardly rejected by relevance theorists. In this way, relevance theorists may be seen as latter-day converts to a view of pragmatics that was already beginning to take shape over 20 years ago.

In order to identify a modular component within our pragmatic knowledge, Kasher must first revise the notion of a 'module' and of 'pragmatics'. Kasher readily accedes to the view that the conversational implicatures of an utterance cannot be determined without appeal to central principles of rationality in intentional action. To this extent, conversational implicatures cannot be represented by an input cognitive module, at least not as that notion is conceived by Fodor: 'We replace the notion of a 'module' as an input cognitive system of certain properties by a notion of a 'module' as a cognitive system that is independent, in several significant respects' (Kasher 1991a, p. 389). According to Kasher, a reconceptualization of pragmatics is also necessary. Every time we speak, Kasher contends, we are performing a basic speech act such as an assertion or a question. To this extent, part of our pragmatic knowledge must be linguistic in nature: 'we have knowledge of basic speech act types, such as assertion and question, which is definitely part of one's knowledge of language' (Kasher 1991a, p. 388). Kasher is able to use these adjustments on the side of both 'pragmatics' and the notion of a 'module' to formulate what he calls the Modularity of Pragmatic Knowledge Hypothesis:

The pragmatic knowledge, of appropriateness relations between sentences and contexts of use, consists of two separate parts:

(I) Modular, pragmatic knowledge, which is purely linguistic and
(II) Central, pragmatic knowledge, which is not purely linguistic (Kasher 1991a, p. 389).

This hypothesis, Kasher contends, commits one to the existence of at least one pragmatic module. Kasher treats it as an open question whether all modular pragmatic knowledge is embodied in a single module, or in several modules. As well as examining possible candidates for this modular pragmatic knowledge, Kasher (1991a, p. 391) delineates other aspects of pragmatic knowledge 'which seem to be related to the general center of cognition'. As one might expect, there are rational intentional processes of the type that allow a hearer to calculate the implicatures of a speaker's utterances (central pragmatics). Additionally, there are a number of interfaces which allow the integration of information from different modules, which can then serve as input to the central system (interface pragmatics). This pragmatic knowledge is the basis upon which we identify referents of indexical expressions such as 'she' and 'there'. In such cases, the output of a language module must be integrated with the output of a perception module, with the central system achieving an integrated understanding of the referent based on information from both sources. Another important component of Kasher's modular pragmatics theory is its attempt to localise each type of pragmatic knowledge in the brain.[8] A proposal for the localization of pragmatic knowledge that is consistent with clinical findings is one in which modular pragmatics is located in the brain's left hemisphere, while parts of central pragmatics are in the right hemisphere. It will be noted that this proposal affords for the first time a significant role in the processing of language pragmatics to the left hemisphere. We will shortly review evidence in support of this proposed localization.

Clearly, the entire edifice of Kasher's modular pragmatics theory rests on the existence of a pragmatics module which is responsible for the processing of basic speech acts. Even more clearly, if Kasher and colleagues cannot bring forward evidence in support of such a dedicated pragmatics module, then the very validity of modular pragmatics theory is in doubt. That evidence derives from a number of sources, as Kasher (1994, p. 314–315) explicitly acknowledges:

> In order to show that a cognitive subsystem is a module we have to demonstrate its independence of other systems on the theoretical level of the principles that govern it, on the psychological level of its information processing, on the neural level of its embodiment in human brain and on the psychological level of its acquisition.

Kasher and his co-workers present evidence across all four areas in support of a modular pragmatics. In the rest of this section, we will examine the substantial support which exists for modular pragmatics theory in investigations of pragmatic skills in clinical subjects. Among the subjects included in these investigations are children with autism[9] and adults with schizophrenia, and left- and right-hemisphere damage. The experimental findings of the latter studies hold particular theoretical significance and will be examined in detail.

Meilijson et al. (2004) found support for a modular category of basic speech acts in a study of 43 patients with chronic schizophrenia. According to Kasher, basic speech acts are performed every time we speak. In fact, one cannot be said to have fully mastered one's language in the absence of pragmatic knowledge of the use and understanding of basic speech acts. Given that every instance of naming or auditory language comprehension is achieved as part of some wider speech act, one might expect to find a relationship between basic speech acts and other language skills (and not just pragmatic language skills). In fact, this is exactly what Meilijson et al. demonstrated in their study. Patients were assessed on Prutting and Kirchner's (1987) pragmatic protocol. The speech acts assessed by this protocol—directive/compliance, query/response, request/response, comment/acknowledgement—are similar to Kasher's basic speech acts and were treated as such by Meilijson et al. Performance on speech acts was found to correlate with all other clusters examined by the protocol (non-verbal, lexical, turn-taking, topic). 'This suggests that speech acts are a necessary basic tool for all other clusters' (Meilijson et al. 2004, p. 707). Kasher's inclusion of basic speech acts within a modular core pragmatics would appear to be confirmed by this finding. Furthermore, given this fundamental role of basic speech acts, one might reasonably expect the appropriateness of these acts to be a good predictor of appropriateness on other clusters. This prediction was also confirmed.

Unlike the above investigation of schizophrenia, the study of subjects with focal lesions of either the left or right hemisphere permits the testing of claims in modular pragmatics theory about the neuroanatomical localization of natural language pragmatics. According to this theory, both hemispheres play a role in the processing of pragmatics. However, these roles are different, with tentative evidence suggesting that modular pragmatic knowledge is localized to the left hemisphere and central pragmatics is localized to the right hemisphere. This was one of the questions addressed by Kasher et al. (1999) in a study of 31 subjects with left-hemisphere damage (LHD) and 27 subjects with right-hemisphere damage (RHD). Along with age-matched normal controls, these subjects completed an implicatures battery that examined verbal and non-verbal implicatures of quantity, quality, relation and manner. Subjects also completed Hebrew versions of the Western Aphasia Battery (Kertesz 1979) and the Right Hemisphere Communication Battery (Gardner and Brownell 1986),[10] a test of basic speech acts, and standard neuropsychological tests.

Several predictions were made about the performance of the clinical subjects in this study based on modular pragmatics theory. Some of these predictions are considered here. Conversational implicatures depend on maxims, which have the status of general rationality principles. These principles are located in the mind's central system, which is indifferent to the modality of information it processes. If modular pragmatics theory is a valid account of pragmatics in the mind/brain, one may expect to find similar deficits in the processing of verbal and non-verbal implicatures (prediction 1). The central system also contains a number of cognitive processes which are measured by the neuropsychological tests used in the study. If implicatures are a central system process, then one may expect to find a relationship between central cognitive abilities and the processing of implicatures (prediction 2). Modular pragmatics theory states that a basic speech act is performed every time we speak. It may therefore be predicted that deficits in these acts should result in deficits in implicatures, but not vice versa (prediction 3).

If modular pragmatic knowledge of the type required for basic speech acts is independent of the language module—as modular pragmatics theory predicts it is—then the processing of implicatures can be expected to be related to basic speech acts, but not to more conventional language skills of the type tested by an aphasia battery (prediction 4). Modular pragmatics theory predicts that both cerebral hemispheres contribute to the processing of natural language pragmatics, but that they do so in different ways. The contribution of the left hemisphere comes in the form of a pragmatic module, while the right hemisphere contributes the general rationality principles that make up the central system. One may expect to find localization of modular pragmatic knowledge (represented by basic speech acts) within a specific area of the left hemisphere, while central pragmatic knowledge is likely to have a more diffuse localization in the right hemisphere (prediction 5).

All five predictions were confirmed for the most part by the findings of this study. In relation to prediction 1, verbal and non-verbal implicatures intercorrelated highly in subjects with LHD, but not in subjects with RHD. There was, therefore, evidence of some processing mechanism based on general rationality principles in the left hemisphere but not in the right hemisphere. This mechanism, which Kasher et al.

call a general implicatures processor, processes verbal and non-verbal information in the same way. There was also broad support for prediction 2. Significant correlations were obtained between standardized neuropsychological tests and implicatures, particularly in subjects with RHD. This confirms implicatures as a central system process along with more general cognitive abilities measured by neuropsychological tests. Prediction 3 was also largely confirmed. In subjects with LHD, most subtests of the implicature battery correlated positively and significantly with most subtests of the basic speech act battery. This is what one would expect if implicatures presuppose some wider basic speech act, as modular pragmatics theory claims is the case. This same pattern was observed in subjects with RHD, but only for the non-verbal components of both batteries.

There was also broad support for prediction 4. Although implicatures correlated positively and significantly with basic speech acts, only some implicatures correlated significantly with only some language functions in the left hemisphere. These language functions were tested by an aphasia battery and included naming, reading and writing in particular. Correlations between implicatures and language functions were even weaker in the right hemisphere. This is exactly the pattern one would expect given that linguistic knowledge is mediated by a distinct language module which is independent of both modular and central pragmatic knowledge. In relation to prediction 5, it was found that both groups of clinical subjects displayed impaired performance on the implicatures battery with the right-hemisphere deficit no more selective or pronounced than the left-hemisphere deficit. This result confirms a role for the left hemisphere in the processing of implicatures, as predicted by modular pragmatics theory. Implicature deficits remained even when the effects of aphasia in subjects with LHD and visuospatial deficits in subjects with RHD were neutralized. This finding is also consistent with modular pragmatics theory, as the modular and central pragmatic knowledge presumed to be involved in the processing of implicatures is independent of the linguistic knowledge embodied by the language module. Neither the left or right hemisphere displayed strong anatomical localization of implicatures (but see below for evidence of the localization of basic speech acts to the left hemisphere).

The central tenets of modular pragmatics theory receive further validation from a study by Soroker et al. (2005), who examined the neuroanatomical localization of basic speech acts in adults with stroke-induced lesions of either the left or right hemisphere. Both groups of clinical subjects performed more poorly than controls on a pragmatics battery that examines basic speech acts. The subjects with LHD not only performed more poorly than subjects with RHD on the processing of basic speech acts—a finding which challenges the idea that the right hemisphere is dominant in the processing of natural language pragmatics—but there was evidence of systematic localization of basic speech acts to the left hemisphere. Specifically, assertions displayed narrow inferior left frontal localization, questions wider left frontal localization, requests left fronto-temporal localization and commands left temporo-parietal localization. With the exception of requests, which were localized to the right middle frontal gyrus, systematic localization was not observed in subjects with RHD.

As well as supporting the predictions of modular pragmatics theory concerning the localization of pragmatics in the brain, Soroker et al.'s investigation supports another key claim of this theory. To the extent that, as Kasher claims, we are performing basic speech acts every time we speak, we might expect to find a relationship between the processing of basic speech acts in the left hemisphere and more conventional language skills of the type tested by clinical aphasia batteries. Just such a relationship was established. Soroker et al. found significant correlations between the four basic speech acts in subjects with LHD and almost all components on the Hebrew version of the Western Aphasia Battery. This finding led Soroker et al. to propose that aphasia batteries assess language functions (e.g. auditory language comprehension) that presuppose control over basic speech acts. The anatomical localization of the language functions tested by aphasia batteries may in part reflect the localization of the basic speech acts that are required to perform those functions. However, to the extent that basic speech acts did not correlate with grammatical ability, it is clear that the localization of basic speech acts does not reflect the localization of the syntactic, semantic or phonological components of those acts.

Like the other cognitively 'strong' pragmatic theories we have examined in this chapter, it emerges that modular pragmatics theory has substantial empirical support among studies of clinical subjects. For the most part, the theory can explain the relationships and dissociations in language and pragmatic skills that we would expect to find if pragmatic processing in the mind/brain were to proceed according to a modular pragmatic framework. Of course, any theory grows in stature when it is shown to predict and explain certain facts, in this case, the facts of utterance interpretation. However, it will not have escaped the reader's attention that all three theories have succeeded in bringing forward experimental evidence in support of their claims. Given that these theories involve competing or opposing claims, one is led to conclude that experimental evidence should not be treated as a final arbiter in an assessment of the validity of theories. It is perhaps appropriate at this point to move the debate onto non-empirical grounds. This is exactly what we will do in the final section of this chapter.

4.4 Critical Evaluation of Pragmatic Theories

In Cummings (2009), it was argued that researchers in clinical pragmatics have typically adopted an uncritical stance to the study of pragmatic disorders. This stance has seen a proliferation of clinical findings with little sense of how these findings are related to each other or to theoretically significant questions. It is not an exaggeration to say that a relentless growth of clinical findings which are largely devoid of theoretical implications has been the dominant trend in clinical pragmatics to date. As long as theory construction, and the critical evaluation that attends such construction, is seen as the concern of others—principally, linguists and philosophers—there is little prospect, I believe, of reversing this dominant trend. Yet, reverse it, we must if clinical pragmatics is not to develop into a field that collects findings in the same way that the geologist collects rock samples or the botanist collects plant species. The hallmark of a mature field of enquiry is that experimental findings are not an end in themselves, but that they enter into further theory development. The critical, reflective processes that are the basis of theory development have been lacking in clinical pragmatics to this point. It is with the aim of establishing these processes as a standard feature of clinical pragmatics that the discussion of this final section is undertaken.

Previously, each of the theories we have examined in this chapter has been critically evaluated on philosophical grounds: relevance theory (see Chap. 4 in Cummings (2005)), cognitive pragmatics theory (see Cummings (2012d)) and modular pragmatics theory (see Chap. 5 in both Cummings (2005, 2009)). Philosophical criticisms can make a substantial contribution to theory construction even in clinically-oriented disciplines such as clinical pragmatics. However, it can sometimes appear that these criticisms have limited relevance for the clinical researchers and practitioners who need to be persuaded by them. Here, the task will be to demonstrate that relevance by conducting a criticism which has both philosophical and clinical components. The philosophical aspect will address if our three theories are able to meet certain conditions in the absence of which, it will be argued, utterance interpretation is not possible. The clinical aspect will consider how these conditions have relevance to the contexts in which clinical researchers and practitioners operate. The result should be a form of theory construction which might have some prospect of taking root in clinical pragmatics.

To establish the essence of any process or activity, one cannot do much better than examine it in action. Utterance interpretation is no exception in this regard. A typical instance of utterance interpretation unfolds as follows:

Hilda: Did Jack come in late last night?
Oscar: His curtains are still drawn.

Hilda will have the same reaction to Oscar's statement as the rest of us: she will take him to be conversationally implicating that Jack did indeed come in late last night. The cognitive and linguistic processes which make it possible for her to derive Oscar's implicature are truly the 'essence' of utterance interpretation. These same processes are also what a theory of utterance interpretation should be attempting to capture. I want to contend that these processes embody certain characteristics which are, in effect, the parameters or conditions under which utterance interpretation is even possible. So central are these characteristics to the very 'essence' of utterance interpretation that a pragmatic theory which fails to capture them is, by virtue of this fact alone, not a pragmatic theory which can be endorsed. Certainly, this fundamental claim is both our starting point and last word in this discussion.

The first thing to notice about the above exchange is that it contains explicable and predictable (i.e. rational) moves on the part of both communicators. It may sound grandiose to say that utterance interpretation involves the exercise of reason or rationality. But this is, indeed, the case. Although she is not aware of it—processes of utterance interpretation only occasionally make it into conscious thought—Hilda is undertaking a number of rational judgements about the situation she is in, her communicative partner, and much else besides. These judgements are what lead her to believe that Oscar is making a relevant, truthful and informative contribution to the exchange (i.e. a cooperative contribution), notwithstanding the superficial irrelevance of his utterance. These same judgements are what lead her to make several inferences linking Oscar's remark about curtains to Hilda's question about Jack's time of return. Specifically, Hilda's line of reasoning can be reconstructed as a series of two linked modus ponens inferences of the form *if p then q, p, therefore q*:

Modus ponens inference 1:

Major premise: If Jack's curtains are drawn, then Jack is sleeping.
Minor premise: Jack's curtains are drawn.
Conclusion: Jack is sleeping.

Modus ponens inference 2:

Major premise: If Jack is sleeping, then he came in late last night.
Minor premise: Jack is sleeping.
Conclusion: He came in late last night.

This series of linked inferences only works because of a proposition in common: Jack is sleeping. But it demonstrates quite clearly that Hilda is engaging in a process of reasoning when she recovers the implicature that Jack came in late last night from Oscar's utterance. This reasoning has been represented by deductive (modus ponens) inferences, but it may equally assume a non-deductive form. The exact form of this reasoning is less important than the fact that it should involve a full-blown or unconstrained rational capacity. This is necessary as it is impossible to say what factors a hearer may bring to the interpretation of an utterance or, indeed, what implicatures a hearer may recover from an utterance. For example, Hilda could have taken Oscar's utterance to implicate 'I don't know if Jack came in late last night. His curtains are drawn and I cannot check if he is in his room'. The exercise of an unconstrained rational capacity applied through one or more processes of reasoning is the first 'condition' which we will be asking our pragmatic theories of utterance interpretation to address.

The second thing to notice about the above exchange between Hilda and Oscar is the intentional character of each of the communicative moves. Hilda's question to Oscar reveals certain of her mental states to him—Hilda *wants* to obtain information about the time of Jack's return and *believes* that Oscar can provide that information. Oscar's response to Hilda also reveals some of his mental states to her—Oscar *believes* Jack returned late and *wants* to convey that information to Hilda. The utterances that are exchanged between Hilda and Oscar are only significant to the extent that they reveal the mental states, and specifically the communicative intentions, of each communicator. These mental states are the basis of the various propositions in Hilda's reasoning which is presented again below.

Contrary to most accounts, it can be seen that mental state attribution is not simply the end point in Hilda's reasoning—the attribution of a particular communicative intention to Oscar—but that the attribution of mental states contributes propositions much earlier in Hilda's reasoning. Many of these propositions capture the content of mental states which Hilda attributes to her own mind (the ability to attribute mental states to one's *own* mind is as important to utterance interpretation as the ability to attribute mental states to the minds of others):

Modus ponens inference 1:

Major premise: If Jack's curtains are drawn, then Jack is sleeping. **Hilda's belief**
Minor premise: Jack's curtains are drawn. **Oscar's knowledge**
Conclusion: Jack is sleeping. **Hilda's belief**

Modus ponens inference 2:

Major premise: If Jack is sleeping, then he came in late last night. **Hilda's belief**
Minor premise: Jack is sleeping. **Hilda's belief**
Conclusion: He came in late last night. **Oscar's communicative intention**

The combination of self- and other-attribution of mental states is what sets utterance interpretation apart from language decoding and a number of other cognitive processes (e.g. perception). Once again, it is not an exaggeration to say that in reflecting on the interpretation of utterances, we are forced to engage with some of the most fundamental issues in the philosophy of mind. Chief amongst them is the question of what it is to have a mind that can represent mental states and states of affairs (intentionality). The intentional character of utterance interpretation is the second 'condition' we will be asking our pragmatic theories to address.

The third thing to notice about the above exchange between Hilda and Oscar is its holistic character. No item of information, however seemingly insignificant or irrelevant, is unavailable to Hilda as she attempts to recover the implicature of Oscar's utterance. Certainly, Hilda draws on the linguistic utterances in the exchange, her understanding of Oscar's mental states, and her knowledge of who Jack is in deriving Oscar's implicature. But this is really only the start of the informational nexus that Hilda will bring to her interpretation of the utterances in this exchange. She will also need to know what curtains are used for, that Jack had been out the night before, and that people who are late to bed are often tired the following day. But then each of these items of information presupposes further items. For example, Hilda can only make sense of what curtains are used for— blocking out daylight—if she further understands that levels of daylight fluctuate during a 24-h period and that daylight can prevent people from sleeping. We do not need to continue in order to demonstrate the point at issue. Utterance interpretation is a truly holistic process which can avail of any, and all, knowledge. Philosophers of different bents have described holism as semantic or epistemic in nature. The exact nomenclature in this case is less important than is the idea of interconnectedness (between thoughts or theoretical statements) that is central to all forms of holism. The holistic character of utterance interpretation is the third 'condition' we will be asking our pragmatic theories to address.

In attempting to capture the 'essence' of utterance interpretation, we have uncovered three philosophical giants: rationality, intentionality, and holism. Each one of these topics has been the focus of numerous books and articles in philosophy. Certainly, in-depth analysis of all three of them is well beyond the scope of the current chapter. What is achievable, and what we will limit ourselves to, is a discussion of how our three pragmatic theories might address the rational, intentional, holistic character of utterance interpretation. Of course, this philosophical discussion of the 'conditions' which must be met by a theory of utterance interpretation is of interest in itself. However, in order that this discussion may also have clinical relevance, we will examine the implications of each of these features for clinical practice. It is only when clinicians can see that some aspect of the assessment or treatment of clients should be done differently as a result of the critical evaluation of pragmatic theories that we can expect theory construction and evaluation to be included as standard in clinical pragmatics.

The rational character of utterance interpretation is variously represented by each of our three pragmatic theories. According to modular pragmatics theory, the rationality of utterance interpretation consists in 'general central principles of rationality in intentional action'. One such principle is the principle of the effective means: 'Given a desired end, one is to choose that action which most effectively, and at least cost, attains that end, *ceteris paribus*' (Kasher 1982, p. 32). It is by means of such central principles, Kasher contends, that we are able to establish the implicatures of utterances. Cognitive pragmatics theory addresses directly the reasoning or inferential mechanism underlying a range of communicative acts. The complexity of communicative acts is characterized in terms of the number of inferences required to link a speaker's expression act to a behaviour game. Each of these inferences is made possible by the operation of base-level inferencing rules. What guides these rules—the closest we come to rationality principles in cognitive pragmatics—are metarules. These metarules 'are capable of driving the inferential process in such a way that all and only those conversational inferences that are relevant may be derived by the partner' (Bara 2010, p. 139). For relevance theory, there is a guiding principle of rationality in the form of the principle of relevance. Rationality is played out through non-demonstrative inference which unfolds in the deductive device. This device processes contextual assumptions according to the logical entries (and deductive rules contained therein) of their constituent concepts. Rationality in this framework thus has a distinctly deductive logical character.

So, there is at least the semblance of rationality in each of our pragmatic theories. The question now is whether this is rationality in more than appearance only. Specifically, we need to interrogate if these theoretical proposals can satisfy the type of full-blown or unconstrained rationality that is integral to utterance interpretation. If we turn to the most explicit of these proposals, relevance theory, there is a case for claiming that they do not. Deductive logical rules of inference are the basis of the relevance processing of contextual assumptions in the deductive device. Yet, these rules can only be applied when a form of rationality which is not represented by deductive logic comes into play. Consider again the exchange between Hilda and Oscar, repeated below:

Hilda: Did Jack come in late last night?
Oscar: His curtains are still drawn.

What makes it reasonable for Hilda to include the following proposition in her reasoning en route to Oscar's implicature: 'If Jack's curtains are drawn, then Jack is sleeping'? It is real-world knowledge of the function of curtains, and of the conditions which must be in place in order for someone to sleep. The reasonableness of this conditional proposition is expressly *not* represented by a deductive logical inference rule such as modus ponens. Such a rule can only be meaningfully applied once it has already been decided that it is reasonable to link the propositions 'Jack's curtains are drawn' and 'Jack is sleeping' by means of the conditional 'if...then' connective. What makes this decision a reasonable one is the operation of some prior form of rationality that is distinct from deductive logic. This prior form of rationality contains a range of informal judgements, all of which must hold in order for the propositions in Hilda's reasoning to be rationally warranted, and none of which can be represented by deductive logical rules of inference. This is what a full-blown or unconstrained communicative rationality looks like. It specifically does *not* look like a relevance-based principle of rationality which is applied through deductive logical rules of inference. The latter is, at best, only scratching the surface of communicative rationality. It emerges that relevance-based rationality à la Sperber and Wilson is largely powerless to explain the reasonableness of the inferential steps taken by Hilda in order to obtain the implicature of Oscar's utterance.

It may seem that by virtue of the more explicit nature of their account, Sperber and Wilson's relevance theory has made itself vulnerable to the above objection. To some extent, this is true. It is easier to understand how Sperber and Wilson construe communicative rationality than it is to grasp the largely implicit sense that Kasher has of the same concept. But, equally, the criticism that has just been levelled against relevance theory could be made of metarules in Bara's cognitive pragmatics theory, for example. The point is the same throughout—communication theorists proceed to examine communicative rationality by instituting boundaries on this notion. These boundaries make it seem that it is possible to describe communicative rationality in toto, without in turn presupposing rationality. But, as the above discussion demonstrates, identifying rationality with deductive inferences or even metarules first requires that we have a form of rationality that is quite unlike deductive inferences or metarules. The largely informal judgements that constitute this prior form of rationality are the essence of communicative rationality, at least as that notion pertains to utterance interpretation. Nor are the pragmatic theories of this chapter alone in mistaking communicative rationality with, at best, one component of that rationality. In other contexts, I described how the same error has been perpetrated by Jürgen

Habermas even as he was trying to counter the restrictive influence of positivism on rationality (Cummings 2002, 2005).

The intentional character of utterance interpretation is also variously captured by our three pragmatic theories. We described above how the representation of mental states, within which we include communicative intentions, lies at the heart of utterance interpretation. Of our three theories, modular pragmatics theory says least about the cognitive processes that are involved in this representation. Kasher (1991a, p. 387) firmly locates beliefs of the form 'S(peaker) believes H(earer) would prefer his doing A to his not doing A' within the mind's central system. These are not beliefs about states of affairs in the world, but beliefs about the contents of another communicator's mind. They are, thus, the type of metarepresentation that is the basis of all utterance interpretation. However, the exact form of that metarepresentation is not specified by Kasher. According to cognitive pragmatics theory, the representation of the mental states of others occurs within a shared belief space. Shared belief is considered to be a primitive in the theory—it is a specific mental state that is not reducible to a conjunction of standard private beliefs. A shared belief takes the form 'A believes p to be shared by A and B', where there is an implicit attribution by A of the belief that p to the individual B. According to (early) relevance theory, the type of metarepresentation that allows us to represent the communicative intentions of others was the function of central, unspecialized inference processes. However, more recently, this metarepresentational capacity has been located within a metacommunicative module which is a specialization of a more general mind-reading module.

So, once again, all three pragmatic theories have something to say about the intentional character of utterance interpretation, where this is understood to be the ability to represent the mental states, and specifically communicative intentions, of others. The question which we must address is whether the proposed mechanisms involved in representing these mental states can adequately capture the type of metarepresentation which is integral to utterance interpretation. Returning to the exchange between Hilda and Oscar, we need to ask what types of cognitive resources Hilda draws upon in order to attribute a particular mental state to Oscar, for example, the mental state that Oscar *knows* that Jack's curtains are drawn. Clearly, her main source of evidence in attributing this knowledge state to Oscar is that he has produced an assertion to the effect that Jack's curtains are drawn. To the extent that assertion of a fact implies true belief or knowledge of that fact on the part of the speaker, it seems reasonable for Hilda to use Oscar's assertion as the basis of her mental state attribution. But, actually, this is not the end of the matter. Because Hilda is using more than Oscar's assertion to attribute a particular knowledge state to him. She is also using her beliefs that Oscar is a reliable informant who can be trusted to report situations and events accurately, that Oscar knows who Jack is and what curtains are, and that Oscar has intact visual perception skills which he has used to describe the state of Jack's curtains. These beliefs, and others like them, are also playing a significant role in Hilda's attribution of a particular knowledge state to Oscar. So, what are the prospects of our theories successfully capturing the representation of these different beliefs?

The prospects are quite poor, in reality. By any account, the beliefs we identified above are only realized by means of belief fixation processes that are located in the mind's central system. It is a feature of these processes that they cannot be constrained in the information that they use to establish beliefs. This is as true of beliefs about the mental states of others (metarepresentation) as it is of beliefs about the world (representation). Central, belief fixation processes, among which are included metarepresentational processes, are noteworthy on account of their informational unencapsulation. Yet, it is this very feature which our pragmatic theories appear largely impotent to capture. The choice we are confronted with seems to be a largely unpalatable one. Either we can, like Kasher and early Sperber and Wilson, look to the belief fixation processes of the mind's central system for some account of how we establish beliefs about the mental states of others, or we can, like late Sperber and Wilson, locate these processes within a specialised metacommunicative module. The reason that this is an unpalatable choice is that the former way leaves us with almost nothing that we can say about these processes, while the latter way only explains metarepresentation by distorting it. To appreciate the first of these difficulties, we need only recall that Hilda could draw upon an indefinable range of beliefs about Oscar's mental states and the world in order to attribute a particular knowledge state to Oscar. It is not an exaggeration to say that a theory of these beliefs is nothing short of a theory of the whole of cognition. Fodor (1983, p. 129) captures the explanatory problem we are facing in the following terms:

> [T]he reason that there is no serious psychology of central processes is the same as the reason there is no serious philosophy of scientific confirmation. Both exemplify the significance of global factors in the fixation of belief, and nobody begins to understand how such factors have their effects.

'Global factors' always go beyond attempts to describe and categorize them, and necessarily so. That is because it is global factors that confer meaning on the beliefs which are established by the central system, a role which they can only perform if they are not part of the description of those beliefs. So, the first way leaves us with an impossible explanatory challenge, the construction of a complete theory of central processes. The second way is no less problematic. That way involves committing metarepresentational processes to a specialized module. One advantage of locating these processes within a module is that a modular mechanism can exploit certain regularities within its domain. In doing so, it can achieve processing efficiencies that are not afforded to a general inferential capacity such as Fodor's central system:

> [A] general-purpose inferential mechanism can only derive conclusions based on the formal (logical or statistical) properties of the input information it processes. By contrast, a dedicated inferential mechanism or module can take advantage of regularities in its specific domain, and use inferential procedures which are justified by these regularities, but only in this domain (Sperber and Wilson 2002, p. 9).

However, these processing gains come at a huge expense, which is nothing less than the distortion of metarepresentation. To see this, consider the type of information that might be found in Sperber and Wilson's metacommunicative module.

As applied to the exchange between Hilda and Oscar, the module may help Hilda determine several of Oscar's mental states, for example, the mental states that Oscar *knows* that Jack is Hilda's brother and that Oscar *believes* that Jack returned late. But these mental states, as we have seen, are only possible given a range of other beliefs. Moreover, not all of *these* beliefs are beliefs about mental states. Some are beliefs about the world such as Hilda's belief that Jack is her brother and her belief that Oscar is a reliable informant. These latter beliefs are not available to a metacommunicative module which is designed to process only intentional data relating to mental states.

The problem is even more acute if we think of the role of non-verbal behaviours in establishing the mental states of others. More often than not, a speaker's mental states can be established on the basis of facial expressions and gestures rather than through what has been uttered or verbalized—the raised eyebrows which indicate disbelief, the shrug of the shoulders which reveal a lack of knowledge or ignorance, for example. Yet, these behaviours are processed by a visual perception module and not by a metacommunicative module. Moreover, given the informational encapsulation of both modules, there is no prospect of this visual perceptual data gaining access to the metarepresentational processes which it needs to influence. At best, a metacommunicative module is representing only one small part of the wider cognitive apparatus by means of which we represent the mental states of others. However, that part is only intelligible to the extent that that wider apparatus is assumed to exist, even if it is not explicitly acknowledged as such in the account of metarepresentation advanced by Sperber and Wilson. In the absence of this apparatus, what we are left with is a type of metarepresentation that is quite unlike the metarepresentational processes at work in utterance interpretation. What we are left with is, in fact, a distortion of those processes.

In summary of this point, it is much easier to acknowledge that utterance interpretation requires a capacity to represent the mental states of others than it is to give a coherent account of how that representation is undertaken. In terms of our pragmatic theories, we appear to be limited to a choice between central belief fixation processes and a specialized, modular metarepresentational capacity. The former processes are global in nature as any item of knowledge or information, however remote or obscure, can play a role in the fixation of beliefs. The global character of belief fixation places this important central process beyond any normal description and explanation. Certainly, any theory of this process is likely to involve nothing short of a theory of the whole of cognition (and even then it would be incomplete). However, a modular metarepresentational capacity fares little better than a central one. By definition, a module can only process data in a circumscribed domain. So it is that a language module only processes linguistic data and a visual perception module only processes visual perceptual data. In exactly the same way, a metacommunicative module of the type proposed by Sperber and Wilson can only process data relating to the mental states of others, at least as those states pertain to communication. But we saw above that metarepresentation, at least as that notion applies to utterance interpretation, involves access to all sorts of data that do not relate to mental states and, importantly, are not even available to a metacommunicative module. It emerged that a modular metarepresentational capacity is at least as problematic, but for different reasons, as a central metarepresentational capacity.

The third essential feature of utterance interpretation is its holistic character. Holism captures the attribute of interconnectedness between the statements in a theory or other body of knowledge. Applied to utterance interpretation, holism describes how the participants in a communicative exchange bring an 'informational nexus' to their interpretation of utterances. Theories of utterance interpretation which make it seem that we can throw a net around one part of this nexus and identify that part as the 'context' of the utterance are misguided, on a holistic approach. For every part of the nexus is connected to every other part. The question now is whether our pragmatic theories are able to capture the holism of utterance interpretation. In modular pragmatics theory, Kasher emphasizes the integration of knowledge or information across modular and central systems. For example, the assignment of a referent to the pronoun 'she' requires that the language module contribute the information that 'she' is used to refer to a human female. The visual perception module must contribute information about the people present during an exchange. Beliefs contained in the central system also play a role in reference assignment. To facilitate this integration of information, Kasher envisages a mental architecture consisting of input modules, a central system and, importantly, two types of interface: an interface between modules and an interface between modules and the central system.

Different types of information are acknowledged in relevance theory. According to Sperber and Wilson, information is stored within the lexical, logical and encyclopaedic entries of concepts. For example, a concept like MOTHER contains a lexical entry which describes linguistic features such as the grammatical category of the word (in this case, a noun). An elimination rule within the logical entry of the concept replaces MOTHER with *female parent*. The encyclopaedic entry of the concept contains world knowledge about mothers. This might include the typical roles mothers assume (e.g. child rearing) and the household duties they perform (e.g. cooking). Also, some concepts may contain one of these entries to the exclusion of others. For example, the concept OR has a logical entry but no encyclopaedic entry, which reflects its role as a logical (disjunctive) operator. In cognitive pragmatics theory, information is processed and organized not according to conceptual entries (as in relevance theory) or domain-specific modules (as in modular pragmatics theory), but according to isolable functional systems. These systems process linguistic and extralinguistic information independently of each other. The information provided by these systems must become equivalent at a certain point in order that central inferencing processes of the type used to reconstruct a speaker's communicative intention can draw upon any item of information.[11] Although Bara explicitly rejects the presence of modules, the similarity between his own central procedures and the central system in a modular view of mind is clear.

So, it can be seen that all three pragmatic theories make quite specific claims about the organization and processing of information that is integral to utterance interpretation. The question now is whether these proposals can accommodate the type of informational holism that we have identified as a key attribute of the interpretation of utterances. All three pragmatic theories propose different types of demarcation in the informational nexus that we bring to utterance interpretation. For relevance theory, that nexus should be demarcated along the lines of lexical, logical and encyclopaedic information. For modular pragmatics theory, the nexus should recognize a distinction between specialized, modularized information of different types (e.g. linguistic data, visual perceptual data) and unspecialized, central information. For cognitive pragmatics theory, the nexus should permit a demarcation of linguistic and extralinguistic information. I want to argue, and will demonstrate, that all such demarcations are antithetical to informational holism and that they serve only to distort the knowledge and information that are the basis of utterance interpretation. To see this, we need to return to the exchange between Hilda and Oscar from above:

Hilda: Did Jack come in late last night?
Oscar: His curtains are still drawn.

We have already described the array of information that Hilda may use in her recovery of the implicature of Oscar's utterance. Hilda uses linguistic information in the form of Oscar's utterance as well as any preceding utterances in the exchange. She also uses non-linguistic information in the form of any facial expressions, gestures and bodily movements performed by Oscar. Hilda can also use information about people, events and states of affairs in the world (real world knowledge). If, as I am claiming, informational holism is a correct characterization of the information and knowledge that language users draw upon in their interpretation of utterances, then there are a couple of observations which we can make about the information that Hilda is using in this case.

The first observation is that we cannot tell in advance which part of the information at Hilda's disposal will be relevant to her interpretation of Oscar's utterance. There is no sense in which Oscar's facial expression, for example, is any less important to Hilda's interpretation of Oscar's utterance than is his linguistic utterance. Indeed, it is quite often the case that a facial expression is more revealing of a speaker's communicative intention than is a linguistic utterance. The speaker who utters 'What a delightful child!' in the presence of a disruptive 5-year-old boy conveys much more about his actual communicative intention through the raising of his eyebrows than through his linguistic utterance. This same facial expression may be important to the interpretation of a sarcastic utterance on one occasion, but may be subordinated to other information (e.g. prior beliefs about the speaker's attitude towards children) on a different occasion. The point is quite simply that knowledge comes to utterance interpretation as a unified whole. If we proceed by demarcating the information that plays a role in utterance interpretation, as our pragmatic theories have done, then we lose sight of a fundamental feature of utterance interpretation—any type of information may be relevant to the interpretation of an utterance, and it is impossible to state in advance which items of information or aspects of our knowledge will hold most sway in a particular case.

The second observation is that Hilda only truly understands the significance of each of these items of information to the interpretation of Oscar's utterance because she has access to other information and knowledge that are not described above. For example, in order for Hilda to understand the significance of Oscar's utterance that Jack's curtains are still drawn, Hilda must have a prior understanding of the function of curtains. That function—to block out daylight—is itself only intelligible given a prior understanding of the way in which daylight fluctuates during a 24-h period. And an understanding of fluctuations in daylight during a 24-h period requires a prior understanding of the concept of time, among other things. In short, it is not possible to place an upper limit on the knowledge or information that is presupposed by the information that Hilda brings to her interpretation of Oscar's utterance. Yet, the type of demarcation pursued by our pragmatic theories suggests that such an upper limit is not only possible but is actually achieved in the case of an encyclopaedic entry of a concept, for example. Any demarcation of the knowledge that is used in utterance interpretation effectively eliminates the prior concepts and understandings that are needed to make sense of that knowledge.

What these observations suggest is that the informational demarcation that abounds in our pragmatic theories is in direct contrast to the informational holism that is characteristic of utterance interpretation. As soon as a boundary of any type is erected within the information that we bring to utterance interpretation, regardless of whether that boundary takes the form of a module, a conceptual entry, or a functional system, we are effectively distorting the informational nexus that is the basis of utterance interpretation. It is only through the interconnectedness of the different parts of this nexus that we can expect to obtain the type of information and knowledge that plays a role in utterance interpretation. By instituting boundaries and demarcations of various kinds within this information and knowledge, this essential interconnectedness is lost and, along with it, any prospect of representing the type of informational holism that is the basis of utterance interpretation.

We have seen that the rational, intentional, holistic character of utterance interpretation is not always successfully captured by each of our pragmatic theories. More often than not, it was demonstrated that these theories end up distorting one or more of these essential attributes of the interpretation of utterances. In demonstrating these failings of pragmatic theories, the aim was not to suggest an alternative theoretical framework which could better address each of these attributes. Rather, it was to demonstrate a type of critical evaluation which must become commonplace if theory development is to assume a more central role in clinical pragmatics. We want to conclude this section by considering the implications of each of these criticisms for clinical practice. If it can be demonstrated that clinicians should approach the assessment and treatment of pragmatic disorders in clients differently as a result of each of these criticisms, then the largely philosophical criticisms of this section will also be shown to have clinical relevance.

It was described above how all utterance interpretation proceeds by means of reasoning. The exercise of a rational capacity sets the interpretation of utterances apart from linguistic decoding—no rational judgement is required in order to apply a syntactic or semantic rule during the decoding of an utterance. Acknowledging that reasoning is fundamental to utterance interpretation is somewhat easier than knowing how to translate this particular feature of interpretative processes into clinical practice. At a minimum, I contend, clinicians need to assess and treat a set of reason-based skills that have been largely neglected in clinical practice to date. These skills include the ability to reflect on factors deemed relevant to the interpretation of utterances, to explore the bases of different interpretations of an utterance and to justify in terms of politeness and other considerations a range of linguistic choices made during the production of utterances. The reflective nature of this work is quite unlike that typically undertaken in speech-language pathology clinics. It also represents a radical departure in terms of the assessment and treatment of pragmatic disorders. This is not the context in which to examine pragmatic assessments and interventions (see Chap. 6 in Cummings (2009) for a detailed discussion). Suffice it to say that pragmatic checklists, which merely note the presence of certain speech acts, and pragmatic interventions, which teach conversational rules, neglect the rational basis of each of these key pragmatic skills.

It was described above how the recognition and representation of mental states, including communicative intentions, lie at the heart of utterance interpretation. The intentional character of utterance interpretation also has implications for clinical practice. One such implication concerns the assessment of pragmatic language skills. Typically, assessments establish if particular skills are part of a client's pragmatic repertoire. For example, clinicians will attempt to establish if a client can comprehend implicatures, formulate polite utterances and develop a topic in conversation. To the extent that these pragmatic skills are present and are performed appropriately, it may be assumed that the client has an adequate appreciation of the communicative intentions that attend each skill. However, when these pragmatic skills are problematic for a client, it would represent a considerable advance in terms of our ability to diagnose pragmatic problems if we knew something about a client's ability to manipulate the mental states underlying each of these pragmatic behaviours. By the same token, simply training a client to use the speech act of request does not develop an appreciation of the mental states associated with this speech act, such as that the speaker *wants* the hearer to undertake a certain action and *believes* that the hearer is capable of performing that action. What these considerations demonstrate is that mental states need to become explicit targets of assessment and intervention rather than, as has been the case to date, implicit components of a client's pragmatic performance which are not assessed or treated. The approach advocated here is not dissimilar to attempts to teach or train theory of mind skills in clients with autism (Swettenham 2000), only applied more generally to all clients with pragmatic disorders.

The holistic character of utterance interpretation also has implications for clinical practice. To the extent that no item of information or knowledge stands alone in informing the interpretation of an utterance, clinicians should give consideration to the connections between different aspects of knowledge when they assess and treat pragmatic language skills. It is too often assumed in a clinical context that failures of pragmatic understanding are related to a lack of knowledge. Clinicians attempt to rectify this knowledge deficit through the training of clients in the use of scripts or schemas to aid comprehension. In reality, many failures of pragmatic understanding are related not to a lack of knowledge, but to difficulties in establishing connections between items of knowledge or information in ways that facilitate utterance interpretation. Hilda can have any amount of knowledge at her disposal in the above exchange. For example, she may know that curtains block out daylight, that people who retire late often do not rise early, and that people sleep best in a darkened room. However, if she does not know how these items of knowledge relate one to another—specifically, that Jack's curtains are still drawn because he is sleeping, and Jack is sleeping because he returned home late the night before—then there is little prospect of Hilda recovering the implicature of Oscar's utterance. It is the connections *between* items of knowledge that are of significance to utterance interpretation. Yet, these interconnections are never examined as part of an assessment of pragmatic language skills or targeted during the remediation of these skills. The holism of utterance interpretation teaches us that from these interconnections a powerful resource for the pragmatic understanding of language proceeds.

4.5 Summary

This chapter has examined theoretical developments which have had an influence on work in clinical pragmatics. It has limited itself to a discussion of three theories which have a 'strong' cognitive orientation. These theories were Sperber and Wilson's relevance theory, Bara's cognitive pragmatics theory and Kasher's modular pragmatics theory. The decision to examine only 'strong' theories was motivated by two considerations. Firstly, a pragmatic theory which lacks a cognitive orientation is of little service to clinical pragmatists who must assess and treat pragmatic disorders often in the context of significant cognitive deficits. Secondly, 'strong' theories have also been extensively tested on clinical subjects and, in turn, have been used to make predictions about the performance of clinical subjects. There is, therefore, substantial empirical support for these theories. As well as describing the main proposals of these theories, we examined clinical findings which are based on them. Finally, a critical evaluation of the theories was undertaken. The aim was to demonstrate that even philosophical criticism has relevance to clinicians when it can be shown to lead to different ways of assessing and treating clients with pragmatic disorders.

Notes

1. Garrett and Harnish (2009) state that experimental work on unspoken contents (what they collectively refer to as 'impliciture') started in the late 1980s.
2. Orjada (2007) examined the processing of implicitures in adults with stroke-induced right-hemisphere damage. Rybarova (2007) examined impliciture

processing in older adults. Although these adults did not exhibit clinical impairment, some adults had high frontal lobe function while others had low frontal lobe function.

3. 'A contextual implication is a special type of logical implication, derived by the use of a restricted set of deductive rules which derive at most a finite set of conclusions from any finite set of premises' (Wilson and Sperber 1991, p. 381).

4. See Chap. 4 in Cummings (2005) for a detailed discussion and criticism of relevance theory. See Cummings (2013c) for a brief overview of the theory.

5. McDonald (1999) uses findings from normal and clinical subjects to assess competing theoretical views (relevance theory vs. traditional model) of the processing of sarcasm. According to relevance theory, hearers recognize sarcasm as a scornful echo of a previous assertion. The traditional model states that hearers derive a counterfactual inference from sarcastic utterances.

6. The concept of explicature receives support from experiments conducted by Gibbs and Moise (1997). These investigators found that when presented with utterances such as *Jane has three children*, subjects treated the pragmatically enriched meaning of this utterance (i.e. Jane has *exactly* three children) as 'what is said' by the speaker. However, Nicolle and Clark (1999) found evidence that when an utterance gives rise to a single strong implicature, this implicature is the paraphrase that subjects select as closest to 'what is said' by the speaker. In other cases, subjects tend to select the explicature of the utterance.

7. It is worth remarking that cognitive pragmatics theory has also been applied to other domains. The theory has provided a conceptual framework for a recently developed pragmatic assessment (Angeleri et al. 2012; Bosco et al. 2012b). Cognitive pragmatics theory has also informed studies of the neural basis of intention (Becchio et al. 2006). These studies include neuroimaging investigations of the theory of mind network in clients with schizophrenia (Walter et al. 2009) and normal subjects (Walter et al. 2004; Ciaramidaro et al. 2007). The effects of intention on action have also been examined from within a cognitive pragmatic perspective (Sartori et al. 2009).

8. Kasher and co-workers have made a significant contribution to the development of the sub-discipline of neuropragmatics. For discussion of this area of work, the reader is referred to Cummings (2010b).

9. Kasher and Meilijson (1996) relate the pragmatic impairments of children with autism to the various components of modular pragmatics theory. The purpose is to present modular pragmatics as a theoretical framework which can account for the core deficits of autism. It is the expressed intention of the authors to test the framework experimentally in a group of subjects with autism using a battery of neuropragmatic tests.

10. Zaidel et al. (2002) investigated if a Hebrew version of the Right Hemisphere Communication Battery examined modular pragmatic language skills. Subjects with LHD or RHD completed the sub-tests of this battery. Zaidel et al. did not find support for a strong modularity hypothesis for the functions of language use tapped by this battery. This was the case whether 'module' was defined in the strict sense of Fodor (1983) or in the wider sense of Kasher (1994).

11. 'At a certain level […] the information acquired through both the functional systems must become equivalent from a processing standpoint; to be exact, at the point at which the actor's communicative intent has to be reconstructed, central inferencing processes use any type of information whatsoever to produce an acceptable meaning' (Bara 2010, p. 39).

Chapter 5
The Impact of Pragmatic Disorders

5.1 Introduction

Pragmatic disorders can have serious, adverse consequences for the children and adults who experience them. Pragmatic impairment in children can lead to educational underachievement, failure to establish social relationships with others, and a range of psychological difficulties. As these children progress into adolescence and adulthood, their problems are frequently compounded by additional difficulties including a lack of vocational opportunity, difficulty forming personal relationships, participation in criminal activity and the development of substance use disorders. Notwithstanding the significant impact of pragmatic disorders on the lives of affected individuals, these various outcomes are seldom the focus of clinicians and researchers who work with this client group. Yet, there are clear reasons why they must be given greater prominence.

Firstly, healthcare providers are increasingly being required to demonstrate the effectiveness of the clinical interventions they offer clients. Speech-language pathology services are no exception in this regard. Clinicians must be able to demonstrate measurable gains in the quality of life of their clients as a result of pragmatic language interventions, and indicators such as improved social and psychological adjustment are often the clearest means of achieving this. Secondly, the considerable cost to individuals, society and the economy of criminal behaviour has prompted discussion of how earlier identification and treatment of those at risk of this behaviour may best be achieved. The increased prevalence of language impairments and pragmatic disorders in detained clients has found clinical language services at the forefront of attempts to prevent and reduce offending behaviour (see Chap. 6). Thirdly, consideration of the impact of pragmatic disorders also develops our knowledge of these disorders, as well as how best to assess and treat them. The science of language pathology thus also stands to benefit from increased awareness of the impact of pragmatic disorders.

It can be seen that there are strong grounds for including a greater emphasis on impact within discussions of pragmatic disorders. In this chapter, I propose to

L. Cummings, *Pragmatic Disorders*, Perspectives in Pragmatics, Philosophy & Psychology 3, DOI: 10.1007/978-94-007-7954-9_5, © Springer Science+Business Media Dordrecht 2014

do just that. In what follows, impact will be addressed along a number of parameters. These parameters include (1) psychological impact, which ranges from minor problems such as low self-esteem through to severe psychiatric disturbances; (2) social impact, which includes problems relating to social adjustment and integration; (3) academic impact, which includes performance on a range of indicators of academic achievement; (4) occupational and vocational impact; (5) behavioural impact, which includes externalizing problems such as conduct disorder; and (6) forensic impact, which includes engagement in juvenile delinquency, the use of illicit substances and other forms of criminal behaviour.

Although I will discuss these different types of impact in isolation from each other, it should be noted that this is merely for descriptive convenience. This is because these various forms of impact are, in reality, closely interrelated. These interrelationships may be causal in nature such as when poor educational achievement on the part of a child with pragmatic disorder reduces his or her vocational opportunities later in life. Alternatively, the co-occurrence of two types of impact may result from the presence of a third type, such as when an individual's low self-esteem makes an independent causal contribution both to his poor academic achievement at school and limited vocational opportunities in adulthood. In short, the reader should be aware that in any particular case, the impact of a pragmatic disorder is likely to involve several components with a complex array of relationships between those components.[1]

Before embarking on an examination of these different types of impact of pragmatic disorders, it is important to introduce a clarification. Pragmatic impairments are a feature of many psychiatric conditions including obsessive–compulsive disorder, avoidant personality disorder and schizophrenia (Cullen et al. 2008; Dreessen et al. 1999; Meilijson et al. 2004). Pragmatic impairments are also found in children with emotional and behavioural problems (Mackie and Law 2010). Pragmatic impairments in these clinical populations were examined in Chap. 2. In that examination, it was assumed that the emotional, behavioural or psychiatric disturbances, in which pragmatic impairments are found, are primary conditions and pragmatic impairments are one clinical feature of these conditions. While this assumption may prove to be incorrect, it is at least consistent with how most clinicians and researchers view the relationship between pragmatic disorders and these clinical conditions.

However, when we describe the emotional, behavioural or psychological impact of pragmatic disorders in this chapter, a quite different relationship between these disorders and a psychiatric condition in an adult or an emotional and behavioural problem in a child is envisaged. Pragmatic impairments are the primary disorder in these cases with psychiatric or other anomalies arising in consequence of these impairments. Accordingly, the reader should not expect to find a discussion of pragmatic disorders in schizophrenia in this chapter—this is one of the clinical populations with significant pragmatic deficits which were examined in Chap. 2. By the same token, the reader of Chap. 2 should not expect to find a discussion of the emotional disturbances that can be caused by pragmatic language impairment (PLI) in children—these affective disturbances are properly addressed in relation to the psychological impact of PLI in children.

5.2 Psychological Impact

There is now substantial evidence that children and adults with language disorders are at an increased risk of developing psychological problems and of experiencing reduced quality of life. Arkkila et al. (2008) studied adults who received a childhood diagnosis of specific language impairment (SLI), and reported a significant difference between them and controls on a measure of distress. Low self-esteem, sometimes in specific domains,[2] has been consistently reported in children with SLI. Lindsay et al. (2010) reported low self-esteem in young people with a history of SLI during adolescence. In a review of studies, Feeney et al. (2012) found evidence that health-related quality of life is compromised in children and adolescents with speech and language difficulties relative to peers. Reduced receptive language skills have been found to be predictive of increased psychosocial difficulties in children aged 4–5 years with hearing loss (Hogan et al. 2011). Adverse psychological outcomes of language disorders have also been reported in adults. Hilari et al. (2010) reported that at 3 months post-stroke, 93 per cent of their subjects with aphasia experienced high psychological distress compared to only 50 per cent of non-aphasic stroke patients. Aphasia severity has been found to affect health-related quality of life in patients post-stroke (Hilari et al. 2012).

Less commonly, clinical studies have examined the psychological consequences of pragmatic impairments in children and adults. These impairments have been linked to a large spectrum of psychological burden including low self-esteem and depression. Some of these psychological problems have minimal implications for a person's sense of well-being; others place serious limitations on an individual's social and occupational functioning and have an adverse effect upon quality of life. In all cases, psychological problems should be considered alongside the pragmatic disorder with which they are associated, as their presence may necessitate referral to other clinical services (e.g. psychiatry). Even in cases where further referral is not judged to be necessary, a pragmatic language intervention may be considered to be only minimally effective if it does not simultaneously achieve a reduction in a client's psychological problems and pragmatic disorder: 'In the treatment of children with language difficulties professional care should aim at reducing or at least dealing with these problems as well' (van Agt et al. 2011, p. 87). Treatments which can reduce the psychological burden of pragmatic disorders will only properly emerge when there is a clear understanding of the psychological sequelae of these disorders. It is to this issue that we now turn.

Several studies have addressed the psychological impact of pragmatic disorders in children. Van Agt et al. (2011) examined the impact of different types of language disorder on the socio-emotional development and quality of life of 8-year-old children. The Child Health Questionnaire—Parent Form 28 (CHQ—PF28) was used to examine health-related quality of life in these children, a concept that includes perceived physical and mental health. All children with language disorder achieved low scores on the following CHQ—PF28 subscales: General Behaviour, Self-esteem, Parental Impact—Emotional, Parental Impact—Time, and Mental health. However, effect sizes were particularly large in those children who were identified as having pragmatic language impairment (see further discussion of this study's findings in Sect. 5.6). Solomon et al. (2008) examined the relationship between formal thought disorder, and stress and anxiety in children aged 8–17 years with ASD. Aspects of formal thought disorder, which is associated with pragmatic language impairments in ASD, were found to be related to parent reports of child stress and anxiety.[3]

Helland et al. to appear examined pragmatic language skills and mental health status in 19 children with SLI, 21 children with ADHD and 19 typically developing children. All children were aged between 6 and 12 years. The parents of these children completed the Children's Communication Checklist-2 (CCC-2; Bishop 2003) and the Strengths and Difficulties Questionnaire (SDQ; Goodman 1999). Helland et al. found that 57.1 % of the ADHD group obtained a negative score on the Social Interaction Deviance Composite of the CCC-2, indicating that pragmatic aspects of communication were disproportionately impaired relative to language. This compared to only 5.3 % of the SLI group and 10.5 % of the typically developing children. The ADHD group also differed significantly from the SLI group on all problem scales of the SDQ as well as on the total difficulties score and the impact score on this measure. This indicated that the children with ADHD had significantly greater mental health problems than the children with SLI. On the SDQ scale measuring emotional symptoms, for example, 81 % of children with ADHD scored in the abnormal/borderline range compared to only 31.6 % of children with SLI. Although Helland et al. did not attempt to relate pragmatic language skills to mental health problems in any of these groups, the presence of significant impairment in both these areas in the children with ADHD is suggestive of a role for pragmatic disorder in the poor mental health of these children.

Silvestre et al. (2007) examined the relationship between conversational competence in the use of pragmatic functions and self-concept in 56 deaf students aged between 6 and 18 years. Data obtained during a conversation with a hearing adult were analysed according to principles suggested by Grice and included an assessment of the adequacy of responses to questions. Conversational difficulties were found to correlate inversely with scores for personal self-concept. In general, the best conversational skills in these students were related to the most positive definitions of self-concept. Silvestre et al. (2007, p. 49) state that '[t]he most outstanding [relationships established] are those that exist between the preference for self-definitions concerning positive psychological traits or psychological traits in general [...] with conversational strategies that represent good conversation management'.

Investigators have also considered the psychological impact of pragmatic disorders in adults. Galski et al. (1998) examined psychological adjustment and discourse skills in 30 adults who sustained traumatic brain injury (TBI). Compared to matched controls, subjects with TBI experienced greater depression, admitted to a poorer general quality of life and reported more symptoms of psychological maladjustment. Poorer quality of life in these subjects was related to the greater use of uninformative language in narrative discourse and failure to repair errors in procedural discourse. The informational content of narrative discourse was one of several areas of pragmatic difficulty reported by Byrne et al. (1998) in a study of 35 adults with chronic schizophrenia. Alongside producing narrative and conversational discourse samples, these subjects completed a criterion-referenced test of pragmatic language. The Global Assessment of Functioning Scale (GAFS) from DSM-IV was used to assess functioning. (The scale requires the assessor to consider psychological, social and occupational functioning on a hypothetical continuum of mental health-illness.) A significant relationship was obtained between these adults' performance on pragmatic language tasks and their functioning on the GAFS.

Sparks et al. (2010) examined the perception of sarcasm and deceit and its relation to functional outcome in 30 outpatients (mean age = 46.1 years) with a diagnosis of schizophrenia or schizoaffective disorder. Compared to 25 healthy controls, subjects with schizophrenia had significantly more difficulty comprehending sarcastic and deceitful exchanges on The Awareness of Social Inference Test (TASIT; McDonald et al. 2003). Also, outpatients with schizophrenia displayed significantly higher personal distress relative to controls on a measure of self-reported empathy, the Interpersonal Reactivity Index (IRI; Davis 1983). Regression analysis revealed that performance on Part 2 of TASIT—simple sarcasm—significantly predicted IRI personal distress in subjects with schizophrenia. This finding demonstrates that subjects with schizophrenia experienced greater personal distress in interpersonal situations on account of their difficulties with the comprehension of sarcasm.

5.3 Social Impact

With so many social interactions and relationships forged through language, it is inevitable that clinical investigators should look to the social domain to establish the impact of pragmatic disorders (Cummings 2011). Social functioning is variously characterized in clinical studies. In some studies, it is captured by the number and quality of friendships and peer relations that a client experiences. In other studies, social functioning is measured by the presence and absence of normal social behaviours such as when clients are described as displaying a lack of prosocial behaviour or reciprocal social behaviour. Other indicators of social impact used in clinical studies include victimization and engagement in recreational activities as well as attributes of the individual, the latter typically expressed through terms such as 'withdrawn'.

Regardless of the concepts and measures used to capture social impact in clinical studies, one thing is indisputable—language disorders invariably cause significant disruption to the social lives of the children and adults who are affected by these disorders. Willinger et al. (2003) found that in a sample of 94 children with language development disorders, 13 % were withdrawn while 8 % exhibited social problems. These social difficulties were not observed in a group of 94 age- and sex-matched control subjects. Social problems have also been reported in adults with language disorders. Among adults who have sustained a first stroke, the loss of friends has been found to be particularly acute in those individuals who have aphasia (Northcott and Hilari 2011). Naess et al. (2009) found that aphasia was associated with social isolation at six-year follow-up in a group of 195 patients who sustained an ischaemic stroke. In this section, we will consider if the social difficulties that attend language disorders in children and adults are also seen in clients with pragmatic disorders.

Social skills problems in children with hyperactivity and inattention have been shown to be mediated by pragmatic language use. Leonard et al. (2011) studied a community sample of 54 children between the ages of 9 and 11 years. Pragmatic language use was found to fully mediate the relation between hyperactivity and social skills problems in these children, and partially mediate the relation between inattention and social skills problems. Moreover, pragmatic language use made a unique contribution to the social skills of these children of 21.6 and 17.2 % above and beyond the contribution of hyperactivity and inattention, respectively.[4] Conti-Ramsden and Botting (2004) examined the social and behavioural status of 242 children with specific language impairment at 11 years of age. These children were first studied at age 7 years. Pragmatic language skills were assessed using the Children's Communication Checklist (CCC; Bishop 1998). Pragmatic difficulties revealed by this checklist were most strongly related to poor social outcome in these children and to expressive language related to victimization.

Eales (1993) studied pragmatic skills in adults who had a diagnosis of either autistic disorders or developmental receptive language disorders in childhood. Difficulty forming appropriate communicative intentions was closely related to impairment of reciprocal social behaviour in both diagnostic groups. St Clair et al. (2011) used the Strengths and Difficulties Questionnaire (SDQ; Goodman 1997) to examine social difficulties in 234 children with SLI at four developmental points between 7 and 16 years of age. Pragmatic skills were assessed at 11 and 16 years using the Children's Communication Checklist (Bishop 1998). These skills displayed a significant linear association with the peer subscale of the SDQ. St Clair et al. (2011, p. 195) concluded that '[w]hat this study makes clear is that pragmatic aspects of language seem to be more directly implicated in peer relation problems in individuals with a history of SLI. Other aspects of language did not reveal statistically significant effects'.

The social impact of pragmatic language impairment (PLI) in a community sample of 1,364 children was examined by Ketelaars et al. (2010). These investigators found moderate to high correlations between peer problems and a lack of prosocial behaviour in these children and their performance on the pragmatic subscales of the CCC. Whitehouse et al. (2009b) examined social outcomes in seven adults with a childhood history of PLI. Over half of these adults (57.1 %) did not have any close friendships at all. Moreover, the quality of friendships in these adults was significantly poorer than in adults who did not have a history of developmental disorder. Half of the adults with PLI experienced a romantic relationship of at least 3 months' duration (less than in adults with histories of SLI or normal development), while none were married or had children.

Botting and Conti-Ramsden (2000) reported that children with complex language impairments—a designation that included pragmatic impairments—had more marked peer interaction problems (as rated by teachers) than either children with expressive language problems or children with mixed expressive-receptive difficulties. Volden et al. (2009) examined socialization and pragmatic language skills in 37 children, aged 6–13 years, who met diagnostic criteria for autism spectrum disorder. Pragmatic skills were assessed using the Test of Pragmatic Language (TOPL; Phelps-Terasaki and Phelps-Gunn 1992). Scores on the TOPL accounted for significant variance in socialization performance as measured on the Autism Diagnostic Observation Schedule (Lord et al. 1999). However, this finding was not replicated in relation to social adaptive functioning on the Vineland Adaptive Behavior Scale (Sparrow et al. 1984).

Interestingly, in a study of 19 children with SLI aged 7–10 years, Marton et al. (2005) reported high social self-esteem scores in a subset of these children who had the lowest social pragmatic scores on a hypothetical scenarios task. This task examined social pragmatic performance in the areas of initiation of interaction, negotiation and conflict resolution. These children's high ratings of their own social competence—they reported coping well socially with their peers—were not reflected in their actual social performance or, indeed, confirmed by the reports of their parents and, to a lesser degree, their teachers. Marton et al. explained this finding in terms of these children's lack of self-awareness and poor social knowledge.

Increasingly, investigators are examining the social impact of pragmatic and discourse deficits in adults. Snow et al. (1998) examined conversational discourse abilities in 26 speakers (mean age 26.2 years) who had sustained a severe traumatic brain injury (TBI). Conversational samples were assessed using the modified version of Damico's Clinical Discourse Analysis (CDA-M; Damico 1985, 1991), an assessment tool which consists of 17 parameters organized according to Gricean maxims of quantity, quality, relation and manner. Psychosocial handicap was assessed using the Craig Handicap Assessment and Reporting Technique (CHART; Whiteneck et al. 1992a, b). At follow-up a minimum of 2 years post-injury, a significant association was obtained between conversation CDA-M scores in 24 speakers with TBI and the social integration subscale of the CHART. Galski et al. (1998) examined social integration and conversational, narrative and procedural discourse in 30 patients with TBI in an outpatient brain injury programme. Five discourse variables predicted 64.5 % of the variance in social integration as measured on the Community Integration Questionnaire (Willer et al. 1993, 1994). These variables included greater wordiness and more topics in narrative and procedural tasks. Additional psychosocial variables such as age, gender, education, quality of life, depression and dementia rating did not add to the variance in social integration achieved by discourse variables.

Verbal underproductivity has been found to predict social skills, social engagement and friendships in chronically institutionalized patients with schizophrenia at 2.5 year follow-up (Bowie and Harvey 2008). Schenkel et al. (2005) studied linguistic context processing in 42 in-patients with chronic schizophrenia. These investigators argued that context processing impairments may be a factor in the poor premorbid social functioning of these patients. In their study of 30 outpatients with schizophrenia or schizoaffective disorder, Sparks et al. (2010) reported significant associations between the comprehension of sarcastic and deceitful exchanges on the TASIT (McDonald et al. 2003) and engagement in recreational activities, as measured on the Longitudinal Interval Follow-Up Evaluation—Range of Impaired Functioning Tool (LIFE-RIFT; Leon et al. 1999). Subjects with schizophrenia who experienced difficulty comprehending sarcastic and deceitful exchanges experienced less engagement in, and enjoyment of, recreational activities.[5]

5.4 Academic Impact

It is well established that language disorders can have marked, adverse consequences for the academic performance of children and adults. Among the academic impact of these disorders are poor literacy skills (reading and writing), truancy and school dropout, and reduced academic attainment, the latter typically measured by the number and level of formal qualifications achieved. In 2000–2001, the U.S. Department of Education (2003) reported that among students aged 14 years and older, 52.3 % of those with speech/language impairments graduated with a standard diploma. This was a lower graduation rate than in six other forms of disability including hearing impairments and traumatic brain injury. Among students with speech/language impairments, 39.7 % dropped out. This dropout rate was higher than that recorded for ten other disabilities including mental retardation and specific learning disabilities. Conti-Ramsden et al. (2009) found that language skills were predictive of educational attainment in adolescents with a history of SLI who were in their final year of compulsory secondary schooling (mean age = 17.4 years).

Such is the strength of the relationship between language functioning and academic performance that adverse academic outcomes of language impairments have been found to persist well into adulthood. Muir et al. (2011) found that maternal-reported speech concerns at age 5 years predicted poorer educational outcomes at 21 years in a sample of 3,193 participants from a birth cohort of 7,223 infants. Young et al. (2002) found that young adults who had been first identified as having language impairment at 5 years of age lagged significantly behind controls on all areas of academic achievement at 19 years of age. Elbro et al. (2011) conducted a 30-year follow-up study of 198 Danish participants who were originally diagnosed with language impairments between 3 and 9 years of age. More than half of these participants reported reading difficulties which had persisted into adulthood (this compares to a figure of only 4.9 % of Danish adults in the population in general). Language measures of verbal memory and productive vocabulary contributed significantly to the variance in this literacy outcome. In this section, we examine the findings of studies which indicate a specific role for pragmatic language skills in academic performance in several clinical populations.

Thagard et al. (2011) examined the relationship between pragmatic language skills and academic success in 81 deaf and hard of hearing students in a school district in a southeastern US state. Regardless of whether the students used spoken language or signed language, a high, positive correlation was found between pragmatic language skills and academic outcomes. In a study of 56 deaf students, Silvestre et al. (2007) reported positive correlations between conversational skills and academic self-concept. Specifically, conversational difficulties that took the form of not responding to questions with all the information required were found to correlate inversely with scores for academic self-concept. The best academic self-concept scores were positively related to fewer requests for the speaker to repeat what they had said and a lower number of inadequate responses throughout the conversation.

Over half of the adults with a childhood history of pragmatic language impairment studied by Whitehouse et al. (2009b) did not achieve five or more passes at GCSE level. (Graduate Certificate of School Education (GCSE) exams are taken by 16-year-old school children in the UK.) Similar pass rates were recorded in adults with a history of SLI or autism spectrum disorder. However, the two adults with PLI who were eligible to take Advanced-Level exams (A-Levels) both went on to complete university degrees. Howlin et al. (2004) reported poor educational attainment and pragmatic language skills in 68 individuals with autism who had a performance IQ of 50 or above in childhood. The majority of these subjects (53.78 %) left school without any formal qualifications. An assessment of pragmatic language skills at 29 years revealed significant impairment, with only 10 % of the group displaying good use of language. However, like Whitehouse et al. (2009b), Howlin et al. did not examine the relationship between the educational attainment of these subjects and their pragmatic language skills. It is conceivable, for example, that poor performance in both areas may be a consequence of a third variable (e.g. impaired socialization).

Reading disability is known to play a key role in the educational attainment of students (Kiuru et al. 2011). Studies are increasingly revealing the presence of significant pragmatic language impairments in students with dyslexia.[6] Griffiths (2007) reported reduced pragmatic competence in the 20 adults with dyslexia in her study compared to adults with no dyslexia adults. Moreover, there appeared to be a correlation between dyslexia and pragmatic impairment in these subjects. Griffiths contends that certain cognitive deficits associated with dyslexia, viz. reduced speed of processing and poor working memory capacity, may also limit individuals with dyslexia in obtaining the intended meaning of a speaker's utterances. This study suggests that as well as playing a direct role in the educational attainment of students, pragmatic language impairment may also operate alongside learning disabilities like dyslexia in predisposing an individual to academic failure and educational under-achievement.

Further evidence that pragmatic disorders can have an impact on a child's academic skills can be gleaned from studies which report academic gains when communication interventions target pragmatic impairments. Adams et al. (2006) describe how teachers reported a demonstrable change in curriculum engagement of children with pragmatic language impairments following a communication intervention. Finally, it should be noted that not all studies have established a relationship between pragmatic language skills and academic outcomes in children. Ben-Yizhak et al. (2011) examined the pragmatic language skills of 35 school-age siblings of children with autism who were at higher risk of developing the broad autism phenotype. Although these children had lower pragmatic abilities than the siblings of children with typical development, school achievements and reading processes were intact.

5.5 Occupational and Vocational Impact

It is well established that language impairments of all types adversely influence the employment prospects of the individuals who have these impairments. Language impaired adolescents and adults are less likely than individuals without language impairment to gain employment. If employment is secured, it is more likely to be in unskilled, manual jobs than in skilled or professional occupations. Language impairment is likely to have a direct relationship and an indirect relationship—the latter via academic attainment—to vocational outcomes. This is because academic achievement, which has a significant influence on one's employment prospects, is also negatively impacted by language impairment (see Sect. 5.4 above). It is no coincidence, for example, that in a study of adults with ADHD and control subjects aged 18–64 years, Biederman and Faraone (2006) reported that statistically fewer adults with ADHD achieved academic milestones and were in full-time employment relative to controls (full-time employment was recorded in 34 % and 59 % of adults with ADHD and control adults, respectively) (see Kuriyan et al. (2013) for further discussion of adult educational and vocational outcomes of children with ADHD). Below, we consider the findings of studies which have found a relationship between language and pragmatic impairments and occupational and vocational outcomes.

Durkin et al. (2012) found that individuals with a history of SLI who were in their final year of compulsory secondary education were more likely to aspire to manual roles. Their typically developing peers aspired to professional roles. Snow et al. (2011) reported that 50 % of a sub-group of young offenders with language impairment undertook some form of vocational training since leaving school compared to 68 % of their counterparts with no language impairment. Among the 198 Danish participants with childhood diagnoses of language impairments studied by Elbro et al. (2011), only 39 % reported that they had entered into post-compulsory education or vocational training (this compares to a figure of 92.4 % in the population in general). Education or vocational training was completed by 30 % of participants (this compares to 82.5 % in the general population). While 84.1 % of people in the same age band as these participants in the general population held a paid job, only 56 % of participants did so. Measures of language, principally verbal memory and productive vocabulary, contributed significantly to the variance in these vocational and occupational outcomes.

Verbal memory is also significantly associated with employment status in adults with bipolar disorder and patients with chronic schizophrenia or schizoaffective disorder (Dickerson et al. 2004; Kaneda et al. 2009). In a study of 195 young patients who sustained an ischaemic stroke between 15 and 49 years of age, Naess et al. (2009) found that aphasia was associated with a loss of employment at six-year follow-up (but see Gil et al. (1996) who found no association between aphasia and occupational outcome in patients with severe TBI). Gasser-Moritz et al. (2012) found that a language measure—naming speed—was significantly correlated with the return to professional activities in adult patients with low-grade gliomas. The remainder of this section will consider if these adverse employment outcomes of language impairment in general are also evident in the case of pragmatic language disorders.

Clegg et al. (2005) studied employment outcomes in 17 men who were diagnosed with a severe receptive developmental language disorder in childhood. These men were assessed in middle childhood, and again in early adult life and in their mid thirties. Significant correlations were obtained between two measures of pragmatic language impairment when these men were in their early twenties, and social adaptation in the mid-thirties. Social adaptation included a measure of continual employment.

Research indicates that approximately 25 % of people with autism are employed (Holwerda et al. 2012). There is evidence that poor employment outcomes in this population are related in part to impoverished pragmatic language skills. Howlin et al. (2004) examined adult outcomes for 68 individuals with autism. These individuals were first assessed at 7 years of age and then again at follow-up at 29 years. At follow-up, almost one third of the group had some form of employment, which mostly took the form of low-level jobs with poor pay. Social use of language (pragmatics) was rated on the Autism Diagnostic Interview (ADI) (Le Couteur et al. 1989). The ADI revealed that only 10 % of the group had good social use of language, while 40 % had severely impaired social use of language. Highly significant and substantial correlations were obtained between almost all adult outcome measures. This included a significant correlation between the social use of language and a social outcome measure which included work placements. Clearly, individuals with autism who had better pragmatic language skills also had the best employment outcomes.

Bearden et al. (2011) examined speech samples elicited from 105 adolescents, 54 of whom were considered to be at clinical high risk for a first episode of psychosis. Speech samples were coded for linguistic cohesion. Adolescents who converted to psychosis at one-year follow-up used significantly less referential cohesion at baseline (i.e. they provided fewer references to events, persons and objects which were mentioned in preceding utterances). Moreover, referential cohesion was a significant predictor of role (work and school) functioning in these adolescents.

Isaki and Turkstra (2000) examined communication abilities and work re-entry in 20 adults with TBI who were 1–4 years post-injury. Three language tests, one of which examined verbal reasoning of the type used in everyday communication, correctly classified 85 % of these subjects as employed or unemployed. Dickinson et al. (2007) found that performance on a social skills assessment, the Maryland Assessment of Social Competence (MASC) (Bellack et al. 2006), was a predictor of vocational functioning in patients with schizophrenia. The four role-play scenarios examined in the MASC required subjects to initiate conversations with new people in the workplace and make requests of a boss, and involved the use of pragmatic language skills.

Klonoff et al. (1990) examined vocational outcomes following rehabilitation in three adults with right-hemisphere damage (RHD). They found that measures of speech and language function tended to underestimate the impact of RHD on the functioning of these patients in a number of domains. Despite having articulate verbal skills, all three patients had marked deficits in pragmatics. These deficits, which were particularly evident in unstructured social situations, included instances of hyperverbality, tangentiality, inappropriate comments and humour, and poor eye contact and turn-taking skills. The colleagues of one patient, who had returned to work as a community college lecturer, identified significant problems, including deficits in pragmatics. This patient had to reduce his participation in lecture activities and was unable to return to his administrative position.

5.6 Behavioural Impact

Investigators have long recognized a link between language disorders and a range of behavioural problems in children including disobedience and defiance, hyperactivity and disruptive classroom behaviour. Keegstra et al. (2010) found that mothers reported more internalizing behavioural problems in children with language problems than in peers in the Dutch population. Coster et al. (1999) examined behavioural problems in 56 children with SLI who were aged 8, 10 and 12 years. Behavioural problems, which included internalizing and externalizing behaviours, were evident in 48 % of these children either at home or in school. Behavioural problems manifested themselves more clearly in these children with SLI as they grew older, with the percentage of these problems increasing with increasing age: 23 % at age 8 (parent rating), 32 % at age 10 (teacher rating) and 48 % at age 12 (parent and teacher rating).

The extended course of the behavioural difficulties in Coster et al.'s children with SLI was not replicated in a study by Whitehouse et al. (2011). These investigators reported that late talkers at age 2 years were at a higher risk for internalizing and externalizing problems than control toddlers. However, late-talking status at 2 years was not related to emotional and behavioural problems at 5, 8, 10, 14 or 17 years. Van Daal et al. (2007) reported significant behaviour problems in 40 % of a sample of 71 five-year-old children with language impairment. Behaviour problems, which included most frequently withdrawn behaviour, somatic complaints, thought problems and aggressive behaviour, were associated with three of four language factors, but not with speech problems.[7]

Clinical studies have also revealed a relationship between language disorders and behavioural problems in patients with adult-onset conditions. Alderman et al. (2002) examined aggressive behaviour in 46 patients with acquired brain injury. Patients with low language function were more likely to physically assault others in the absence of identifiable antecedents. Moreover, these assaults were more severe and required more intrusive intervention to manage them than assaults with identifiable antecedents, or aggression displayed by patients with better language function. Language difficulties are also known to be a risk factor for agitation in patients with schizophrenia (Lambert and Naber 2011). This section will consider if behavioural problems are also related to impairments of pragmatic language skills in children and adults.

Van Agt et al. (2011) reported significant behavioural problems among the 8-year-old children with pragmatic disorder in their study. The personality characteristics and classroom behaviour of these children were assessed using the School Behaviour Checklist—Revised (SCHOBL-R). Children with pragmatic disorder had unfavourable scores on the SCHOBL-R factor Attitude to School Work, which indicated that they displayed more disobedient or distracted behaviour compared to children without language disorders or children with other types of language disorder. These children also had significantly lower mean scores on the SCHOBL-R factor scale Agreeableness, indicating that there was more selfish or cold or teasing behaviour in children with pragmatic disorder compared to children without language disorders.

Lindsay and Dockrell (2000) examined the behaviour of 69 children aged 7–8 years with specific speech and language difficulties (a general designation which included pragmatic difficulties). On two measures of behaviour—the Strengths and Difficulties Questionnaire (SDQ) and the behaviour subscale of the Junior Rating Scale (JRS)—these children were rated as having significantly more problems than standardization samples. Parents and teachers rated 36.7 and 30.2 % of children, respectively, in the 'abnormal' category on the SDQ total difficulties score. Four to ten times more children than expected were rated by teachers at the most extreme score on the Behaviour and Social Interaction items on the JRS. Parents and teachers indicated problems with hyperactivity in approximately 44 % of children. It is noteworthy that a measure of narrative production— the information component of the Bus Story Test (Renfrew 1997)—was the only language measure with a significant correlation to the teachers' SDQ total score. St Clair et al. (2011) reported a significant linear association between pragmatic language skills at 11 and 16 years in 234 children with SLI and ratings on the hyperactivity and conduct subscales of the SDQ.

Ketelaars et al. (2010) examined the behavioural impact of pragmatic language impairment in a community sample of 1,364 children with a mean age of 4.11 years. Dutch versions of the Children's Communication Checklist and the Strengths and Difficulties Questionnaire were used to assess pragmatic language skills and behavioural problems in these children, respectively. Hyperactivity/ inattention on the SDQ showed a high correlation with CCC subscales measuring pragmatic competence. Pragmatic competence was also a good predictor of behavioural problems. The structural language skills of these children did not predict their behavioural problems. Farmer and Oliver (2005) found that ratings of hyperactivity on the SDQ were significantly correlated with pragmatic difficulties on the CCC in a clinically diverse group which included children with SLI and pervasive developmental disorder.

Lindsay et al. (2007) examined language skills and their relation to behavioural problems in 69 children (mean age 8.3 years) with specific speech and language difficulties. The pragmatic language skills and behaviour of these children were assessed using the CCC and SDQ, respectively. Scores on the CCC at 10 years were a significant correlate of behaviour (measured as SDQ total difficulties) both concurrently (at 10 years) and predictively (at 12 years). This was the case both for parent and teacher ratings on the SDQ. Additionally, the Bus Story information—a measure of narrative production—at 8 years of age was a significant correlate of SDQ total difficulties at 8, 10 and 12 years for both parent and teacher ratings. Botting and Conti-Ramsden (2000) found that 53 % of their children with complex language impairments—a designation that included pragmatic impairments—had a clinical level of behavioural difficulty. These studies clearly indicate that pragmatic language impairments can have a significant, adverse impact on the behaviour of children, in some cases over many years.

Fontenot et al. (2011) examined language and pragmatic skills in 11 adolescents aged 13–16 years who attended an alternative education setting because of behaviour problems. All 11 participants had behaviour problems which were rated as either moderate or severe, and which often involved fighting with or without the use of weapons. The Comprehensive Assessment of Spoken Language (CASL) (Carrow-Woolfolk 1999) was used to assess a wide range of language skills. Several CASL subtests examine pragmatic language skills: Non-Literal Language; Meaning from Context; and Pragmatic Judgement. On two of these subtests—Meaning from Context and Pragmatic Judgement—no standard score for any of the 11 participants was within 1 standard deviation of the mean. Pragmatic difficulties on the Pragmatic Judgement subtest were apparent on items that required a request for clarification or information, and polite introductions or declines. Responses were inappropriate (not impolite) to test criteria and often lacked specificity. Participants very quickly reached a ceiling on the Meaning from Context subtest, producing 'I don't know' responses.

To a lesser extent, the behavioural impact of pragmatic disorders in adults has also been studied. Alderman (2007) examined the causes of aggressive behaviour shown by 108 patients in a neurobehavioural unit. Most patients (82 %) were male and had sustained a closed head injury (64.8 %). Poor communication, which included a measure of pragmatics, was the largest single factor contributing to aggression, accounting for 23.8 % of the variance in aggressive behaviour. Given the relationship between theory of mind and pragmatics, it is pertinent to ask if the presence of ToM deficits in adults with TBI (Havet-Thomassin et al. 2006) might not be related to the often severe behavioural problems of these clients. At least two studies suggest that this is not the case. In an investigation of 33 patients with TBI, Milders et al. (2008) reported that the severity of impairments in the understanding of other people's intentions (i.e. theory of mind) was unrelated to the severity of behavioural problems in these clients. Bach et al. (2006) found that ToM ability did not predict behavioural disturbance in 20 patients with TBI.

It is well established that language impairment is related to abusive and aggressive behaviour in adults with dementia (Hall and O'Connor 2004; Volicer et al. 2009). Impaired language comprehension in particular has been shown to be correlated with aggression against other people (as opposed to objects) (Welsh et al. 1996). However, most studies in this area fail to distinguish pragmatic language impairments from general language impairments, making it difficult to draw conclusions about the relationship between pragmatics and aggression in this population. A notable exception is a study by Talerico et al. (2002) who investigated correlates of aggression in 405 older nursing home residents with evidence of dementia. In an effort to use measures 'that make a conceptual distinction between pragmatic communication and cognitive processes' (171), Talerico et al. employed two items from the behaviour subscale of the Psychogeriatric Dependency Rating Scale (Wilkinson and Graham White 1980). A language measure of naming ability was also included in the study. Impaired communication was the only resident characteristic that was consistently associated with aggression. The failure to interpret the communicative intentions of others is proposed as an explanation of the aggressive behaviour of clients with dementia (Welsh et al. 1996).

5.7 Forensic Impact

The forensic impact of pragmatic disorders includes any behaviour that brings an individual into contact with the criminal justice system. This behaviour may take the form of illicit drug use, damage to property, and offences involving violence towards others. The forensic impact of pragmatic disorders has received relatively little attention from clinical investigators. The dearth of research in this area is related to a number of factors. Language impaired clients in correctional facilities frequently do not receive language services. Pragmatic language skills are not assessed and treated in these clients even though they can experience clinically significant levels of language impairment. Also, clients in correctional facilities often have a range of additional difficulties including drug dependence and psychiatric disturbances. These difficulties make it particularly difficult to identify, assess and treat pragmatic deficits in this population.

Notwithstanding the lack of research in this area, there are strong grounds for believing that pragmatic impairments may have a significant forensic impact. Firstly, there is now clear evidence that adolescents and adults in correctional facilities have marked pragmatic impairments (see Sect. 6.3 in Chap. 6). These impairments may or may not contribute directly to offending behaviour. At the very least, they are likely to compromise engagement with the verbally mediated rehabilitation programmes that are aimed at reducing reoffending. Secondly, studies have demonstrated a relationship between language impairment, offending

behaviour and substance use disorders (Beitchman et al. 1999, 2001; Brownlie
et al. 2004; Linares-Orama 2005). Indeed, such is the relationship between language and offending behaviour that significant correlations have been reported
between criminality and language development in boys at 6, 18 and 24 months
(Stattin and Klackenberg-Larsson 1993). These considerations give investigators
reasonable grounds for examining the forensic impact of pragmatic disorders.

Snow and Powell (2011) examined the general language and pragmatic skills
of 100 young offenders who were completing custodial sentences in Victoria,
Australia. Offenders were divided into two sub-groups in accordance with their
scores on violent and non-violent offending scales of the Cormier-Lang Crime
Index (Quinsey et al. 1998). The group with high scores on both these scales performed more poorly on all language measures compared to the sub-group whose
scores were not high on these scales. Importantly, there was a statistically significant difference between these groups on the figurative language sub-test of the
Test of Language Competence–Expanded Edition (Wiig and Secord 1989), with
the high-offending sub-group performing significantly more poorly on this pragmatic measure. While Snow and Powell (2011, p. 487) emphasize that 'no causal
or temporal inferences can be drawn about the role that a developmental history
of language impairment plays in later engagement in crime', it seems reasonable
to conclude that pragmatic language skills represent an area of particular vulnerability in this population of clients (see Sect. 6.3 in Chap. 6 for further discussion).

There is some evidence that impaired pragmatic language skills in children may
increase their liability for a substance use disorder. Najam et al. (1997) examined
the language abilities of 135 children who were the offspring of men diagnosed
as having a substance use disorder. These children, who were judged to be at
high risk of drug abuse, were compared at baseline (10–12 years) and follow-up
(16 years) to 208 children whose fathers had no psychiatric disorder or substance
use disorder (low risk children). High risk children obtained significantly lower
scores than low risk children on subtests of the Test of Language Competence
(Wiig and Secord 1989) which assess pragmatic language skills. Specifically, the
tests in question examined these children's ability to assign meaning to ambiguous sentences, comprehend metaphorical language, and express intents. At follow-
up at age 16 years, high risk children were still significantly poorer than low risk
children at comprehending ambiguous sentences and expressing intents. Najam
et al. (1997, p. 78) concluded that '[i]mpaired linguistic ability, especially in those
facets which involve the interpretation of abstract information [...] appears to contribute to the liability for a substance use disorder'.

It appears likely that the relationship between pragmatic language disorders and
the forensic impact of these disorders is mediated by a number of other factors
that have been examined in this chapter. Many of these factors are linked to pragmatic language impairments, and place individuals at an increased risk of committing actions which bring them into contact with the criminal justice system.
For example, the relationship between pragmatic disorders and forensic impact
may be mediated by aggressive behaviour which, as we saw in Sect. 5.6, is linked
to pragmatic language impairment in subjects with TBI. (It is worth noting that

there is an increased prevalence of TBI in adult male offenders; Williams et al. 2010). Similarly, the relationship between impaired pragmatic language skills and poor academic achievement is unlikely to terminate in a reduced number of formal qualifications. Rather, the limited vocational opportunities of young people who have not experienced academic success expose these individuals to an increased risk of offending behaviour and incarceration. (ADHD, a disorder which has adverse implications for educational attainment, and marked pragmatic impairments, has been reported to occur in 40 % of adult male longer-term prison inmates; Ginsberg et al. 2010). So, even in those cases where pragmatic language disorders cannot be demonstrated to have a direct forensic impact, it is still likely that these disorders have severe forensic implications for affected individuals through a number of mediating variables.

Finally, theory of mind (ToM) or mentalizing deficits have been linked to violent crime and other offending behaviour in adolescents and adults. Many of the tests that are used to assess ToM are tests of pragmatic language skills such as the interpretation of sarcasm or irony, and the attribution of intentions to agents (see Cummings (2014b) for discussion of ToM tests of pragmatics). Studies which link mentalizing deficits to criminal behaviour are thus also suggestive of a link between pragmatic impairments and offending behaviour. Individuals with Asperger's disorder are over-represented in forensic criminal settings (Haskins and Silva 2006). When offending does occur in clients with Asperger's disorder, it typically takes the form of arson and sexual abuse (Mouridsen 2012). ToM deficits are implicated in the criminal behaviour of these clients (see Burdon and Dickens (2009) and Lerner et al. (2012) for discussion). ToM findings in forensic patients with schizophrenia have been inconclusive. Abu-Akel and Abushua'leh (2004) found that violent patients with paranoid schizophrenia have better mentalizing abilities than non-violent patients with schizophrenia (a finding which Proctor and Beail (2007) replicated in offenders with intellectual disability). However, Majorek et al. (2009) found that when 'excitement' was covaried out, forensic patients with schizophrenia are as impaired as non-forensic patients in their ability to infer mental states (see Bo et al. (2011) for further discussion). The reader is referred to Sect. 3.3 in Chap. 3 for a detailed discussion of the role of ToM deficits in pragmatic disorders.

5.8 Limitations of Impact Studies

Investigations into the impact of pragmatic disorders on the lives of clients are beginning to reveal a burden of disability that has been largely overlooked to date by clinicians and researchers. Pragmatic disorders, it emerges, are more than just communication or language disorders. Rather, these disorders have the potential to disrupt different aspects of clients' lives, in some cases for many years beyond the point when these disorders were first diagnosed and treated by clinicians. In order to mitigate the pernicious consequences of pragmatic disorders, clinicians must have a better understanding of the impact of these disorders than has been the case to date. This will require that researchers substantially increase the number of investigations that examine impact—studies which address impact still constitute a small propor- tion of all clinical investigations into pragmatic disorders. However, it will also require that investigators think in a critical fashion about how studies in this area have been conducted, and identify ways in which these studies can be improved.

In the rest of this chapter, a critical examination of some of the studies dis- cussed above will be undertaken. Some studies contain methodological and other flaws that compromise their conclusions, or at least reduce the significance of these conclusions. These flaws can be broadly classified as (1) the use of samples of children (and, to a lesser degree, adults) which are clinically and linguistically heterogeneous, (2) the use of small numbers of subjects, (3) the use of general rather than specific impact measures, (4) the use of language measures which fail to distinguish pragmatic language skills from more general language skills, and (5) the use of parent reports to assess pragmatic skills and other abilities. Additionally, a number of clinical populations, which have not featured in impact studies to date, will be considered. By drawing attention to these weaknesses and omissions in some of the studies that have been undertaken thus far, it is hoped that impact studies will employ a more rigorous approach in the future.

Many clinical studies investigate groups of children which are not sufficiently homogeneous to permit claims to be made about the impact of pragmatic disor- ders. This lack of homogeneity is evident both in the linguistic and clinical char- acterizations of subjects. For example, Botting and Conti-Ramsden (2000) studied behavioural problems in 77 children with so-called 'complex language impair- ments' (CLI). Over half these children (53 %) were found to have a clinical level of behavioural difficulty. However, the designation CLI included children with pragmatic language impairments as well as children with 'complex combinations of lexical impairment' (the latter corresponding to Rapin's 'higher-order process- ing' group). Given the linguistic heterogeneity of the children with CLI in this study, it is difficult to relate these children's behavioural problems to their pur- ported difficulties with pragmatics.

A linguistically heterogeneous sample of adults with aphasia was used by Hinckley (2002) in a study of vocational and social outcomes. In an already small sample of just 20 clients with aphasia (see below), Hinckley recruited adults with three different forms of aphasia: nonfluent (14 subjects), fluent (3 subjects) and global aphasia (3 subjects). These forms of aphasia have quite different linguistic features which are likely to have a significant influence both on the ability of the person with aphasia to return to work and to achieve social integration. Moreover, two subjects with aphasia developed aphasia as a result of a traumatic brain injury and a right-hemisphere cerebrovascular accident. Both forms of brain damage are associated with marked pragmatic and discourse difficulties (see Chap. 2), and so some degree of impairment in these areas could be present in these cases. In short, there is likely to be considerable linguistic heterogeneity in these subjects with aphasia. This may account for the unexpected findings obtained, particularly in relation to vocational outcome.[8]

As well as the linguistic heterogeneity of child and adult samples, there is also substantial heterogeneity in the clinical conditions of the subjects who are included in these samples. The following studies examine the impact of language impairment in children on a range of domains: Lindsay and Dockrell (2000), Van Agt et al. (2011), Mackie and Law (2010), Hall and Segarra (2007), and Jerome et al. (2002). However, these studies vary considerably in the children that are included in, and excluded from, their respective samples. Lindsay and Dockrell (2000) exclude children with autism from their clinical sample. However, Van Agt et al. (2011) include children with autism, excluding only those children who have intellectual disability or who have fully foreign-language parents.

Mackie and Law (2010) go further still and exclude children for whom English is an additional language, as well as children with a diagnosis of autism or autism spectrum disorder, and children who have a neurological impairment or sensorineural hearing loss. The most exclusive criteria of all these studies are adopted by Hall and Segarra (2007) and Jerome et al. (2002). Hall and Segarra, for example, go beyond Mackie and Law in excluding children with orofacial anomalies, emotional disturbance, any hearing loss (not just sensorineural hearing loss) as well as any child in whom there is not a 15-point discrepancy between non-verbal IQ and language quotient. In all but one of these studies (Hall and Segarra), the relationship between childhood language impairment and social performance is examined. Yet, the heterogeneity of the clinical samples of children used in these studies precludes any direct comparison of their findings in relation to social function.

Many clinical studies involve such small numbers of subjects that it is difficult to see how any meaningful conclusions can be drawn from them. For example, in their study of psychosocial outcomes in adults who had received a range of childhood diagnoses, Whitehouse et al. (2009b, p. 511) state that '[t]he PLI group tended to obtain higher levels of education and work in 'skilled' professions'. However, upon closer examination it emerges that this statement is based on the education levels and professional status of only two and three subjects with PLI, respectively.

The problem of small sample sizes is also evident in a study conducted by Hinckley (2002) of vocational and social outcomes in adults with chronic aphasia. Of 20 subjects who completed all assessments in the study, only 13 were non-retirement age respondents who could be considered in an analysis of vocational outcome. Among these 13 respondents a gainful employment rate of 62 % was obtained. Hinckley (2002, p. 554) reported that '[t]his sample of respondents displayed relatively positive ultimate outcomes, particularly for vocational status'. But when we consider that this employment rate was calculated on the basis of the vocational status of only 13 respondents, it is difficult to say with any conviction if this rate is positive or otherwise. The same pattern emerges time and time again in studies of the impact of pragmatic and language disorders: conclusions about the impact of these disorders are based on such small samples of subjects that they are of dubious merit. The reward for devoting more time, effort and resources to the recruitment of larger samples of subjects in future impact studies will be the knowledge that conclusions based on the results of these studies are robust in a way that many conclusions advanced to date have not been.

Often, measures of a client's general functioning subsume many different domains, making it impossible to relate pragmatic impairments to specific types of impact. In this way, Byrne et al. (1998) succeeded in demonstrating in adults with schizophrenia a moderately strong relationship between scores on the Test of Pragmatic Language (TOPL; Phelps-Terasaki and Phelps-Gunn 1992) and ratings of conversational discourse, on the one hand, and scores on the Global Assessment of Functioning Scale (GAFS; DSM-IV), on the other hand. However, GAFS scores—a single numerical code from 0 to 90—are calculated on the basis of a client's functioning in psychological, social and occupational domains, making it impossible to relate pragmatic impairments during conversation and on the TOPL to any one of these domains.

Similarly, in a study of men with a childhood history of receptive developmental language disorder, Clegg et al. (2005) demonstrated a significant correlation between pragmatic language impairment scores in the mid-twenties and social adaptation in the mid-thirties. However, the social adaptation composite used in this study included several different outcome categories including continual employment, relationships, independent living and friendships. With such a broad spectrum of social, emotional and occupational outcomes subsumed within social adaptation, it is difficult to draw meaningful conclusions about the impact of pragmatic impairment on specific domains of functioning.

By the same token, language measures may not be sufficiently refined to permit conclusions to be drawn about the impact of pragmatic disorders. Snow and Powell (2008) examined the oral language abilities of 50 juvenile offenders. Although these offenders performed significantly worse on all language measures than 50 non-offending controls, impaired language in the offenders was not shown to be related to either type of offending (property or violent) or self-reported substance misuse. However, language impairment was based on a language composite score that included the results of tests that examined structural language, pragmatic and narrative discourse skills. Even if pragmatic impairment was related to offending behaviour and substance use in these offenders, it is unlikely to be revealed as such on the basis of a general language composite score.

A further problem of some impact studies is that language measures may not accurately capture a client's language and pragmatic skills. This is a particular problem when language ratings and scores are based on parent report, as often occurs in studies which examine the impact of language disorders. For example, Hall and Segarra (2007) used a parent report instrument—the Communication Domain of the Vineland (Sparrow et al. 1984)—to assess the communication skills of 35 preschool children with language impairment. Although this measure was found to be the best predictor of these children's academic abilities in reading, writing and mathematics at 9 years of age, this measure displayed only weak-to-moderate significant relationships with some language measures and non-significant relationships with other language measures. These additional language measures were completed by professionals and their disparity with a measure based on parental report suggests that parents and professionals may have been rating the language skills of these children differently.

This disparity is also evident in how parents and professionals rate children's pragmatic language skills. Bishop and Baird (2001) reported low correlations (0.30–0.58) between parental and professional ratings on the individual pragmatic scales of the Children's Communication Checklist, with a correlation of 0.46 for the pragmatic composite. In a later study by Bishop et al. (2006), similarly low correlations between parent and professional ratings on the CCC were obtained. These investigators found that interrater reliability between parent and teacher ratings was generally weak with correlations exceeding 0.5 on non-pragmatic scales such as syntax. My point is not that parent reports and ratings have no place in an assessment of pragmatic language skills. Clearly, they do. Rather, it is that if we are to use such reports and ratings in impact studies of pragmatic disorders, we must be sure they are accurately measuring the behaviours which clinicians and other professionals would identify as pragmatic in nature.

Studies which have examined the impact of pragmatic disorders have tended to focus on a rather small number of conditions to the exclusion of other clinical populations. These conditions include specific language impairment, autism spectrum disorder, aphasia, traumatic brain injury and schizophrenia. However, there are reasons to believe that an equally strong case can be made for the adverse impact of pragmatic disorders by examining a number of other clinical populations, including children with selective mutism, children and adults who stutter, and adults with right-hemisphere damage (RHD). Individuals with these disorders have (often unrecognized) pragmatic impairments in the presence of significant psychological problems such as anxiety and depression. This section concludes with a brief examination of these clinical groups.

It appears likely that anxiety and pragmatics are related in selective mutism. Anxiety is a consistent feature of selective mutism in children. Children with selective mutism have greater social anxiety than both normal controls and children with anxiety disorders (Manassis et al. 2007; Carbone et al. 2010). Moreover, social anxiety is predictive of more severe mutism in these children (Manassis et al. 2007). Although there is evidence of receptive and expressive language impairments in children with selective mutism (Cohan et al. 2008), these impairments appear not to account for the severe difficulties with communication of these children. Indeed, in DSM-5 (American Psychiatric Association 2013), where selective mutism is classified under social anxiety disorder (social phobia), language impairment must be excluded as a source of these children's communication difficulties ('failure to speak is not better accounted for by stuttering or expressive language problems in communication disorders'). To the extent that the communication problem is manifested only in certain contexts and settings (e.g. at school), there is likely to be a pragmatic component in the disorder. Of course, this still leaves open the question of the exact nature of the relationship between pragmatics and anxiety in selective mutism. The findings of Manassis et al. suggest that anxiety may contribute to pragmatic problems in selectively mute children.

It has been known for some time that situational and context factors exacerbate dysfluency in children and adults who stutter. For example, Brundage et al. (2006) found that the communication style of an interviewer affected the frequency of stuttering during virtual reality interviews, with more stuttering observed during challenging than supportive interviews. This feature of stuttering has led some clinicians to consider a role for pragmatic language impairment in stuttering (Weiss 2004). A large range of psychological problems, including anxiety, depression, low self-esteem and reduced quality of life, have also been consistently documented in individuals who stutter (Blood et al. 2011; Koedoot et al. 2011; Tran et al. 2011). Of course, pragmatic and psychological anomalies may simply co-exist in individuals who stutter without one set of problems contributing to the other. However, as more becomes known about the pragmatic problems of this clinical population, and the specific influence of communicative context on speech fluency, clinicians will increasingly have to consider the contribution of pragmatics to the adverse psychological outcomes of people who stutter.

Finally, depression and pragmatic deficits frequently co-occur in adults with right hemisphere damage (RHD). However, the exact nature of the relationship between these clinical features is unclear. Lehman Blake (2003) states that depression is one of several RHD-related conditions which may exacerbate problems with humour appreciation in these adults. The status of depression and mood disorders in right hemisphere stroke is an area of ongoing clinical investigation (Carota and Bogousslavsky 2012). This research may eventually make it possible to establish what relationship, if any, these sequelae of stroke have to the significant pragmatic deficits that attend RHD (see Sect. 2.5.2 in Chap. 2 for discussion of these deficits).

5.9 Summary

It has been argued in this chapter that pragmatic language disorders have some of their most pernicious effects on an individual's ability to function competently in a range of domains beyond communication. These domains include the formation and maintenance of social relationships, participation in occupational roles, and the attainment of educational and academic goals. One's success or otherwise in these areas has a direct bearing on perceptions of quality of life. Additionally, pragmatic disorders may cause, or contribute to, a number of aspects of psychological maladjustment including poor self-esteem, depression and anxiety. With such wide-ranging and adverse consequences emanating from impairment of pragmatic language skills, much more research, it has been argued, must now be undertaken into the impact of pragmatic disorders on the lives of the children and adults who are affected by these disorders. That research must be pursued in a methodologically rigorous fashion to avoid the pitfalls of some impact studies that have been conducted to date. In particular, investigators must aim to examine the impact of pragmatic disorders on specific domains in large, clinically well-defined samples of children and adults. It is only with such a systematic research effort that clinicians can hope to achieve an improved understanding of the impact of pragmatic disorders and the development of interventions which do more than merely remediate deficient language skills.

Notes

1. These interrelationships are amply demonstrated in a recent study by Wadman et al. (2011) of emotional health symptoms (depression and anxiety) in 16-year-olds with specific language impairment. These investigators found that adolescents with SLI experienced significantly more depressive and anxiety symptoms than typically developing 16-year-olds. Also, compared to typically developing controls, adolescents with SLI had significantly lower academic achievement (measured as GCSE/GNVQ points), significantly higher behaviour scores (indicating conduct problems, hyperactivity and peer problems), and reported significantly more bullying. While receptive language ability was weakly correlated with depressive symptoms in these adolescents with SLI, stronger correlations were obtained between depressive symptoms and academic achievement, hyperactivity, conduct problems, peer problems and bullying and depressive symptoms in these subjects. Clearly, each of these separate impacts of specific language impairment contributed to the development of depressive symptoms (psychological impact) in these adolescents with SLI.

2. Jerome et al. (2002) reported significantly poorer self-esteem in 34 children with SLI aged 10–13 years than in a group of typically developing children. Low self-esteem in the children with SLI was most evident in the domains of scholastic competence, social acceptance and behavioural conduct. Language impairment accounted for 62, 22 and 15 % of variability in self-esteem ratings in these domains, respectively. There were no significant differences in self-esteem ratings between typically developing children and younger children with SLI aged 6–9 years.

3. The specific feature of formal thought disorder (FTD) which was found to be related to parent reports of child stress and anxiety in this study was loose associations. However, Solomon et al. (2008) relate FTD more generally to pragmatic impairments when they state that 'FTD is in many ways similar to the pragmatic language impairments and unusual verbal behavior that is part of the core diagnostic criteria for autism' (1475). For discussion of the pragmatic character of FTD in the context of schizophrenia, the reader is referred to Cummings (2013b).

4. A similar finding is reported by Bruce et al. (2006). In a study of 76 children diagnosed with ADHD, Bruce et al. (2006, p. 52) stated that '[p]roblems with language and pragmatics [...] seem to be associated with the typical problems with learning and social skills in children with ADHD'.

5. It is worth noting that the ability to represent the mental states of others—a key cognitive skill required for the pragmatic interpretation of utterances—has also been found to be related to social functioning in adults with schizophrenia (Lysaker et al. 2011). For detailed discussion of the role of theory of mind in pragmatic interpretation, the reader is referred to Cummings (2013a).

6. There is also evidence of literacy difficulties in children who have a primary diagnosis of pragmatic language impairment. Freed et al. (2011) examined

literacy skills in 59 primary school-aged children with pragmatic language impairment. Impaired reading accuracy ability was identified in just over 40 % of these children. On reading comprehension ability, 40.7 % of children with PLI attained attained scores that were at least one standard deviation below the mean. Written expression scores at least one standard deviation below population norms were identified in just over 40 % of these children. Freed et al. (2011, p. 345) concluded that '[t]he clinical implication [...] is that in a subgroup of children (PLI) with mainly normal structural language abilities, there is still considerable risk of literacy difficulties'.

7. Significant language impairments have also been reported in children with behaviour problems, raising interesting questions about the nature of the relationship between language disorder and behavioural difficulties. Ripley and Yuill (2005) studied 19 boys aged 8–16 years who had been excluded from school. Exclusions were related to verbal and physical aggression, failure to follow rules and possession of an offensive weapon, among other things. Excluded boys performed significantly more poorly on measures of expressive language (but not receptive language) than a control group of non-excluded boys. Among excluded boys, those attending primary school had poorer auditory working memory than controls.

8. It will be recalled that a gainful employment rate of 62 % was obtained in the subjects with aphasia in this study. Hinckley (2002, p. 554) remarked that this 'employment rate was [...] unusually high compared to other reports for adults with chronic aphasia'.

Chapter 6
Pragmatic Disorders in Complex and Underserved Populations

6.1 Introduction

Not all pragmatic disorders have received the level of clinical study of the populations examined in Chap. 2. While the pragmatic impairments of clients with right-hemisphere damage or traumatic brain injury are well characterized, relatively little is known about the pragmatic language skills of children with emotional and behavioural disorders or adults with non-Alzheimer's dementias. These children and adults belong to 'complex' populations by virtue of the fact that their pragmatic disturbance occurs in the presence of significant psychiatric and cognitive disorders. Similarly, certain groups of clients with pragmatic impairments are beyond the reach of, or are overlooked by, clinical language services. These groups include adolescents in juvenile detention facilities and adults in prison. These clients belong to an 'underserved' population to the extent that their language needs are inadequately assessed and treated. Although these different clients have not been the focus of extensive academic research or clinical services to date, what is clear is that an array of factors means complex and underserved populations are likely to become an increasingly important part of the caseload of speech and language therapists in years to come. With this consideration in mind, an examination of the pragmatic impairments of these clients now seems timely.

6.2 Emotional and Behavioural Disorders

The population of children with emotional and behavioural disorders (EBDs) poses a number of challenges for educationalists and clinicians. Chief amongst these challenges is how best to define and classify these disorders. Even a brief survey of the literature in this area reveals that there is a distinct lack of unanimity among academics and clinicians on how to define this group of disorders. This situation makes it difficult for investigators to estimate the prevalence of these

L. Cummings, *Pragmatic Disorders*, Perspectives in Pragmatics, Philosophy & Psychology 3, DOI: 10.1007/978-94-007-7954-9_6, © Springer Science+Business Media Dordrecht 2014

disorders and plan the specialist services that these children require.[1] In the UK, the Department for Education and Employment (1994, p. 7) states that 'emotional and behavioural difficulties range from social maladaptation to abnormal emotional stresses. They are persistent (if not necessarily permanent) and constitute learning difficulties. They may be multiple and may manifest themselves in many different forms and severities. They may become apparent through withdrawn, passive, aggressive or self-injurious tendencies'.

In arguing for an updated, standard definition of emotional/behavioural disorders, Brauner and Stephens (2006) place emphasis on behaviours listed in the Diagnostic and Statistical Manual of Mental Disorders (DSM). The diagnostic criteria in DSM will be important to the discussion of the three emotional and behavioural disorders to be examined in this section—attention deficit hyperactivity disorder (ADHD), conduct disorder and selective mutism. In some cases, these diagnostic criteria refer to impaired communicative functioning in certain contexts or environments (selective mutism is a case in point). In other cases, these criteria describe behaviours which help explain certain communication difficulties in children with EBDs (the impulsivity of children with ADHD, for example, may contribute to their inappropriate initiation of turns in conversation). In discussing each of these EBDs, we will examine their prevalence and general language features before considering what is known about pragmatic impairments in these children.

Attention deficit hyperactivity disorder is one of the most extensively studied emotional and behavioural disorders in children. In the fifth edition of the Diagnostic and Statistical Manual of Mental Disorders (DSM-5; American Psychiatric Association 2013), ADHD is diagnosed when there are either six (or more) symptoms of inattention and/or six (or more) symptoms of hyperactivity and impulsivity. These symptoms must have persisted for at least 6 months to a degree which is inconsistent with developmental level and which impacts on social and academic/occupational activities. Several inattentive or hyperactive-impulsive symptoms must be present by 12 years of age. Also, symptoms must be apparent in two or more settings (e.g. at home and school), and should not occur exclusively during the course of schizophrenia or another psychotic disorder or be better accounted for by another mental disorder (e.g. anxiety disorder). DSM-5 recognizes three types of ADHD depending on the pattern and duration of inattentive and hyperactive/impulsive symptoms: combined presentation; predominantly inattentive presentation; and predominantly hyperactive/impulsive presentation.

Using prevalence data from 102 studies comprising 171,756 subjects from all world regions, Polanczyk et al. (2007) reported a worldwide-pooled prevalence of ADHD of 5.29 %. Data from the US National Survey of Children's Health (2003) reveal that ADHD was diagnosed in 8.8 % of children aged 6–17 years (Blanchard et al. 2006). ADHD is found more commonly in boys than in girls with male-to-female ratios ranging from 3:1 in community samples to 10:1 in clinic-referred samples (Biederman et al. 2002). The condition is associated with cognitive impairments including inhibition deficits, slower processing speed, impaired social perspective-taking and reduced visual-spatial short-term memory (Cardy et al. 2010; Kibby and Cohen 2008; Marton et al. 2009; Schoemaker et al. 2012).

Increasingly, investigators are examining language impairments in children with ADHD. Some of these impairments have been related to cognitive deficits in ADHD. Engelhardt et al. (2009) examined the production of grammatical sentences in adolescents and adults with ADHD. These investigators hypothesized that poor inhibitory control in ADHD would lead these subjects to produce ungrammatical sentences when presented with two pictures and a verb. Subjects with ADHD combined subtype were particularly prone to producing ungrammatical sentences, a finding which was related to their tendency to begin speaking before they had planned how to produce a grammatical utterance. Language comprehension is also impaired in ADHD. Wassenberg et al. (2010) examined complex sentence comprehension in 15 children and 15 adolescents with ADHD combined subtype. These children and adolescents were found to be slower and less efficient than matched controls in comprehending complex sentences.

DaParma et al. (2011) examined receptive and expressive language skills in 100 children with ADHD between 6 and 16 years of age. Between 6.6 and 20.2 % of subjects with ADHD had impairments on various receptive language skills. Up to 15.7 % of these subjects had impairments on expressive language skills. Similar language scores would be expected in only 2 % of the normal population. Receptive language impairments included problems understanding spoken language, following directions and understanding concepts and grammatical relationships. Impairments of expressive language were evident in sentence formulation, speed of word recall and word association tasks. Literacy difficulties, including poor reading comprehension, word decoding, spelling and written language disorder, have also been reported in children with ADHD (Asberg et al. 2010; Yoshimasu et al. 2011). Asberg et al. (2010) reported at least one reading and writing disorder in 56 % of the girls with ADHD examined in their study.

DSM-5 defines conduct disorder as a repetitive and persistent pattern of behaviour in which major age-appropriate societal norms or rules, or the basic rights of others are violated. For a diagnosis of conduct disorder to be made, three or more of the following criteria must be present in the past 12 months (at least one criterion must be present in the last 6 months): aggression to people and animals; destruction of property; deceitfulness or theft; serious violations of rules. Clinically significant impairment in social, academic or occupational functioning must be caused by the behaviour disturbance. Criteria for antisocial personality disorder must not be met in individuals aged 18 years or older. There are three subtypes of conduct disorders based on age of onset: childhood-onset type; adolescent-onset type; and unspecified onset. Conduct disorders may be diagnosed as mild, moderate or severe in nature.

Conduct disorders are the most common reason young children are referred to mental health services (Richardson and Joughin 2002). As might be expected, these disorders are more prevalent in boys than in girls. In 5–10 year-olds, the prevalence of conduct disorders is 6.5 % for boys and 2.7 % for girls (Richardson and Joughin 2002). Cognitive deficits have been widely documented in children and adolescents with conduct disorder. Olvera et al. (2005) reported impairments in cognitive ability, set shifting/inhibition, planning and verbal memory-language functioning in the incarcerated subjects in their study who met criteria for conduct disorder. Children with conduct disorder who are low on callous-unemotional traits display deficits in cognitive and affective perspective-taking (Anastassiou-Hadjicharalambous and Warden 2008). Toupin et al. (2000) found executive function deficits in their sample of 57 children with conduct disorder after ADHD symptoms and socioeconomic status were controlled.

The language skills of children with conduct disorder have been consistently shown to be below those of same-age normal peers. Déry et al. (1999) found significantly lower verbal skills in 59 adolescents with conduct disorder compared with controls. The lower verbal performance of these adolescents was not explained by the presence of ADHD symptoms (see below for a role for inattention in ADHD in literacy problems in conduct disorder). Speltz et al. (1999) found that verbal tests distinguished a clinic group of preschool boys with early onset conduct problems from matched comparison boys. Even after controlling for general vocabulary knowledge, the clinic boys in this study had poorer vocabularies for describing affective states than comparison boys. Giancola and Mezzich (2000) reported that performance on tests of language competence was significantly poorer in female adolescents with conduct disorder, or conduct disorder with comorbid substance use disorder (SUD), than in normal controls or in female adolescents with SUD only.

Specific literacy difficulties have been reported in children with conduct disorder, although the nature of this relationship is unclear. Carroll et al. (2005) investigated the relationship between specific literacy difficulties and psychiatric disorder in a large-scale national sample of children aged 9–15 years. Among children identified as having specific literacy difficulties, 13.8 % had conduct disorder. The relationship between reading problems and conduct disorder in these children was shown to be mediated by inattention (conduct disorder and ADHD were strongly associated in the sample). Bennett et al. (2003) reported that an eight point increase in reading scores in kindergarten and grade one children resulted in a 23 % decrease in the risk of conduct problems 30 months after school entry. These investigators recommend further research to establish if reading problems have a causal role in the development of conduct problems.

In DSM-5, selective mutism is classified for the first time as a social anxiety disorder (SAD), following recommendations that the disorder be viewed as a developmental variant of SAD (Bögels et al. 2010). For a diagnosis of selective mutism to be made, a child must exhibit a consistent failure to speak in specific social situations where this is expected (e.g. at school), despite speaking in other situations. Selective mutism is the least prevalent of the emotional and behavioural disorders examined in this section. In a review of prevalence studies, Viana et al. (2009) stated that prevalence estimates oscillate in the range 0.47–0.76 % of the population. Selective mutism is slightly more common in girls than in boys. However, this difference may be related to research limitations such as small sample populations (Wong 2010). The mean age of onset ranges from 2.7 to 4.1 years, although children are often older before a diagnosis is made (Viana et al. 2009).

Language and other communication deficits have been reported in children with selective mutism, although they are unlikely to be a significant factor in the aetiology of the disorder (Bögels et al. 2010). In a study of 54 children with selective mutism, Kristensen (2000) found mixed receptive-expressive language disorder and expressive language disorder in 17.3 and 11.5 %, respectively. Phonological disorder was present in 42.6 % of this sample. Speech difficulties were reported in almost 50 % of children with elective mutism studied by Andersson and Thomsen (1998). In a study of young adults who had selective mutism in childhood, Steinhausen et al. (2006) found premorbid speech and language abnormalities in 30.3 % at presentation. Cohan et al. (2008) reported scores in the clinically significant range for syntax problems on the Children's Communication Checklist-2 (CCC-2; Bishop 2003) in 130 children with selective mutism.

Pragmatic disorders have not been extensively characterized in children with EBDs. This is despite the fact that diagnostic criteria in DSM-5 for at least one of the emotional and behavioural disorders—attention deficit hyperactivity disorder—indicate that pragmatic language skills (specifically, conversational skills) are likely to be an area of difficulty for these children. In this way, the child or adult with ADHD and inattention may have difficulty remaining focused during conversations, and often does not seem to listen when spoken to directly. The hyperactive-impulsive individual often talks excessively, blurts out an answer before a question has been completed (or completes people's sentences and 'jumps the gun' in conversations), and/or interrupts or intrudes on others (e.g. frequently butts into conversations). These conversational difficulties are evident in the following exchange between an adult and an 8-year-old boy who has received a diagnosis of ADHD (Tannock 2005, p. 45). The exchange occurs 20 min after the start of a psychoeducational assessment:

Child: "What are we gonna do next? Huh? What's in there? What's that?"
(interferes by grabbing test materials)

Adult: "You'll see in a sec"
(adult reaches into case for next set of test materials)
—a few minutes later, child interrupts testing—

Child: "Where's the um…the things…um…where's the um…bugs?"
(climbs on seat to peer into case)

Adult: "Pardon? What bugs? There are no bugs here. Now, tell me what –"
—child interrupts again—

Child: (loud unmodulated voice) "—The bugs. You said I'll see the bugs. I don't wanna do this. I wanna see the bugs…the…um…secs…the insecs!"

In this short exchange, the child interrupts the adult's conversational turn on two occasions and creates two further, non-verbal interruptions (he grabs test materials and climbs onto the seat). His verbal contributions consist largely of questions which are delivered in quick succession and do not wait for responses from the adult. Even when presented with a direct command ('Now, tell me what…'), it is clear the child disregards the adult's instruction and continues to pursue a topic (the bugs) which the adult has indicated has no relevance to the exchange (the adult explicitly states 'There are no bugs here'). These conversational and pragmatic anomalies can be seen to reduce the child's compliance with the psychoeducational assessment and will have adverse implications for his academic functioning.

Several studies have attempted to characterize pragmatic skills in children with ADHD. Bishop and Baird (2001) used the Children's Communication Checklist to assess pragmatic language skills in children with ADHD, and compare these skills to those found in children with Asperger's syndrome or pervasive developmental disorder, not otherwise specified (PDD, NOS). On the basis of combined parent and professional ratings, the 132 cut-off point indicative of pragmatic impairment on the CCC was recorded in 73 % of children with ADHD. This compared with 77 % and 61 % of children with Asperger's syndrome and PDD, NOS, respectively. Particularly poor scores were recorded for children with ADHD on the CCC scale which measures inappropriate initiation. A later study by Geurts et al. (2004) confirmed the poor pragmatic skills of children with ADHD on the CCC, but this time in relation to normal controls.

A community sample of boys with ADHD and normal language skills studied by McInnes et al. (2003) were found to have comprehension deficits when listening to spoken expository passages. Although these boys were able to comprehend as well as normal children the factual details in expository and narrative passages, they had significantly more difficulty making inferences from expository information than normal children (see also Berthiaume et al. 2010). Bignell and Cain (2007) found impairments in pragmatic aspects of communication in 7–11-year-old children with problems of inattention and hyperactivity. Most notably, these impairments included difficulty with the comprehension of figurative language. Studies have also demonstrated a close association between pragmatic impairments and hyperactive-inattentive behaviours in children (e.g. Farmer and Oliver 2005). Pragmatic language skills have been found to mediate the relation between hyperactive-inattentive behaviours and social skills problems in children (Leonard et al. 2011).

There has been little systematic study of pragmatic language skills in children with conduct disorder. Those studies which have been conducted indicate that pragmatics is compromised in children with this disorder. Pragmatic abilities were investigated by Gilmour et al. (2004) in 142 referred children, 55 of whom had a predominant diagnosis of conduct disorder. The CCC was used to characterize the pragmatic skills of these children along with those of children with an autism spectrum condition and children with typical development. Among the children with conduct disorder, two-thirds displayed pragmatic language impairments and other behavioural features similar to those found in autism. Similarity with autistic symptomatology was also evident in a study of 26 persistently disruptive children examined by Donno et al. (2010). These children displayed poor pragmatic language skills and mentalising (theory of mind) abilities. Nine children (35 %) met diagnostic criteria for atypical autism or Asperger's syndrome.

Adams et al. (2002) used children with severe conduct disorder as a control group in their study of conversational behaviour in Asperger's syndrome. They found that these children were more likely to let the researcher contribute the first part of a conversational pair (e.g. the question in a question–answer pair) during social-emotional conversations than during non-routine conversations (about a trip out, for example). This finding, Adams et al. (2002, p. 687) argue, confirms the clinical impression that 'it is hard to develop a flowing conversation with most adolescent individuals with a diagnosis of conduct disorder, particularly on emotional topics'. These studies demonstrate that further investigation into the pragmatic skills of this clinical population is warranted, particularly if researchers are to address issues such as the status of pragmatic impairment in children with conduct disorder and comorbid autism spectrum disorder.

Of the three emotional and behavioural disorders examined in this section, there has been least investigation into the pragmatic language skills of children with selective mutism. Yet, there are reasons to believe that children with this disorder experience difficulty with pragmatic aspects of language. Firstly, studies have demonstrated a link between pragmatic impairments and disorders related to selective mutism such as shyness and social phobia (Coplan and Weeks 2009; Scharfstein et al. 2011). Secondly, most interventions for selective mutism aim to reduce children's anxiety about speaking in certain contexts or social situations. To this end, they target social-pragmatic skills rather than structural language skills in these children. The success of these interventions suggests that they must be remediating compromised pragmatic language skills in children with selective mutism. Thirdly, there is evidence that children with selective mutism experience problems with the production of narratives (e.g. McInnes et al. 2004). Many of the skills required to produce a coherent narrative are pragmatic in nature.

It is thus incumbent on researchers to undertake a comprehensive investigation into the pragmatic language skills of children with selective mutism alongside other emotional and behavioural disorders. Such an investigation will only be truly revealing if it engages with pragmatic skills in large samples of these children. For example, the finding by Mackie and Law (2010) that a referred group of children with EBD scored significantly lower than a control group on all subscales of the CCC-2 that measure pragmatic language skills is certainly interesting. But to the extent that this finding is based on the completed checklists of only 11 referred children, it is clear that we must be cautious in using such a study to draw conclusions about the pragmatic skills of this population. Empirical studies of this type will not be quickly amassed. Yet, as this section clearly demonstrates, an important first step has been taken in this direction.

6.3 Prison Population

There is now clear evidence that adolescents and adults in a range of correctional facilities have significant language impairments. The language needs of these clients range from problems with literacy to deficits in oral language comprehension and expression. Notwithstanding the often severe language disorders of this population, it is widely acknowledged that detained clients do not receive the clinical language services that are normally readily accessed by other people. In a study of incarcerated female adolescents, Sanger et al. (2003, p. 480) remarked that '[i]t would appear that the traditional referral and eligibility system for determination of eligibility for services did not well serve students in this population. New realizations regarding the failures of the current system in serving many students may include benefits for retraining professionals to consider the possibilities of language deficits and disorders in this troubled population'.[2]

In this section, we begin by examining studies which have revealed the presence of significant language impairments in adolescents and adults in detention. We then turn to consider the evidence that exists for pragmatic deficits in this population of clients. Although the clinical literature in this area is not particularly well developed, studies that have examined pragmatic language skills in detained clients reveal quite clearly that this aspect of language function is at least as impaired as structural language skills. Finally, it is argued that a much better understanding of pragmatic skills in detained clients is necessary given the emphasis on pragmatics and the social use of language in corrective programs that are targeted at these clients.

The importance of good language skills among detainees in correctional facilities cannot be over-estimated. The ability to comprehend and express oneself through language allows detainees to participate in verbally mediated interventions that are designed to reduce re-offending and encourage social reintegration. Also, language is the basis upon which we negotiate relationships (including conflict) with others and receive validation from others. In the absence of good language skills, detained persons report poor communication with others and experiencing feelings of worthlessness and failure.[3] Poor language skills are also a cause of academic underachievement in detained persons with all the adverse consequences (e.g. unemployment) that this entails.[4] Boys with language-learning disorders who have been in juvenile institutions are also at greater risk of developing a serious substance abuse disorder (Linares-Orama 2005). For these reasons, it is important to consider the nature and extent of language disorders in adolescents and adults who are detained in correctional facilities.

Studies which have examined language in detained clients have revealed that language disorders are particularly prevalent in this group and are well in excess of that expected based on rates in the general population. In a survey of 10 % of the young offenders in one institution, Bryan (2004) reported that 43 % scored at a level significantly below acceptable limits for their age on the Boston Naming Test (Kaplan et al. 1983). Acceptable limits based on age were not achieved by 73 and 23 % of young offenders on grammatical competency and language comprehension, respectively. On picture description, 47 % of young offenders received more than one rating of moderate impairment. Gregory and Bryan (2011) examined the language skills of 72 persistent and prolific young offenders who were sentenced to an Intensive Supervision and Surveillance Programme. The language skills of the group were lower than those of the general population. Language difficulties which might benefit from speech and language therapy intervention were found in 65 % of the young offenders, and 20 % were judged to be 'severely delayed' on standardized assessment.

Bryan et al. (2007) reported below average language skills in 66–90 % of a group of 58 juvenile offenders with 46–67 % of these offenders in the poor or very poor category. No subject reached age equivalence on the British Picture Vocabulary Scale (Dunn et al. 1997). Snow and Powell (2004) found poorer oral language processing and production skills in a group of 30 male juvenile offenders than in a demographically similar comparison group. Svensson et al. (2001) reported reading and spelling problems in more than 70 % of 163 Swedish juvenile delinquents studied, with 11 % displaying serious difficulties. Literacy difficulties have also been reported among Texas prison inmates (Moody et al. 2000). On the basis of these findings, it is clear that language impairment is a sufficiently widespread and serious problem among detained clients to warrant further consideration by speech and language therapists and other prison personnel.

Pragmatic skills are rarely the focus of investigation among detained clients. The reasons for this lack of study are unclear, and may include a dearth of formal pragmatic assessments, inadequate time in which to conduct informal pragmatic assessments and the traditional stronghold that structural language skills have exerted in academic research and clinical practice. When pragmatic skills are examined, an interesting picture emerges. There is some evidence, for example, that detained clients display an understanding of the pragmatic rules that govern communicative interactions, but that they apply those rules inadequately during interactions. This metapragmatic awareness may allow detained clients to pass pragmatic assessments, while still experiencing significant pragmatic problems during communication with others.

In this way, the incarcerated female adolescents examined by Sanger et al. (2003) were able to pass the Pragmatic Judgment subtest of the Comprehensive Assessment of Spoken Language (Carrow-Woolfolk 1999). However, these subjects still reported significant communication problems that were pragmatic in nature. For example, one female adolescent described how she failed to grasp jokes told by others: "Some jokes I don't get the point. I just feel really dumb and I just laugh at them [jokes] even though I don't understand them" (Sanger et al. 2003, p. 476). This ability to pass assessments while still exhibiting significant pragmatic impairments may be contributing to the neglect of the language needs of those detained in correctional facilities, as Sanger et al. (2003, p. 478) remark:

> It is speculated that knowing the rules and performing within normal limits on the Pragmatic Judgment subtest would not guarantee the youth could apply this information during on-going conversations. Moreover, it may be yet another reason these types of individuals are overlooked for language services—they appear to have some metapragmatic awareness of rules governing listening, turn taking, maintaining a topic, etc. but at least for some are unable to apply that information in conversational interactions. Perhaps this discrepancy between their awareness of the rules and their actual performance has camouflaged their need for language services. Unfortunately, they might be labelled "lazy" or "out of control" when in actuality they should be considered for language services.

In the few studies that have examined pragmatic skills in detained clients, a wide range of pragmatic deficits has been described. Humber and Snow (2001) examined language skills in 15 community-based young offender males between the ages of 13 and 21 years. Narrative discourse ability was assessed using a six-frame black and white cartoon which was sequentially organized. Pragmatic skills were examined using subtests of the Test of Language Competence—Expanded Edition (Wiig and Secord 1989). These skills included explanations of lexical and structural ambiguities in sentences (e.g. John was looking up the street), the ability to make inferences from incomplete information in order to select plausible story outcomes, and the comprehension of figurative language. The young offender males in the study performed significantly worse on all these tests than a comparison group of 15 male students aged 15–17 years who were drawn from government high schools.

During the narrative task, young offenders produced significantly fewer story grammar elements and omitted important information. (The ability to appreciate a listener's information requirements, and devise utterances according to those requirements, is a key pragmatic skill.) The young offenders' reduced ability to decode ambiguous and figurative utterances also indicates the presence of a pragmatic deficit. Young offenders were more likely to interpret figurative and metaphorical utterances in a literal fashion. For example, when asked to describe the meaning of the expression 'There is rough sailing ahead of us' in the following scenario—two students move to a new town and one says to the other 'There is rough sailing ahead of us'—one young offender responded 'They're in a boat', and another replied 'It's going to be pretty rough, with waves and the wind' (Humber and Snow 2001, p. 8). The impaired pragmatic skills of this group of young offenders, it was argued, disadvantage these males in conversational interactions, police interviews and legal cross-examinations.

A subsequent study by Snow and Powell (2005) examined the narrative discourse skills of male juvenile offenders in more detail. In this study, the story telling abilities of 30 male young offenders were compared to those of 50 male non-offenders attending government high schools. The same six-frame cartoon sequence used in Humber and Snow (2001)—known as the 'Flowerpot Incident'—was employed to elicit narrative samples which underwent story grammar analysis. In this story, a man is walking his dog along the street when he is struck on the head by a flowerpot that has fallen from the balcony of a house occupied by an old woman. The man is angry and enters the building to remonstrate with the woman. However, she placates him by giving his dog a bone and they part on good terms. Although juvenile offenders did not produce significantly fewer story grammar elements in their narratives than non-offenders—unlike in Humber and Snow (2001)—their narratives were nevertheless qualitatively deficient compared to those produced by non-offenders. The three story grammar elements that were most impaired were:

(1) *a plan*—an intention on the part of the character in the story to act/react because of the effects of the initiating event
(2) *direct consequences*—the outcome of an action taken by the character in order to respond to the initiating event
(3) *resolution*—a description of the way in which events are resolved or reconciled between the characters

Snow and Powell (2005) offer an explanation of why these story elements are particularly impaired. Their explanation emphasizes the failure of the juvenile offenders in the study to make certain 'links' between actions and events in the story. In the case of the *plan* story element, that explanation runs as follows:

> Being able to include some information about a protagonist's plan requires the ability to make extrapolations from information which is only implicit in the stimulus. It also requires the ability to extrapolate and articulate a link between an internal response (in this case anger) and a subsequent action (going inside to sort things out). In general, the young offenders did not make this link, and tended instead to describe the pictures on a frame-by-frame basis (2005, p. 246).

To the extent that the young offenders in the study did not articulate these links, it is accurate to describe their linguistic behaviour in the terms used by Snow and Powell. However, I want to suggest an alternative explanation of the narrative discourse skills of these offenders which is based on (probable) deficits in a particular cognitive capacity. That capacity has been variously described as theory of mind (ToM) or mind-reading and is the ability to attribute mental states to one's own mind and to the minds of others. Snow and Powell do not mention ToM in their account of the limited narratives produced by their young offenders. Yet, even a cursory glance at their explanation of the narrative failure of their subjects suggests that a ToM-based account is needed.

Establishing that a subject is having a certain 'internal response' to an event—in this case, that the man is experiencing anger in response to being struck on the head by a falling flowerpot—is a type of first-order reasoning about the mental states of another person. Similarly, deciding that the old woman in the story wishes to placate the man by offering a bone to his dog requires that juvenile offenders can attribute certain mental states to this particular character in the story—the woman *wants* to make some form of reparation to the man, the woman *believes* that she will be able to do this by offering a bone to his dog, etc. In short, in order for the juvenile offenders in this study to make the type of links described by Snow and Powell, they must first be able to engage in mental state attribution or ToM reasoning. This is the more powerful explanatory framework that is overlooked by Snow and Powell when they proceed to characterize the narrative failure of their subjects in terms of 'missing links'. This point warrants further discussion.

The ability to narrate a story requires much more than a set of linguistic skills. Certainly, a story teller must be able to use syntactic constructions and make correct lexical selections if anything meaningful is to be conveyed to the listener. However, these linguistic processes are preceded by a set of cognitive processes which may be loosely characterized as mind-reading skills. These skills make it possible for the narrator to establish why the characters in a story perform the actions they do. In the case of the flowerpot story, for example, the man enters the building because he *wants* to remonstrate with the woman, and the woman gives the man's dog a bone because she *wants* to make reparation for the injury the man has sustained. These motivations on the part of the characters in this story are only comprehensible to the person who is able to attribute mental states (in this case, desires) to the minds of these characters.

If Snow and Powell's juvenile offenders are unable to attribute mental states such as desire, belief and knowledge to the minds of the characters in this story, then they are likely to represent the actions of these characters as a series of disconnected events (which is, in effect, how Snow and Powell characterize the narrative performance of their subjects when they describe them as failing to make 'links'). Of course, Snow and Powell do not test the ToM skills of their juvenile offenders. Therefore, it cannot be stated with certainty that poor mind-reading skills account for the deficient narratives produced by these subjects. However, the presence of poor ToM skills in several other incarcerated groups requires that we at least consider the role of ToM in the impoverished narrative performance of juvenile offenders.[5] Certainly, this cognitive explanation has more to offer an account of the narrative performance of these subjects than one based on 'missing links'.

Pragmatic language skills in detained clients are likely to become the focus of much greater academic research in years to come. This is because these skills are increasingly being included in interventions designed to improve social behaviour in these clients. In this way, Sanger et al. (2003, p. 479) remark that '[p]ragmatic and social use of language...is the focus of most newly developed programs designed to prevent violence in youth' (see Sanger et al. (2002) for discussion). Such are the links between pragmatic language skills and social skills that the development of improved social behaviour in offenders seems an unattainable goal in the absence of full consideration of these key language skills. In the rest of this section, we discuss how pragmatics might contribute to the development of social skills in detained clients. We also examine the results of empirical research which demonstrate that pragmatic language skills and social skills are interrelated in this client group.

Many of the behaviours that we recognize as social silks are, in essence, linguistic interactions (see Chap. 7, this volume). Social skills such as the ability to greet someone appropriately and to establish rapport with others are verbally-mediated interactions through and through. The contribution of pragmatics to these social skills is evident in the range of pragmatic concepts that may be used to characterize these social behaviours. To perform a *speech act* of greeting, for example, a speaker must select an appropriate *term of address* (e.g. 'Good morning, Mr Smith'; 'Hi there, Bill'). This selection must be sensitive to features of *context* such as the formality of the setting in which the greeting occurs, and the social relationship between speaker and hearer. Similarly, social rapport is most often established between interlocutors by means of humour and banter, two forms of linguistic interaction that make extensive use of *non-literal utterances* (e.g. implicature, indirect speech acts). Additionally, socially rewarding interactions are those in which participants are able to develop conversations around *topics* of interest to others.

In short, the behaviours we identify as part of a person's social repertoire are heavily dependent on pragmatic language skills. It is to these skills that we must turn if the goal of rehabilitative interventions is to achieve improvement in the social skills of offenders. A model for how those interventions might proceed can be found in the pragmatic treatments that have been used for some time, and with a degree of success, in various clinical populations (see Chap. 6 in Cummings (2009) for extensive discussion). These treatments employ techniques such as the teaching of conversational 'rules' and role-playing exercises, in which clients can practice how they would respond to the pragmatic demands of different conversational exchanges. Although they will require some adaptation to a population of offenders, these pragmatic treatments represent the best prospect of effecting improvement in the social skills of these clients.

Alongside the development of effective rehabilitative interventions based on pragmatics, there needs to be further research conducted into the nature of the relationship between pragmatic language skills and social skills in young offenders and prison detainees. Such research is necessary in order to validate the links discussed above between pragmatic behaviours on the one hand and aspects of social skill performance on the other hand. At least one study has attempted to examine the relationship between pragmatic language skills and social skills in young offenders. Snow and Powell (2008) studied oral language and social skills in 50 male juvenile offenders who were completing community-based orders. The same language measures adopted by Humber and Snow (2001) were used to assess pragmatic and discourse skills in these subjects. Social skills and non-verbal intelligence were also assessed.

The juvenile offenders in this study performed significantly worse on all language and social skill measures than a control group of 50 non-offending boys attending a local government high school, a difference which was not accounted for by IQ. However, the oral language skills of the juvenile offenders did not correlate significantly with their social skills (in the control group, the correlation between these skills was moderately strong and statistically significant). Snow and Powell attribute the lack of a correlation between language and social skills in the juvenile offenders in this study to a floor effect. Nevertheless, they argue that 'the potential for such a relationship warrants further examination especially in the light of prior research that suggests strong links between language impairment and antisocial behaviour' (2008, p. 24).

6.4   Non-Alzheimer's Dementias

Most studies of pragmatic deficits in dementia have focused on clients who have Alzheimer's disease. A recent review by Rapp and Wild (2011) confirms the dominance of Alzheimer's dementia in these studies. Of 25 studies identified in a comprehensive literature search, most investigated the comprehension of non-literal language (i.e. proverb, metaphor, metonymy, idiom, sarcasm) in clients with Alzheimer's disease. This emphasis on Alzheimer's dementia is to a large extent warranted. Alzheimer's disease is the most common cause of dementia, accounting for 53.7 % of 2,346 dementia cases identified in 11 European cohorts (Lobo et al. 2000). However, there are compelling reasons why it is now timely to give attention to pragmatic impairments in other forms of dementia not caused by Alzheimer's disease.

Firstly, communication disorders are of considerable diagnostic value in assisting clinicians to discriminate among dementia subtypes (Reilly et al. 2010). Detailed clinical characterizations of these subtypes, including language and pragmatic features, will assist clinicians in arriving at reliable diagnoses of these disorders. Secondly, although less common than Alzheimer's dementia, other forms of dementia still form significant clinical populations. For example, vascular dementia accounts for 15.8 % of dementia cases in 11 European cohorts (Lobo et al. 2000) and 29.5 % of cases in a population of Japanese elderly (Matsui et al. 2009). Thirdly, several diseases, in which dementia is a clinical feature, will have an increasing prevalence in years to come. These diseases include Parkinson's disease (PD),[6] HIV infection[7] and variant Creutzfeldt-Jakob disease (vCJD).[8] In short, there are strong reasons why clinicians and researchers should re-direct some of their focus onto the non-Alzheimer's dementias. This section makes a small contribution in this regard by examining the pragmatic features of these conditions.

Neuropathologies other than Alzheimer's disease are associated with dementia. A proliferation of Lewy bodies in the cerebral cortex is found in both Parkinson's disease dementia and dementia with Lewy bodies (Ash et al. 2011). Damage to the brain's vascular system can cause vascular dementia. In an era of combination antiretroviral therapies, classical HIV-associated brain pathology (e.g. HIV encephalitis) may be less prevalent, while other forms of brain injury (e.g. loss of synapses and dendrites) are still common (Woods et al. 2009). A number of different neuropathologies can give rise to frontotemporal dementia (FTD), which includes behavioural variant FTD (bvFTD), semantic dementia and progressive non-fluent aphasia (PNFA). In a study of 60 patients with FTD, Kertesz et al. (2005) identified the following histological varieties at autopsy: motor neurone disease, corticobasal degeneration, Pick's disease, progressive supranuclear palsy, Alzheimer's disease, Lewy body variant, prion disease and vascular dementia. Rohrer et al. (2010) identified parkinsonism, Alzheimer's disease and mutations in the progranulin (GRN) gene (a major cause of frontotemporal lobar degeneration) in a study of 24 patients with PNFA.

Not all neuropathologies that cause dementia are detectable during brain imaging. For example, magnetic resonance imaging (MRI) has a relatively low sensitivity for bvFTD, with many patients with bvFTD presenting with a normal MRI (Koedam et al. 2010). The presence or absence of lobar atrophy on MRI is thus not a reliable indicator of the clinical phenotype of FTD. Also, neuroanatomical abnormalities may only be taken to indicate specific dementia subtypes in the very early stages of disease. Rogalski et al. (2011a) studied 13 patients who fulfilled research criteria for logopenic, agrammatic and semantic dementia subtypes. After 2 years, cortical atrophy had spread beyond the distinctive neuroanatomical locations that characterized these subtypes to encompass all three major components of the language network: the inferior frontal gyrus, the temporoparietal junction and the lateral, temporal cortex.

What these latter findings demonstrate is that a diagnosis of dementia cannot proceed on the basis of neuropathological and neuroanatomical anomalies alone.

Detailed cognitive and linguistic characterizations of the dementias are also necessary in order that clinicians may arrive at reliable diagnoses of these disorders. In fact, the cognitive and linguistic deficits of clients with dementia are so strongly interrelated that it is not possible to consider one group of these impairments in isolation from the other group. In the same way, the pragmatic disorders of clients with non-Alzheimer's dementias can only be examined alongside the cognitive deficits of these clients. It is for this reason that the non-Alzheimer's dementias represent a 'complex' population for clinicians aiming to characterize the pragmatic disorders of this clinical group.

Although a detailed discussion of cognitive and language deficits in the non-Alzheimer's dementias is beyond the scope of this chapter, we begin by giving a brief overview of these deficits in some of these dementias. We then turn to examine what is known about pragmatic disorders in non-Alzheimer's dementias. Although still relatively undeveloped, the literature in this area is growing. As further studies examine the pragmatic language skills of these clients, it is likely that pragmatic disorders will assume the type of diagnostic significance that is more commonly seen in relation to aspects of structural language (e.g. syntax, semantics). A first step in establishing pragmatic language 'markers' of different types of dementia must surely be a clear summation of our current knowledge of the pragmatic features of these disorders. This section will attempt just such a summation.

Although a more common form of dementia than previously believed to be the case, frontotemporal dementia is still relatively rare compared to Alzheimer's disease. In a UK study of 185 subjects with dementia onset before 65 years, Harvey et al. (2003) reported FTD and AD in 12 and 34 % of cases, respectively. FTD is most prevalent between the ages of 60 and 70 years (van Swieten and Rosso 2006). The condition involves pathological changes in the temporal and frontal cortices of the brain. Non-cognitive symptoms of FTD include impairment in social behaviour (disinhibition, aggressiveness), loss of insight and inappropriate acts (Valverde et al. 2009).

Specific cognitive deficits were investigated in a study of 35 patients with bvFTD conducted by Torralva et al. (2009). Compared to paired controls, patients with bvFTD displayed significantly poorer performance on a neuropsychological battery that evaluated attention, memory, visuospatial abilities, language and executive functions. Additionally, patients with bvFTD performed significantly more poorly than controls on theory of mind tests and tests of real-life executive functioning and complex decision-making. The language variants of FTD—semantic dementia (SD) and progressive non-fluent aphasia (PNFA)—are classified along with logopenic progressive aphasia as primary progressive aphasia (PPA). Clients with PPA have marked language impairments in the absence of, at least initially, significant deficits in other cognitive domains including episodic memory, visuospatial abilities and visuoconstruction (Diesfeldt 2011; Reilly and Peelle 2008; Rogalski et al. 2011b). Kertesz et al. (2010) reported intact visuospatial function and relatively preserved episodic memory in the 48 patients with SD in their study.

Language deficits in PPA are wide-ranging in nature and include impaired word retrieval and sentence repetition, the presence of phonemic errors, problems with spelling and reading irregular words (surface dyslexia), impaired comprehension of complex sentences and receptive prosodic deficits (Ash et al. 2010; Diesfeldt 2011; Rohrer et al. 2012; Sepelyak et al. 2011). In a study of eight patients with SD, Meteyard and Patterson (2009) reported the substitution and omission of open class words, the substitution (but not omission) of closed class words, the substitution of incorrect complex morphological forms and the production of semantically and/or syntactically anomalous sentences. Wilson et al. (2010) found increased proportions of closed class words, pronouns and verbs, and higher frequency nouns in their patients with SD. Circumlocution errors have been reported in patients with the semantic variant of PPA (Budd et al. 2010).

A combination of spared and impaired language processes characterizes the logopenic variant of PPA (Henry and Gorno-Tempini 2010). Gorno-Tempini et al. (2008) reported preserved grammar and articulation in six patients with logopenic variant PPA. However, speech rate was slow with long word-finding pauses. Naming was impaired as was sentence repetition and comprehension. Circumlocution errors are also present in this subtype of PPA (Budd et al. 2010). Some of these same language features are also observed in patients with PNFA. In a study of 15 patients with PNFA, Knibb et al. (2009) reported an increase in grammatical and speech sound errors and simplified syntax during conversational speech relative to controls. Slow speech was a common feature. Impairments in picture naming and syntactic comprehension were present in almost all patients.

Investigations into the pragmatic skills of patients with FTD and PPA are slowly beginning to emerge. Rousseaux et al. (2010c) studied verbal and non-verbal communication in patients with bvFTD, Alzheimer's disease and dementia with Lewy bodies. The most severe pragmatic impairments were found in patients with bvFTD, particularly in responding to open questions, presenting new information, logically organising discourse, adapting to interlocutor knowledge and emitting feedback. Kertesz et al. (2010) reported pragmatic disturbance in 75.7 % of his 37 patients with probable SD. Pragmatic difficulties included perseveration, failure to switch speaker roles and failure of topic maintenance. Excessive garrulous output was recorded in 21.6 % of these patients (one might expect this output to violate Gricean quantity and relevance maxims). A further four patients (11 %) were described as having empty speech output which had some coherence and conversational relevance. The speech output of one patient was described as being 'tangential'.

Ash et al. (2006) examined narrative production in patients with FTD. Three aspects of narrative performance—global connectedness, maintenance of a search theme and local connectedness—were particularly impaired in a group of patients with FTD and right frontotemporal disease. All three narrative dimensions are dependent on pragmatic skills (see further discussion below). Moreover, global connectedness[9] in these patients with FTD correlated with scores on a test of executive resources. The use of profanity by patients with dementia reveals a lack of awareness of the linguistic forms that are appropriate in a particular context.

Ringman et al. (2010) found profanity, specifically the use of 'fuck' during a letter fluency task, distinguished the patients with FTD in their study from those with Alzheimer's dementia. The only patients to use this expletive had bvFTD, progressive nonfluent aphasia or semantic dementia.

Certain of the above findings emphasize the strong link that exists between cognitive impairments in FTD—and non-Alzheimer's dementias more generally—and the linguistic features of this type of dementia. In much the same way that the narrative performance of Ash et al.'s patients with FTD was related to executive function deficits, the use of profanity is also likely to be related to the wider cognitive deficits of patients with FTD. These deficits include disinhibition and problems with impulse control (Torralva et al. 2009). It is likely that a further cognitive deficit in these clients—their problems with mental state attribution or theory of mind—will also have special significance for the pragmatic language skills of individuals with FTD (Fernandez-Duque et al. 2009; Kipps and Hodges 2006).

Shany-Ur et al. (2012) studied the ability of 102 patients with one of four neurodegenerative diseases—bvFTD, Alzheimer's disease, progressive supranuclear palsy (PSP) and vascular cognitive impairment—to comprehend two types of insincere communication: lying and sarcasm. The interpretation of sarcasm is a ToM skill in essence, as the hearer must be able to establish that the speaker entertains a belief which is the opposite of that expressed by the utterance. Videos of interactions involving deceptive, sarcastic or sincere speech were shown to all patients. Compared to healthy, older control subjects, patients with bvFTD displayed impaired comprehension of lies and sarcasm, even though their comprehension of sincere remarks was intact. While subjects with bvFTD and PSP had impaired ToM skills, only patients with bvFTD were impaired on perspective-taking and emotion reading. Shany-Ur et al. (2012, p. 1329) concluded that 'bvFTD patients show uniquely focal and severe impairments at every level of theory of mind and emotion reading, leading to an inability to identify obvious examples of deception and sarcasm'. Clearly, further investigations of the cognitive substrates of pragmatic impairments in clients with FTD are warranted by these findings.

Of course, FTD is just one type of non-Alzheimer's dementia, albeit a significant type. Dementia is also a common clinical feature of several other conditions including Parkinson's and Lewy body disease, Huntington's disease, multiple sclerosis, Creutzfeldt-Jakob disease, vascular disease, HIV infection and alcoholism. In a German epidemiological study of 1,449 patients with Parkinson's disease, 28.6 % met DSM-IV criteria for dementia (Von Reichmann et al. 2010). The prevalence of dementia with Lewy bodies (DLB) ranges from 0 to 5 % in the general population, and from 0 to 30.5 % of all dementia cases (Zaccai et al. 2005). Renvoize et al. (2011) estimated the prevalence of dementia in Huntington's disease in the 45–64 age group in an English health district to be 2.4 per 100,000 population. In a population of 20,561 residents with a diagnosis of MS who were admitted to nursing facilities between January 1998 and June 2003, Buchanan et al. (2005) calculated that 11 % had some type of dementia.

In a study of 624 patients with suspected sporadic CJD, Gao et al. (2011) reported that progressive dementia was the most common presenting symptom and affected 45.6 % of patients. In a population of 3,201 individuals who sustained a first-ever stroke, Béjot et al. (2011) recorded that 20.4 % had poststroke dementia. Mild dementia was recorded in 87.5 % of elderly patients with HIV infection studied by Brito e Silva et al. (2011). The prevalence of alcohol-related dementia in the 45–64 age group was recently estimated to be 10.9 per 100,000 population (Renvoize et al. 2011). These figures reveal that non-Alzheimer's dementias apart from FTD constitute significant clinical populations. To this extent, their language and cognitive phenotypes warrant investigation. In the rest of this section, we briefly discuss language and cognitive deficits in these non-Alzheimer's dementias. We conclude this section by examining what is known about pragmatic language skills in clients with these dementias.

Parkinson's disease dementia (PDD) is characterized by impairment in attention, memory and executive and visuo-spatial functions (Emre et al. 2007). Even in the absence of dementia, patients with PD have language impairments including receptive language deficits and impaired production of grammatical sentences (Murray 2000; Walsh and Smith 2011). In dementia with Lewy bodies (DLB)—a condition which differs clinically from PDD in that there is a later onset of motor disorder—there are deficits of attention, memory and executive function which can be more severe than those in PDD (Park et al. 2011). Difficulty processing syntactic ambiguities has been shown to correlate with measures of executive control in clients with DLB (Grossman et al. 2012).

Cognitive deficits are widely reported in Huntington's disease, even among pre-clinical individuals who have the HD mutation (Lawrence et al. 1998). In early Huntington's disease, there is progressive impairment in attention, executive function and immediate memory (Ho et al. 2003). Expressive language of patients with Huntington's disease displays grammatical errors and errors in confrontation naming (Frank et al. 1996; Jensen et al. 2006). Chenery et al. (2002) found impaired performance in their subjects with HD during lexico-semantic tasks (e.g. naming), and in single-word and sentence-level generative tasks. Dawes et al. (2008) describe a 'prototypical pattern' of neuropsychological results in patients with HIV infection. This pattern involves impaired executive functioning, motor skills, speed of information processing and learning with intact memory retention, most language skills and visuospatial functioning. However, as cognitive impairment progresses to the stage of dementia, some of these intact areas also deteriorate. In this way, the patients with HIV and mild dementia investigated by Brito e Silva et al. (2011) displayed language deficits, dyscalculia and visual-spatial change.

There is substantial evidence of cognitive and language impairments in clients with multiple sclerosis (MS). Nocentini et al. (2006) reported cognitive deficit in 31 % of patients with relapsing-remitting MS in their study. Within this figure, 15, 11.2 and 4.8 % had mild, moderate and severe cognitive impairment, respectively. Information processing speed was the most compromised area followed by memory. Tur et al. (2011) found that patients with primary progressive MS performed worse than controls on tests of attention/speed of visual information processing, delayed verbal memory and executive function. Episodic memory and linguistic expression were especially affected in patients with chronic progressive-type MS studied by Mackenzie and Green (2009). Language difficulties were recorded in 63.3 % of patients with MS studied by Klugman and Ross (2002). Lexical access problems have been reported in clients with MS (Sepulcre et al. 2011).

Working memory and executive functioning deficits have been reported in clients with vascular dementia (McGuinness et al. 2010). The language deficits of these clients include problems with auditory comprehension and picture naming as well as the use of semantic units (themes) during narrative production (Vuorinen et al. 2000). Clients with alcohol-related dementia display executive control and memory deficits as well as language disorder in the areas of confrontation naming and verbal concept formation (Schmidt et al. 2005). Cognitive deficits are commonplace in CJD. Cordery et al. (2005) reported verbal and visual memory impairments, perceptual impairment, executive dysfunction and impaired nominal skills in patients with variant and sporadic CJD. Language disorders have been documented in clients with CJD including conduction aphasia, alexia and verbal perseveration (Adair et al. 2007; Snowden et al. 2002; Song et al. 2010).

Pragmatic language skills are also commonly disrupted in clients with these dementias. Impairment of these skills is most often examined during the production of narratives and other forms of discourse.[10] McCabe et al. (2008) described the language and communication skills of a 36-year-old man known as Warren who was diagnosed with AIDS dementia complex by an AIDS specialising neurologist. Neuropsychological testing revealed average working memory, psychomotor speed, visuo-construction and verbal fluency performance. However, Warren's attention in complex simultaneous processing tasks was significantly impaired. During a semi-structured interview conducted in his own home, Warren was observed to be verbose, unable to maintain topic, self-focused and unaware to a large extent of the needs of his listener. Although Warren displayed word-finding difficulties and produced circumlocutions, his language disorder was described as pragmatic in nature rather than a high-level aphasia. His pragmatic deficits are evident in the following exchange which is taken from the initial interview between Warren (W) and the researcher (R):

R: So you'd be 34 then?

W: I've been 34 for the last 3 years

R: ah, OK so you're actually?

W: Oh what happened was I added a year and a year at my birthday, didn't celebrate it so therefore I forgot about it. In September as a halfway between two ages I start saying what the next one is

R: Uh huh?

W: So I've added there as well and the years come along and I didn't remember doing either of the first two so I did it again when I was 32

R: Oh dear

W: Someone pointed out that I was 34 last year and 33 last year and I went "no, I'm not I'm 34", I'm gonna get me a calculator and a new set of batteries that were still in the package so that guaranteed the calculator was working properly 'cause it kept telling me I was 33 and I could'a swore it was lying to me.

R: What year were you born in?

W: '64

R: '64

W: The odd thing was, was I was filling out doctors' forms and hospital forms and all sort of things, putting down the date of birth as xxth of xxxx of '64 and my age was 34 but a diversional therapist in a nursing home was the only person who actually noticed that there was something wrong with this picture. I thought "well, it's fairly obvious I'm in it" so there's your problem (McCabe et al. 2008, pp. 208–209).

Warren's linguistic output displays problems with topic maintenance. On the one hand, he tends to perseverate on the topic of age. The result of this topic perseveration is that his language displays considerable informational redundancy. On the other hand, within each of his extended utterances, he can also veer off topic such as when he discusses points like the calculator and batteries and gives a detailed account of how he determines his age. The inclusion of these points and other unnecessary details finds his verbal output violating conversational maxims of relevance and quantity and confirms the initial clinical impression of verbosity. Of course, as he engages in each of these extended turns, he is also denying his interlocutor opportunities to take turns in the conversation. Indeed, the researcher is confined to taking minimal turns after her initial questions.

Warren's use of reference is also impaired in this exchange. For example, it is difficult for the listener to determine the referents of several of the pronouns and adverbs that Warren uses (e.g. 'it's fairly obvious I'm in *it*'; 'So I've added *there* as well'). The effect of Warren's failure to manage reference in language is that the listener must work harder to make sense of his utterances. This suggests poor awareness on Warren's part of how referential difficulties in his own output are increasing the burden of comprehension for his listener. McCabe et al. attribute at least some of these pragmatic problems to Warren's reduced cognitive executive functioning.

Problems with the management of reference are also evident during narrative production in clients with dementia with Lewy bodies (Ash et al. 2011). The following extracts are taken from narratives produced by patients with DLB who were tasked with telling the story depicted in a wordless children's picture book *Frog, Where are You?* (Mayer 1969). An 80-year-old man with a 10-year history of DLB is attempting to describe a scene in which a boy and his dog are both searching for their lost frog. In their search, the dog shakes a hive down from a tree, and bees are emerging from the hive. Meanwhile, the boy is climbing a tree and looks into a hole in the trunk. The man with DLB states:

(a) It's a ... it's an ug- bees, from- from the one hive, I guess.

(b) Oh! By golly there's another one.

(c) Uh that's t- about midway the- halfway up the tree, where the tree is- the base is broken (Ash et al. 2011, p. 33).

In (c), the demonstrative pronoun 'that' refers to the boy who has climbed halfway up the tree. However, given that he has been newly introduced into the narrative, he should have nominal reference ('the boy'). Moreover, the tree that the boy is climbing is also new to the story and should therefore have an indefinite determiner ('a tree'). Ash et al. describe these referential anomalies as a failure of local connectedness. Difficulties with local connectedness among the patients with DLB in this study correlated with deficits on measures of executive function including working memory and mental search.

The production of a comprehensible narrative places pragmatic demands on the narrator beyond the management of reference. The narrator must not only decide what information the listener needs to be given, but also the order in which that information should be presented. If the listener receives too little information, information that is false or inaccurate or information that is presented in a way which does not reflect causal and temporal relations between events, there are grounds for doubting the narrator's mastery of Gricean maxims (viz., quantity, quality and manner maxims, respectively). Exactly these difficulties with the presentation and sequencing of information are present in the following narrative produced by a 76-year-old male patient with DLB. This patient's narrative unfolds as follows:

Page 1:   (a) There's a boy, his little dog and his frog sitting up by the boy's bed.
Page 1/2: (b) And it's nighttime.
Page 2:   (c) Boy's fallen asleep.
Page 2:   (d) The frog is getting out of his … container.
Page 2:   (e) and the dog is with the boy, I believe.
Page 3:   (f) Yep, then uh there's a boy, in the bed with the dog on top of him.
Page 3:   (g) and he's about ready to fall asleep I believe.
Page 4:   (h) Boy's playing with his boots.
Page 4:   (i) The dog's crawling into the … container.
Page 4:   (j) The boy's looking in the boots (Ash et al. 2011, p. 33).

This patient with DLB successfully sets the scene in (a)–(c). He also manages to describe the problem in (d), the resolution of which is the whole point of the story. However, in (e) the patient returns to setting the scene by adding information that is repetitive on (a), and which is therefore largely redundant. There is further repetitiveness in (f) when the patient describes again that there is a boy and a dog in bed. No new information is contributed by the patient in either (e) or (f) with the result that the listener is unable to develop his understanding of this narrative beyond the original description of the scene and the statement of the problem to be addressed. In (g), the patient has produced an inaccurate description of the scene on page 3—it is in fact morning and the boy is surprised to discover that his frog has disappeared.

In (h)–(i), the patient appears not to appreciate the significance of the depicted activities in relation to the wider purpose of the story, which is an account of how the boy and his dog search for the lost frog. So the boy is not 'playing with' his boots so much as looking into them to see if the frog has crawled inside them. Similarly, the dog is crawling into the container with a view to searching for the lost frog. This loss of the purpose or goal of the narrative suggests further pragmatic disturbance, as this patient appears to lose the very communicative intention that was his motivation for producing the narrative in the first place. As with local connectedness, this patient difficulty in maintaining the search theme of the narrative correlated with impaired executive functioning, in this case mental search and inhibitory control.

Through the absence of listener participation, narrative production tasks lack the ecological validity of conversation as a context in which to examine pragmatic language skills. Clients who have dementia with Lewy bodies have also been found to have difficulties with aspects of conversational discourse. Perkins et al. (1998) examined several conversational exchanges involving patients with DLB and their relatives. The patients displayed difficulty with turn-taking and topic initiation. In each case, these problems were related to the cognitive impairments of the patients. Clients with Parkinson's disease with and without dementia have also been reported to have pragmatic deficits. Berg et al. (2003) reported particular problems in making inferences and comprehending metaphors and ambiguities in four subjects with Parkinson's disease who had different degrees of cognitive dysfunction. A further 26 subjects with Parkinson's disease and normal cognitive status had significantly worse performance than control subjects on tests assessing inferences.

Pragmatic disorders have also been described in clients with Huntington's disease. Saldert et al. (2010) examined the comprehension of complex information in 18 patients with Huntington's disease. Tasks required complex cognitive processing and assessed a range of pragmatic language skills. Subjects were required to comprehend metaphors and ambiguous sentences (the latter containing lexical ambiguities), draw elaborative inferences based on general knowledge and the content of narratives, disambiguate words in order to make a narrative coherent and make inferences about a character's attitudes and motivations. Subjects with HD and controls performed similarly on basic tasks requiring language comprehension and production. However, on more complex tasks requiring pragmatic skills, the performance of subjects with HD was significantly worse than that of controls. Clearly, clients with cognitive dysfunction and dementia in conditions other than Alzheimer's disease can display significant pragmatic impairments. These impairments are evident in different types of discourse as well as during structured language testing.

6.5 Summary

In the rush to characterize pragmatic disorders in certain clinical populations, investigators have neglected other populations in which there are significant pragmatic impairments. While the reasons for this neglect are understandable— a lack of clinical expertise and misunderstanding of the prevalence of disorders are certainly among them—this chapter has undertaken to give prominence to three populations that are likely to assume increasing prominence in clinical pragmatics in years to come. These populations include children with emotional and behavioural disorders, adolescents and adults in correctional facilities and adults with non-Alzheimer's dementias. A range of factors, such as the increasing health burden of the dementias and a growing appreciation of the reduced life chances of children and adolescents with language disorders, means that clinicians and researchers can no longer afford to overlook these client groups.

However, the study of these groups will not be easy. In some of these clients, pragmatic impairments exist alongside significant psychiatric and cognitive disorders (so-called 'complex' populations). In other clients, pragmatic disorders have been overlooked on account of societal prejudices about who warrants clinical language services (so-called 'underserved' populations). However, if clinical pragmatics is to continue to develop in ways that are of benefit to people with pragmatic disorders, it must engage with these new and challenging groups of clients. As the discussion of this chapter demonstrates, the first steps in this process are already underway.

Notes

1.   Brauner and Stephens (2006, p. 304) state that '[e]stimating the prevalence of emotional/behavioral disorders in children is critical to providing the mental health services they need. This is extremely difficult, however, given the lack of a "standard" and correct inclusive definition for a minimum functional level of impairment in some or all domains for an agreed-upon duration'.

2.   In an earlier study of 78 female juvenile delinquents in a correctional facility, Sanger et al. (2000) reported that 17 (22 %) were candidates for language services. However, none of these girls had received language services. Similar findings were reported in a subsequent study of 67 female adolescent delinquents (Sanger et al. 2001). Thirteen girls (19.4 %) performed sufficiently poorly on language assessments to qualify for language services. Although six (46.15 %) of these thirteen subjects had received special education services, none of these six had received services for speech and language.

3.   In a study of 13 female adolescents who resided in a correctional facility, Sanger et al. (2003, p. 481) reported that issues relating to poor communication with others and low self-worth emerged during interviews conducted with these girls. One teenager described communication with her friends in the following terms: 'In our group no one wants to listen what the other person has to say. She's telling me something and I don't want to hear it. I'll just start talking faster'.

4.   Snow and Powell (2008: 16) state that '[p]oor academic performance in turn carries the risk of early school departure, inadequate further education and training, chronic unemployment and dependence on welfare and/or continued criminal activity'.

5.   Jones et al. (2007) reported social cognitive deficits—specifically, a failure to recognize the facial expression of anger—in the male young offenders in their study. ToM deficits have also been reported in child sex offenders (Elsegood

and Duff 2010). Additionally, several clinical conditions, in which ToM deficits are found, tend to be over-represented in the criminal justice system. These conditions include schizophrenia, autism spectrum disorder and antisocial personality disorder. (Cashin and Newman 2009; Dolan and Fullam 2004; Haskins and Silva 2006; Rautanen and Lauerma 2011).

6. The prevalence of Parkinson's disease increases with age. In a study of a general elderly population in the Netherlands, de Rijk et al. (1995) reported the following prevalence figures for different age groups: 0.3 % (55–64 years), 1.0 % (65–74 years), 3.1 % (75–84 years), 4.3 % (85–94 years). As people live longer, it is to be expected that that the number of PD cases, and dementia cases related to PD, will also increase.

7. As HIV drug therapies improve and become more widely accessible, the number of people living with HIV infection (HIV prevalence) will increase. Dementia is one of the neurological complications of HIV infection. It might therefore be expected that the number of cases of HIV-associated dementia (HAD) will also increase. However, alongside the marked increase in survival rates of HIV-infected persons since the introduction in 1996 of combination antiretroviral therapies (Woods et al. 2009), there has also been a large decrease in the number of cases of HAD as a direct consequence of these therapies (Vivithanaporn et al. 2011).

8. Dementia is one of the clinical features of vCJD, a recently identified form of CJD that has been caused by the transmission of BSE in cattle to humans. A study which attempted to estimate the number of people who are incubating this disease suggests that vCJD will become a more significant cause of dementia in years to come. Hilton et al. (2004) tested samples of appendix and tonsil tissue from 16,703 patients for the accumulation of prion protein, which is believed to be indicative of vCJD. From the tissues identified as containing prion protein, an estimated prevalence of 237 per million was calculated. This is equivalent to 1 person in 4,219 population believed to be incubating vCJD.

9. An example of how the narratives of these patients lacked global connectedness can be seen in the following description of one of the scenes in the story. The patient with FTD who produced this extract failed to make any connection between one of the two frogs in the scene and the frog that escaped from the jar at the start of the story (Ash et al. 2006, p. 1409):

Dog—or boy's.. over log
Dog's over the log too
Um … they're on the log
See two frogs
See the mom and … dad and a mom frog
And you got one, two, three, four, five .. seven little—eight little toads.

10. Perkins et al. (1998, p. 33) state that 'research into pragmatic behaviour has primarily been carried out through the analysis of the ability of the person with dementia to produce different forms of discourse, including picture description, story telling, procedural discourse and clinical interviews'.

Chapter 7
Pragmatic Disorders and Social Communication

7.1 Introduction

Communication between people performs several vital functions. There is, of course, a fundamental need on the part of each of us to receive information from, and convey information to, other people. We must also communicate with each other in order to satisfy our needs for food and shelter and to gain assistance with a host of different tasks. While important, functions such as the exchange of information are not the only evolutionary purpose for which humans have developed a capacity for communication. As social beings, humans must establish mutually sustaining, interpersonal relationships. Social communication is the principal mechanism by means of which this is achieved. Indeed, it is to social communication that all other functions of communication are ultimately subordinated. Even the simplest exchange of information, for example, requesting the time from a passer-by, can only be conducted between participants for whom there is a pre-existing social relationship (in the case of a request for the time, a social relationship is first established by means of a greeting (e.g. 'Good morning') or other opening remark).

This chapter examines in detail the nature of social communication. It will be shown that a range of language and cognitive skills underlie this important form of communication. Chief among these skills is pragmatic competence in the use and understanding of linguistic utterances. However, social communication is broader than pragmatics alone and includes a number of other key competences, each of which will be examined. To the extent that pragmatics plays an important role in social communication, we may expect social communication to be disrupted in clients with pragmatic language disorders (see Chap. 2, this volume and Cummings (2005, 2009, 2012a, 2014d) for discussion of these disorders). We will see that this expectation is confirmed by studies that have investigated social communication skills in clients with clinical conditions in which there are marked pragmatic impairments (e.g. autism spectrum disorder). These studies complement findings of significant social dysfunction, including social exclusion and withdrawal,

L. Cummings, *Pragmatic Disorders*, Perspectives in Pragmatics, Philosophy & Psychology 3, DOI: 10.1007/978-94-007-7954-9_7, © Springer Science+Business Media Dordrecht 2014

in child and adult clients with pragmatic disorders (see Chap. 5, this volume and Cummings (2011) for discussion of the social impact of pragmatic disorders). A previously neglected area of clinical need, social communication is increasingly finding its way into the assessment and treatment of clients with pragmatic disorders. The chapter examines some of the instruments and techniques which are used for this purpose. Finally, the chapter concludes with a discussion of how future research can usefully contribute to an understanding of social communication, both on its own terms and as a clinical construct.

7.2 The Scope of Social Communication

It was described above how a range of linguistic and cognitive skills are the basis of the behaviour which we are referring to as 'social communication'. In this section, each of these skills will be identified and examined. The view of social communication which will be developed is one in which social communication is emergent upon functioning in three main areas.[1] These areas are (1) language pragmatics, (2) social perception, and (3) social cognition. The pragmatics of language appears in most definitions of social communication. Indeed, there has been a reasonably consistent tendency among investigators to identify social communication *with* pragmatics.[2] This is evident in the following definition of social communication provided by one Special Educational Needs and Psychology Service in the UK:

> Social communication is the skill of getting a message across to another person and accurately interpreting their response. We can get our messages across through speech but body language, facial expression, gestures, tone and intonation of speech are also important (SENaPS Central Area Team 2005, p. 6).

This definition characterizes social communication in terms of the production and interpretation of utterances (i.e. pragmatics). It is undoubtedly the case that in the absence of intact pragmatic language skills, a speaker will not function as, or be perceived to be, a competent social communicator. At a minimum, such a speaker will experience a significant reduction in his or her opportunities for social communication. A speaker cannot forge opportunities for social communication when the utterances he produces are perceived by others to be impolite or in other ways pragmatically anomalous (verbose, irrelevant, under-informative, etc.). By the same token, a hearer who consistently misses the pragmatic point of an exchange by, for example, failing to recover the intended meaning of a speaker's utterances, will quickly experience a reduction in the conversational interactions through which social communication is enacted. Each of these pragmatic failures leads to the social devaluation of the speakers and hearers who commit them, with consequent reduction in the number and frequency of opportunities for social communication.

Clearly, pragmatics is integral to social communication. However, competence in pragmatics must exist alongside a number of other skills if social communication is to be achieved. The above definition hints at one of these skills when it describes how facial expressions may be used to convey messages. The identification of a speaker's emotional states (e.g. anger, happiness) by means of the recognition of his or her facial expression is an important social perceptual skill. The ability to perceive, and attribute significance to, a large range of subtle, mostly non-verbal behaviours is fundamental to social communication. For example, it is the lapse in eye contact that tells a speaker it is time to change the topic of a conversation. Also, the fall in intonation at the end of an utterance is a cue to other participants that they can assume the conversational turn. Although these behaviours appear inconsequential—they are, after all, largely beyond the conscious awareness of communicators—in their absence significant social communication problems result. This is demonstrated by the fact that impaired social perceptual skills (e.g. impaired recognition of facial expressions) in children and adults with ASD contribute significantly to the social communication problems of these clients. We will say more about this in the next section.

Although pragmatics and social perception are necessary for social communication, they are not sufficient by themselves to confer full social communicative competence on a speaker. The remaining skill set involves a group of interrelated abilities that are grouped under the label 'social cognition'.[3] Chief among these abilities is the cognitive capacity to attribute mental states both to one's own mind and to the minds of others, a cognitive capacity known as theory of mind (ToM). ToM skills have been extensively studied in normal and clinical populations (see Cummings (2013a) for a review). There is also a growing literature on the role of these skills in pragmatics and utterance interpretation (see Cummings (2013a, 2014b, d) for discussion). The contribution of ToM to social communication is no less than an understanding of the mind of the communicator, who is only producing linguistic utterances and performing other behaviours with a view to making certain mental states manifest to others. An understanding of the inferential and reasoning skills by means of which this is achieved is the chief concern of ToM investigators. We will see in the next section that ToM deficits are a significant source of social communication problems in children and adults with a range of clinical disorders.

So, we have thus far delineated the three cognitive and linguistic domains that make a significant contribution to social communication. The aim has been to show that social communication cannot be reduced to any one of these domains without the loss of important skills. In reality, the three domains are so intertwined that it is impossible to achieve a strict demarcation between them. Certain interdependencies between pragmatics, social perception and theory of mind demonstrate this to be the case. All utterance interpretation (pragmatics) only succeeds to the extent that a hearer is able to attribute a certain communicative intention to the mind of the speaker (theory of mind). A hearer's lapse in eye contact with the speaker (social perception) will be a largely meaningless behaviour in the absence of inferences about the hearer's mental states (theory of mind). It is only those inferences—and the particular inference that the hearer *wants* the topic of conversation to be changed—that confers significance on this behaviour. And the recognition of facial expressions and other non-verbal behaviours (social perception) serves to moderate utterance interpretation processes (pragmatics) in ways that are still largely indefinable. These interdependencies reveal that social communication is emergent on the interaction of these domains rather than the outcome of any one of them. At least this will be the guiding assumption of the discussion in the rest of this chapter.

On account of its component processes, social communication can be disrupted as a result of impairment in more than just one underlying domain. This means that a range of clinical scenarios is possible. The adult with schizophrenia can present with social communication difficulties as a result of impairment in ToM skills. The child with autism spectrum disorder can also exhibit social communication difficulties on account of social perceptual deficits (although ToM impairments are also likely to be a significant cause of these difficulties in a client with ASD). Finally, the adult with right-hemisphere damage (RHD) may also have social communication difficulties, but this time caused by a pragmatic disorder which affects the interpretation of non-literal language. The fact that all three of these clients have social communication difficulties in the presence of different contributing factors has implications for the assessment and treatment of clients. At a minimum, assessment needs to consider a client's skills in all three underlying domains—intact functioning in one domain cannot be taken as evidence of intact functioning in other domains. Also, treatments need to target the specific source of a client's social communication difficulties—a pragmatic therapy will be ineffective if ToM deficits are the source of the problem. Each of these issues will be addressed more fully in Sect. 7.4.

In the next section, we examine what is known about social communication in clients with a range of clinical disorders. Clinical studies of social communication skills are still relatively small in number. However, shifting agendas in healthcare in recent years have conferred greater prominence on social communication. This is because social communication is one aspect of wider social functioning which is increasingly used to assess levels of disability[4] and determine the efficacy of clinical interventions. As the above discussion demonstrates, in examining impairments of social communication, we have to throw our net more widely than pragmatic disorders alone. Specifically, we also have to address the contribution of ToM impairments and social perceptual deficits to social communication difficulties in children and adults. Reflecting the centrality of pragmatic disorders in this chapter, the impact of ToM impairments and social perceptual deficits on social communication will be discussed first and then only relatively briefly. A more detailed examination of the consequences for social communication of a range of developmental and acquired pragmatic disorders will then be undertaken.

7.3 Social Communication in Clinical Studies

That social communication has come of age as a clinical construct is indicated by its appearance for the first time in the fifth edition of the Diagnostic and Statistical Manual of Mental Disorders (DSM-5) (American Psychiatric

Association 2013). In DSM-5, social communication disorder[5] is characterized as follows:

> [A] primary difficulty with pragmatics, or the social use of language and communication, as manifested by deficits in understanding and following social rules of verbal and non-verbal communication in naturalistic contexts, changing language according to the needs of the listener or situation, and following rules for conversations and storytelling. The deficits in social communication result in functional limitations in effective communication, social participation, development of social relationships, academic achievement, or occupational performance. The deficits are not better explained by low abilities in the domains of structural language or cognitive ability (American Psychiatric Association 2013, p. 48).

Social communication disorder is intended to supersede a number of other diagnostic labels which have been used in the clinical literature to describe children with pragmatic disorders. These labels include semantic-pragmatic disorder and pragmatic language impairment (PLI). Given this most recent reincarnation of the population of children with developmental pragmatic disorders, it is unsurprising that among the studies to be examined in this section are findings of significant social communication difficulties in children with PLI. But before embarking on an examination of social communication difficulties in children and adults with pragmatic disorders, something must be said about the part played by ToM impairments and social perceptual deficits in these difficulties.

7.3.1 Theory of Mind and Social Communication

Studies have consistently shown that failure to attribute mental states to the minds of others—impaired ToM—is related to impoverished social communication skills in children and adults. One clinical condition in which this relationship between ToM and social communication has been clearly demonstrated is autism spectrum disorder (see Cummings (2008, 2014a) for discussion of ASD). Hale and Tager-Flusberg (2005) examined ToM and social communication in 57 children with autism. Social communication skill in these children was assessed in terms of their ability to maintain an ongoing topic of conversation during a parent–child interaction. Hierarchical regression analyses revealed that ToM skills contributed unique variance to individual differences in the contingent discourse ability of these children, and vice versa. The authors concluded that 'theory of mind and contingent discourse are reciprocally related, indicating that there is a dynamic interaction between social cognition and social communication among children with autism' (173). Theory of mind was one of three domains of social communication handicap identified by Roberston et al. (1999) in a study of 51 children with ASD. Specific aspects of social communication, such as teasing behaviour, have also been found to be related to ToM in children with autism (Heerey et al. 2005).

Donno et al. (2010) examined ToM and social communication in a study of 26 persistently disruptive children. The Children's Communication Checklist (CCC) (Bishop and Baird 2001) was used to assess social communication deficits in these children. Significantly more disruptive children than comparison children obtained scores in the clinical range on the pragmatic composite scale of the CCC. Disruptive children also had poorer ToM skills than comparison children. However, no attempt was made to correlate mentalising abilities with social communication skills in these children. Hong et al. (2011) reported reduced social competency and impaired ToM skills in girls with Turner syndrome. Social competency was rated in these girls using the Social Responsiveness Scale (Constantino and Gruber 2005), which examines reciprocal social communication among other social competencies. Findings of social communication difficulties in children with congenital visual impairment (Tadić et al. 2010) and attachment disorders (e.g. reactive attachment disorder, Sadiq et al. 2012), both of which have associated ToM deficits (Minter et al. 1998; Colvert et al. 2008), lead one to suspect that many more social communication impairments in childhood will be shown ultimately to be related to ToM.

ToM is also related to social communication difficulties in adults with acquired or adult-onset clinical disorders. McDonald and Flanagan (2004) examined social communication skills and ToM abilities in 34 adults with severe traumatic brain injury (TBI). Second-order ToM judgements (e.g. Mary believes that Bill wants to go home) were shown to be related to social communication ability in these subjects.[6] Bora et al. (2006) examined the relationship between ToM and social Functioning in 50 patients with schizophrenia. ToM performance was assessed by means of a mental state decoding task and a mental state reasoning task. The Social Functioning Scale (SFS) (Birchwood et al. 1990) was used to assess the social functioning of patients. (The SFS contains a number of communicative items within its social withdrawal and relationships subscales, e.g. How often will you start a conversation at home? How easy or difficult do you find talking to people at present?) Bora et al. found that mental state decoding was the best predictor of social functioning in these patients. Shany-Ur et al. (2012) examined the relationship between ToM and social communication in patients with neurodegenerative disease. Patients with behavioural variant frontotemporal dementia and progressive supranuclear palsy obtained significantly poorer scores than normal controls on ToM measures. Moreover, these patients' ToM scores were significantly related to their performance on a social communication task. The task in question required subjects to answer questions about videos that depicted social interactions involving deceptive, sarcastic or sincere communication.

7.3.2 Social Perception and Social Communication

Social perceptual deficits have been examined in a number of clinical conditions including autism spectrum disorder, schizophrenia and the dementias. These deficits involve impairments in the recognition of social behaviours such as facial expressions (and related emotions) and eye gaze. Tanaka et al. (2012) reported that subjects with ASD performed reliably worse than typically developing control participants on the recognition of five facial emotions during an experimental task. The emotions in question were happiness, sadness, disgust, fear and anger.

Subjects with ASD were also found to recognize the mouth feature of faces holistically but the eyes as isolated parts. Along with other gaze processing problems, children with autism have been shown to display an insensitivity to gaze direction (Pellicano and Macrae 2009). Adults with schizophrenia have been found to display overperception of eye contact, a behaviour which is associated with more severe negative symptoms in the disorder (Tso et al. 2012). Mutual gaze, i.e. when two individuals make eye contact, is disrupted during conversations with partners who have frontotemporal dementia (FTD) (Sturm et al. 2011). Fernandez-Duque and Black (2005) reported impaired recognition of negative facial emotions in patients with FTD. Phillips et al. (2010) reported impaired emotion decoding performance in subjects with Alzheimer's disease, particularly when relatively subtle facial expressions were presented to these individuals.

While social perceptual deficits have been consistently demonstrated in clinical subjects across a large number of studies, few studies have attempted to relate these deficits directly to social communication problems. That problems with the perception of eye gaze are related to social communication difficulties in individuals with ASD is undeniably the case. Itier and Batty (2009, p. 858) state that:

> Taken together, studies in ASDs suggest no general impairment in visual attention or specific impairment in gaze orienting *per se* but rather a deficit in the perception of social cues and a possible impairment in direct/mutual gaze discrimination. The main deficits seem to lie in the incapacity to extract relevant information from the eye region necessary for social communication.

Pexman et al. (2011) reported significant differences in eye gaze behaviour during an irony comprehension task between children with high-functioning ASD and typically developing children. These differences reflect processing strategies on the part of children with high-functioning ASD which, Pexman et al. argue, may 'involve less elaborate simulation of other minds' (2011, p. 1110). Impaired facial emotion recognition is also a source of social communication difficulties in children with ASD, as Baron-Cohen (2012, p. 115) states below:

> Children with autism spectrum conditions have major difficulties in recognizing and responding to emotional and mental states in others' facial expressions. Such difficulties in empathy underlie their social communication difficulties.

Social perceptual deficits have also been related to social communication problems in other clinical conditions. John and Mervis (2010) examined the ability of pre-schoolers with Williams syndrome (WS) or Down's syndrome (DS) to use eye gaze shift to recognize a partner's communicative intent. Both groups of pre-schoolers had more difficulty inferring communicative intent from eye gaze alone than from eye gaze paired with a pointing gesture. However, these difficulties were more pronounced in the pre-schoolers with WS than in the pre-schoolers with DS. John and Mervis (2010, p. 958) concluded that '[t]his pattern of findings provides further evidence of sociocommunicative difficulties for children with WS and relative strength in sociocommunicative abilities for children with DS'. Hooker and Park (2002) found a relationship between affect recognition and social functioning in 20 chronic, medicated patients with schizophrenia. Social functioning was assessed using the Social Dysfunction Index (SDI) (Munroe-Blum et al. 1996), which contains a specific communication subscale.[7] Watts and Douglas (2006) reported a significant relationship between the ability to interpret facial expressions and perceived communication competence in 12 individuals with severe TBI. Communication competence was assessed through the use of the close-other form of the La Trobe Communication Questionnaire (Douglas et al. 2000).

It should not be overlooked that problems in the *use* (and not just perception) of eye gaze and contact, and facial expressions are also a source of social communication difficulties for children and adults with clinical disorders. Klein-Tasman et al. (2007) reported socio-communicative deficits and eye contact and gaze anomalies in 29 children with Williams syndrome. On the communication domain of the Autism Diagnostic Observation Schedule (Lord et al. 1999), 72 % of these children attained cut-offs for 'autism spectrum' or 'autism'. More than half of these children (52 %) displayed unusual eye contact and 34 % displayed either some abnormality or definite abnormality in the integration of eye gaze and other behaviours during social overtures. (See Riby et al. (2008) who reported superior eye gaze *perception* in subjects with Williams syndrome compared to individuals with autism.)

Dickey et al. (2011) studied facial affect display in 55 subjects with schizotypal personality disorder (SPD). Although raters were able to identify the facial expressions of subjects with SPD and healthy controls equally well, they were less confident in their determinations of the expressions used by subjects with SPD. The facial expressions of these subjects were judged to be more odd, more ambiguous, less attractive and less approachable than those of control subjects. These factors contributed to an important finding with regard to social communication, that raters were less comfortable at the prospect of meeting subjects with SPD compared to normal controls. This finding appeared to be related to how attractive these subjects were to the rater. Clearly, the presentation of subjects with SPD, including their facial emotion expression, placed them at risk of reduced opportunities for social communication.

7.3.3 Pragmatics and Social Communication

It was argued above that pragmatics is merely one competence underlying social communication and, as such, should not be identified with social communication. However, it was also described how many investigators fail to draw any distinction between these domains and, in so doing, end up treating social communication and pragmatics as interchangeable terms. This latter tendency has created some clinical anomalies. One such anomaly is that investigators often treat a narrow aspect of pragmatics (e.g. comprehension of implicatures) as representative of the domain of social communication in general. Obviously, such a characterization of social communication is problematic when it is the relationship between pragmatics and this wider form of communication that is the focus of discussion in this section. However, with this cautionary note in mind, this section discusses the findings of clinical studies that have attempted to examine the relationship between pragmatics and social communication.

The relationship between pragmatics and social communication has been examined in a number of developmental disorders in children. Leonard et al. (2011) studied pragmatic language use and social skills in 54 children with hyperactivity and inattention. Pragmatic language use was assessed using the Children's Communication Checklist (Bishop 2003). Social skills were rated using the Social Skills Rating System (SSRS) (Gresham and Elliott 1990). Although the SSRS does not include a specific social communication subscale (see note 7), several items included in its four subscales contain items that assess aspects of social communication, e.g. 'acknowledges compliments or praise from friends', 'politely refuses unreasonable requests from others'. Leonard et al. reported that pragmatic language use made a unique contribution to the social skills of these children of 21.6 and 17.2 % above and beyond that made by hyperactivity and inattention, respectively.

Volden et al. (2009) found that pragmatic language scores on the Test of Pragmatic Language (Phelps-Terasaki and Phelps-Gunn 1992) accounted for significant variance in communication and socialization performance on the Autism Diagnostic Observation Schedule (ADOS) (Lord et al. 1999) in 37 high-functioning children with ASD. (The ADOS assesses the amount of reciprocal social communication within its reciprocal social interaction domain.) Better pragmatic skills were linked to fewer symptoms in social and communicative domains in these children. Eales (1993) reported that higher rates of pragmatic inappropriacy were associated with greater impairment of social interaction, as measured on the reciprocal social interaction domain in ADOS, in adults who had received a childhood diagnosis of autism. Tadić et al. (2010) reported significantly poorer pragmatic language skills, as measured on the CCC-2 (Bishop 2003), in children with congenital visual impairment than in typically developing sighted children of similar age and verbal ability. The performance of visually impaired children on the Social Communication Questionnaire (SCQ) (Rutter et al. 2003) significantly correlated with non-verbal communication, one of four pragmatic subscales on the CCC-2. Tadić et al. argue that the relationship between SCQ scores and non-verbal communication suggests a specific vulnerability in non-verbal aspects of pragmatics in the social communication difficulties of visually impaired children.

Aside from specific measures of social communication, studies have revealed associations between pragmatic language skills and social functioning more generally in children with developmental disorders. Conti-Ramsden and Botting (2004) found significant correlations between the pragmatic score of the CCC (Bishop 1998) and measures of social and behavioural functioning in 242 children with specific language impairment who were aged 11 years at the time of study. These investigators stated that 'poor pragmatic language skills go "hand in hand" with social difficulties' (159). Laws and Bishop (2004) reported significant levels of pragmatic language impairment, as measured on the CCC (Bishop 1998), and difficulties with social relationships in 19 children and young adults with Williams syndrome. One area of pragmatic competence that was particularly affected in these subjects—inappropriate initiation of conversation—is a feature of the social phenotype of Williams syndrome. This same feature was addressed by an item on the social relationships scale of the CCC, with the majority of parents of subjects with Williams syndrome agreeing that the statement 'talks to anyone and everyone' applied to their son or daughter. Although pragmatic language skills and social relations are impaired in individuals with Williams syndrome, performance in these domains is still superior to that of children with autism spectrum disorder (Philofsky et al. 2007).

The relationship between pragmatic skills and social communication has also been examined in disorders which have their onset in adolescence. In a study of adolescents at high risk for a first episode of psychosis,[8] Bearden et al. (2011) examined the association of linguistic cohesion and formal thought disorder with social and role functioning at one-year follow-up. Social functioning was assessed by means of the Global Assessment of Functioning: Social Scale (Auther et al. 2006) which describes communicative features alongside other social behaviours. A feature of formal thought disorder (viz., poverty of content of speech) was found to be significant predictor of social functioning in these adolescents (see Cummings (2012b) for discussion of the pragmatic attributes of poverty of content in schizophrenia).

Adolescence is a time of considerable social communicative vulnerability for the client with TBI who has pragmatic language disorder, as Turkstra et al. (1996, p. 329) have remarked: 'Deficits in pragmatic communication ability have a significant impact on functional outcome from traumatic brain injury, particularly during adolescence, when sophisticated social communication skills are developing'. A range of social communication deficits were identified post-TBI in three adolescents examined by Turkstra et al. These deficits included, in the case of one adolescent with TBI known as B.W., a lack of eye contact, disengagement from a group when he was not directly spoken to, and the introduction of topics and requests at inappropriate times. Of the three adolescents studied, B.W. was the only statistically significant outlier when his performance on a pragmatic assessment protocol was compared to that of control subjects.

Finally, studies have addressed the relationship between pragmatic language skills and social communication in adults with a range of clinical disorders.[9] Yamaguchi et al. (2011) investigated the contribution of pragmatic language skills to the social communication difficulties of individuals with dementia. These investigators stated that 'it is often observed that even patients with preserved lexical-semantic skills might fail in interactive social communication. Whereas social interaction requires pragmatic language skills, pragmatic language competencies in demented subjects have not been well understood' (2011, p. 205). Sixty-nine subjects with dementia were asked the meaning of a familiar proverb categorized as a figurative expression. Subjects also completed a test of cognitive inhibition. Proverb comprehension decreased significantly as dementia progressed, with the erroneous, literal interpretation of the proverb related to cognitive disinhibition in demented subjects.[10]

De Carvalho et al. (2008) examined functional communication ability in six patients with Alzheimer's disease (AD) and eight patients with frontotemporal lobar degeneration (FTLD). Functional communication was assessed in these patients using the Functional Assessment of Communication Skills for Adults (Frattalli et al. 1995). This assessment contains a Social Communication domain, in which there are several pragmatic items. Although the social communication performance of patients with AD was generally superior to that of patients with FTLD, it was only significantly better on one item—understands non-literal meaning and inference. De Carvalho et al. attribute the superior social communication performance of patients with AD to their enhanced ability to compensate for difficulties in communication.

Social communication is increasingly a topic of investigation in clients with aphasia. Davidson et al. (2006) used data from a number of sources (e.g. qualitative interviews, social network diaries) to examine social communication in three older people with stroke-induced aphasia. Two discourse and pragmatic aspects of language—storytelling and humour—were found to play a particularly important role in the daily social communication of these clients. Irwin et al. (2002) examined the relationship between pragmatic performance and functional communication[11] in 20 adults who were aphasic subsequent to a first, single thromboembolic stroke. Pragmatic performance was assessed by means of the Pragmatic Protocol (Prutting and Kirchner 1987). The Rating of Functional Performance (RFP) was used to assess functional communication. The RFP is an adaptation by Wertz et al. (1981) of the Functional Communication Profile (Sarno 1969). Irwin et al. found that the severity of pragmatic performance in these patients was significantly related to the severity of functional communication at only 1 month postonset.

Pragmatic language skills have also been linked to social communication abilities in adults with schizophrenia. Bowie and Harvey (2008) examined the relationship between two communicative behaviours—disconnected speech and verbal underproductivity—and social and adaptive functions in a sample of 317 chronically institutionalized patients with schizophrenia (see Cummings (2012b) for discussion of the pragmatic attributes of disconnected speech and poverty of speech in schizophrenia). Functional disability was assessed on the Social-Adaptive Functioning Evaluation (SAFE) (Harvey et al. 1997). Bowie and Harvey were specifically concerned to examine if disconnected speech and verbal underproductivity had differential relationships to the social-interpersonal domain of SAFE. This domain comprises six social behaviours: Communication, Conversation, Social Skills, Social Politeness, Social Engagement and Friendships. At 2.5 years follow-up, disconnected speech was a significant predictor of four of these behaviours, including the three most closely identified with social communication (i.e. communication, conversation and social politeness). Verbal underproductivity was a significant predictor of five social behaviours, including communication and conversation. Bowie and Harvey (2008, p. 246) concluded that '[a]cquisition of social skills may require efforts to address communication disorder, above and beyond attempts to alleviate clinical symptoms or remediate neurocognitive dysfunction'. In the next section, we say something about how one set of social skills, those involved in social communication, may be addressed during clinical remediation.

7.4 Assessing and Treating Social Communication

Social communication disorders are more than just an interesting clinical phenomenon. These disorders are part of, and pose significant challenges to, the daily lives of many children and adults.[12] In an effort to mitigate the adverse effects of social communication disorders, clinicians have sought to manage these disorders in several ways. The two principal ways in which this is achieved is through the assessment and treatment of these disorders.

Clinical literature regularly exhorts those with a professional interest in social communication disorders to give greater priority to the assessment and treatment of these disorders. For example, Pexman et al. (2011, p. 1110) state that 'particular emphasis should be given to the social functions of ironic language when devising strategies to help children with high-functioning ASD to deal with this complex aspect of everyday communication'. Yet, the specific features of the assessment and treatment techniques that are available to clinicians suggest that the management of social communication disorders may display many of the same problems that have beset clinical studies of social communication. This is not the context in which to undertake a detailed review of techniques and approaches used in the assessment and treatment of social communication disorders. Such reviews have been undertaken elsewhere and will not be repeated here.[13] Nor is it the context in which to develop a critical evaluation of assessment and treatment approaches (see Cummings (2007b, 2009, 2012c) for such an evaluation). This section will limit itself to the more realistic goals of describing the features of social communication assessments and therapies, and of making critical remarks where these are judged to be necessary.

7.4.1 Social Communication Assessments

The assessment of social communication skills presents clinicians with a unique set of challenges. These skills are put into practice when a client embarks on a communicative interaction with one or more partners in settings as diverse as the home environment, the workplace and social venues. To gain an understanding of a client's social communication skills in these different contexts, clinicians must abandon the formal assessment protocols which permit structural language skills to be examined, and adopt in their place a range of informal techniques. These techniques require the involvement of communicative partners, with all the issues of informant reliability that this dependency entails.[14] Also, to the extent that it is not possible to examine social communication skills in every setting, decisions must be made about which settings to select in order to obtain samples of these skills. Any selection inevitably raises issues about the representativeness of the social communication skills that are sampled in these settings. Finally, the data gathered in these settings cannot be meaningfully analysed in quantitative terms (or, at least, not only in these terms), and must be subjected to a qualitative analysis. Such analysis is often time-consuming and labour-intensive and, more often than not, is not practicable within busy speech-language pathology clinics. These various challenges have seen social communication skills subordinated to the assessment of other language and communication skills, a point acknowledged by Landa (2005) when she states that '[w]hile social communication is perhaps one of the most important skills for peer acceptance, these skills are often overlooked in language evaluation with children' (247).

Notwithstanding these various challenges, clinicians and researchers have developed a range of instruments to assess social communication skills in children and adults. Some of these instruments require the assessing clinician to conduct interviews with the carers or parents of the client (e.g. Diagnostic Interview for Social and Communication Disorders, Wing et al. 2002). Other instruments involve carers and professionals completing checklists of behaviours that only people familiar to the client can reliably describe. For example, the Children's Communication Checklist-2 (Bishop 2003) may be completed by a caregiver, a speech-language pathologist or a teacher. Still other tools require a clinician or other professional to observe and rate a client's behaviour in clinic or in educational settings (e.g. Social-Communication Assessment Tool, Murdock et al. 2007). Several of the instruments in use display good psychometric properties. In this way, Skuse et al. (2005) reported excellent internal consistency (0.93), high test-retest reliability (0.81) and good discriminant validity (sensitivity 0.90; specificity 0.69) for the Social and Communication Disorders Checklist (originally developed to measure social-behaviour deficits in Turner's syndrome, James et al. 1997). Some social communication assessments have been developed for use with specific client groups. This is particularly true of autism spectrum disorder (e.g. Social Communication Assessment for Toddlers with Autism, Drew et al. 2007), where many social communication assessments also contribute to the screening and diagnosis of ASD (e.g. Social Communication Questionnaire, Rutter et al. 2003).

Although several of the above instruments have versions which can be used with adults[15], these social communication assessments are intended primarily for use with children who have developmental disorders such as the ASD. However, social communication assessments have also been developed for use with clients who have adult-onset conditions such as aphasia, traumatic brain injury (TBI) and schizophrenia. With the growing prominence of a social model of disability in the management of aphasia, clinicians have been increasingly concerned to assess the communication skills of adults with aphasia from a social perspective (see Whitworth et al. (2014) for discussion). Simmons-Mackie and Damico (1996) describe one such assessment procedure, the Communicative Profiling System (CPS), and demonstrate its use by means of a case study. The assessment derives data from ethnographic interviews supplemented by participant observations. The CPS has not been described as a measure for use with adults with TBI. However, Coelho et al. (2005b) state that it has 'great potential' for documenting the decreased socialization that frequently follows TBI.

A social communication assessment which has been used extensively in adults with TBI is the La Trobe Communication Questionnaire (Douglas et al.

2000). This 30-item questionnaire measures perceived communication ability from different sources including the self-perceptions of the client with TBI and the perceptions of those with whom he or she converses regularly (e.g. family members, friends, clinicians). Respondents are required to rate items, which describe verbal and non-verbal aspects of communication, as occurring never or rarely, sometimes, often, or usually or always. Many items are squarely within the domain of pragmatics. For example, conversational relevance is assessed by means of items such as 'Get 'side-tracked' by irrelevant parts of the conversation?' and 'Give answers that are not connected to the question?'. The questionnaire displays good psychometric properties in adults with severe TBI (Douglas et al. 2007) and has been found to distinguish adolescents with severe TBI from neurologically normal adolescents (Douglas 2010b). This social communication measure has also been found to contribute significantly to social integration outcomes in adults with TBI (Struchen et al. 2011).

Notwithstanding the significant communicative impairments of clients with schizophrenia, no dedicated instrument exists to assess the social communication skills of this clinical population. This is not to say, however, that the assessment of language and communication skills is overlooked in adults with schizophrenia. An assessment of considerable significance in clinical practice and research, with translations into other languages (Bazin et al. 2002; Andreou et al. 2008), is the Scale for the Assessment of Thought, Language, and Communication (TLC) (Andreasen 1986).[16] Although the TLC contains a comprehensive set of clearly defined and illustrated disorders, and has very high inter-rater reliability (Mazumdar et al. 1991; Andreasen 1986), it is doubtful whether features such as 'pressure of speech' and 'tangentiality' can reveal much, either in isolation or in combination, about a client's social communication skills.

Of somewhat greater clinical value in this regard are assessments of functional capacity and social skills in schizophrenia. Many of these assessments contain communication sub-scales or require subjects to undertake tasks (e.g. social role-plays) that demand competence in social communication. For example, the UCSD Performance-Based Skills Assessment (UPSA) (Patterson et al. 2001a) examines a client's functioning in five areas: household chores; communication; finance; transportation; and planning and recreational activities. The communication domain requires subjects to engage in a role-play task that involves the use of the telephone. In one scenario, subjects are given a medical appointment confirmation letter to read and are then asked to call the hospital to reschedule the appointment. The UPSA can be administered in 30 min, has excellent inter-rater reliability (Patterson et al. 2001a) and has been shown to predict independent living status in patients with chronic schizophrenia-related conditions (Mausbach et al. 2008). A brief version of the assessment has been found to be useful in assessing functioning in people diagnosed with schizophrenia and bipolar disorder (Mausbach et al. 2010).

The Social Skills Performance Assessment (SSPA) permits direct observation of social skills performance in two role plays, one involving introduction to a stranger and the other demanding assertive behaviour with a landlord. The SSPA has been used to measure social functioning in middle-aged and older outpatients with schizophrenia (Sitzer et al. 2008) where it has proven utility over self-report measures (Patterson et al. 2001b). The assessment takes approximately 12 min to complete, has excellent inter-rater reliability and has good test–retest reliability (Patterson et al. 2001b).

As the instruments above indicate, there is an extensive range of social communication assessments available to the clinician. However, these tools vary widely in how they construe social communication and the extent to which they probe the skills of clients in this domain. The Social and Communication Disorders Checklist is a 12-item scale, with only three of these items examining behaviours related to communication: (1) does not seem to understand social skills, e.g. persistently interrupts conversations, (2) does not pick up on body language, and (3) cannot follow a command unless it is carefully worded. At the other end of the scale, the Diagnostic Interview for Social and Communication Disorders (DISCO) contains 91 items, 14 of which fall under communication (three of these, bizarrely, describe aspects of play). Some DISCO items capture specific features of autistic language (e.g. echolalia, pronoun reversal) or pragmatic aspects of language (e.g. content of speech is irrelevant), while other items describe more general attributes of communication (e.g. communication is one-sided).

There are also DISCO items for the social perception and cognition domains in social communication, although these domains are not identified as such in the schedule. For example, the interviewer rates clients' social perceptual and social cognitive skills using items such as 'eye contact poor', 'stares too long and hard', and 'lack of awareness of others' feelings'. In between these assessments lies the Social-Communication Assessment Tool, in which social communication is examined in terms of performance in four core domains: (1) verbal initiations, (2) verbal responses, (3) joint attention, and (4) non verbal communication attempts. These domains are selected because they represent 'the most thoroughly researched and potentially the most striking indicators of the discrepancies in social language between children with ASD and their typical peers' (Murdock et al. 2007, p. 162).

Even from this briefest of surveys of social communication assessments, it is apparent that there is considerable variability in the operational definitions of social communication that are in current clinical use. In fact, so great is this variability that it is only rarely possible to trace a particular social communicative behaviour from assessment to assessment. The lack of a standard set of behaviours across assessments is a direct reflection of the lack of a standard definition of social communication among clinicians and researchers. This issue is not without significant consequence. For not only does a particular construal of social communication affect how clinicians assess and treat clients with social communication disorders, but a lack of comparability between assessment protocols has severely limited the extent to which we can compare the results of research studies.

To the extent that studies are assessing different behaviours when they claim to examine social communication, it is difficult to characterize social communication problems in clients, even in clients within a single clinical population. This accounts in large part for the less well developed clinical descriptions of social communication problems in clients with a range of disorders in comparison with other areas of language and communication (e.g. phonology, syntax). The only corrective to this situation is for proper clarity to be achieved by investigators on the nature and extent of social communication. To this end, future research in the area of social communication must involve greater conceptual and theoretical deliberation on what this notion may reasonably be taken to include (see Sect. 7.5).

What this survey of assessments also reveals is that there are more and less accurate ways of assessing social communication. Self-reports of social communication skills are likely to be of little value in patients who have conditions which result in limited insight into their own abilities and levels of functioning (e.g. schizophrenia and TBI). At a minimum, these reports need to be corroborated by independent assessments undertaken by clinicians. Also, the use of parents and spouses as informants about an individual's social communication skills often results in different (usually better) ratings of those skills than the evaluations arrived at by clinicians (see note 14). It is a paradox that in attempting to solicit the views of the people who, on account of their familiarity with the client, are best placed to give an accurate account of social communication skills, clinicians may actually be receiving an excessively positive assessment of those skills.

But, by far the greatest difficulty with social communication assessments in current clinical use is that many distort social communication through the implementation of inappropriate tasks and exercises. It is doubtful, for example, that asking a client to assume a certain role in the rather contrived assessment scenarios described above is in any way faithfully reproducing the social communication processes which are at work in naturalistic contexts. Yet, it is these processes, and only these processes, which should be the target of assessment and intervention efforts. Clearly, there is still much work to be done before clinicians can claim to have instruments at their disposal that are truly revealing of a client's social communication skills.

7.4.2 Social Communication Interventions

Like social communication assessments, interventions for social communication disorders involve an equally eclectic mix of techniques and approaches. For ease of discussion, these techniques and approaches can be categorized into two main types of intervention. The first type of intervention employs a notion of social communication which is similar to the one we have been adopting throughout this chapter. That is, several cognitive and linguistic domains are assumed to contribute to social communication performance and intervention proceeds by targeting each of these domains. This type of intervention is exemplified by the recent Social Communication Intervention Project (SCIP) of Adams and colleagues (Adams 2012a, b). A key rationale of SCIP intervention is that social communication consists in, or emerges from, the interaction of social, cognitive and linguistic domains. A number of other interventions also claim to remediate social communication skills directly. These interventions have been implemented in research studies (Braden et al. 2010) and some are available as commercial packages (Alarcon and Rogers 2007). However, it is debatable whether these interventions embrace the same notion of social communication that motivates SCIP intervention and that is the essence of this first type of social communication intervention.

The second type of intervention is represented by approaches that address one or more of the component domains of social communication. These domains are targeted either in isolation (teaching of theory of mind skills, for example), or alongside other behaviours that are not typically included in social communication (in social skills training, for example). Interventions of this second type make no explicit claim to remediate social communication skills. Instead, it is assumed (correctly or incorrectly) that an improvement in social communication skills will be one of the beneficial consequences of the particular intervention that is undertaken. Interventions in this category can take the form of social skills training (see Kopelowicz et al. (2006) for review), the teaching of conversational skills to clients (e.g. Chin and Bernard-Opitz 2000) and direct remediation of emotion recognition (e.g. Williams et al. 2012) and theory of mind skills (see Swettenham (2000) for discussion). In this section, both of these main approaches to social communication intervention will be discussed. The techniques employed by clinicians as part of these interventions will be briefly described. Not all of these interventions are equally effective in remediating social communication problems in clients. Accordingly, the section concludes with an examination of the findings of studies that have considered the effectiveness of social communication interventions.

Few clinical interventions address the full gamut of competences which, it has been argued in this chapter, are integral to social communication. A notable exception is the Social Communication Intervention Project (SCIP) of Adams et al. (2012a, b). Adams acknowledges the combined contribution of several linguistic and cognitive domains to social communication performance.[17] These domains include social interaction, social cognition, pragmatics, and language processing. Therapy content in SCIP addresses each of these domains. In this way, the language processing aspect of SCIP aims to remediate impairments in semantics and high-level language skills; the pragmatics aspect addresses pragmatic difficulties using principally metapragmatic therapy; and the social understanding and social interaction aspect addresses limitations of social interaction and social cue interpretation.

Each of these three aspects contains five components which, in turn, contain therapy targets linked to a set of therapeutic activities. For example, the second component of the pragmatics aspect—understanding information requirements—contains five main therapy targets: too much/too little information; excess information; seeking relevant information; sabotaging information; and personalizing information. Methods used in SCIP include modelling, role play, sabotage (the therapist deliberately makes errors to draw attention to a communicative act), and sabotaged role play. Therapy activities are conducted in one-to-one sessions of one hour each (up to a maximum of 20 h), and are carried out in the classroom or at home. Adams and her colleagues performed SCIP intervention in children with complex pragmatic communication needs (Adams et al. 2012b) with or without features of ASD (Adams et al. 2012a).

Social skills training (SST) is used extensively in clinical practice. The content of such training can be very broad indeed.[18] However, as a recent definition of SST demonstrates, communication lies at the heart of this type of intervention: 'social skills training utilizes behaviour therapy principles and techniques for teaching individuals to communicate their emotions and requests so that they are more likely to achieve their goals and meet their needs for affiliative relationships and roles required for independent living' (Kopelowicz et al. 2006, p. S12). The clinician works with the client to identify behaviours that serve as obstacles to his or her social functioning. These behaviours are then the basis of goal-setting. Role plays are used to practice alternative behaviours which will help the client attain his goals. The clinician provides positive and corrective feedback on role plays and models behaviours, where appropriate. The use of homework assignments ensures generalization of newly acquired social skills to non-clinical contexts.

Although SST can be conducted with individuals, it is more typically undertaken in groups. As well as being more cost effective, group therapy provides an invaluable opportunity for skills to be modelled and reinforced by the client's peers. There is also an opportunity for clients to learn from the real-life experiences of others and to receive peer support. SST is particularly widely employed with clients who have schizophrenia. In this way, Chien et al. (2003) undertook SST in patients with schizophrenia that focused on conversation and assertiveness skills. Park et al. (2011) used traditional and virtual reality role-playing in SST of inpatients with schizophrenia. However, SST has also been used in other clinical populations, including clients with autism spectrum disorder (e.g. Gantman et al. 2012), attention deficit hyperactivity disorder (e.g. Storebø et al. 2012) and acquired brain injuries (e.g. McDonald et al. 2008). Sanger et al. (2006) argue for the inclusion of pragmatics in SST for female delinquents.

As well as forming one component of social skills training, conversational skills can also be the sole focus of a social communication intervention. The teaching of conversational skills can include the use of appropriate turn-taking in conversation, topic management (that is, the introduction, development and termination of topics), and practice in employing appropriate opening and closing remarks in conversation. Direct teaching of conversational skills has been implemented with a range of clinical subjects. Chin and Bernard-Opitz (2000) undertook teaching of conversational skills to three high-functioning children with autism. These children were taught how to initiate a conversation, listen attentively, take turns during a conversation, and maintain and change a conversation topic appropriately.

Some conversational skills training can involve instruction on the use of specific moves in conversations that are identified to be of functional value to clients. For example, Mechling et al. (2005) taught students with intellectual disabilities how to verbally respond to questions and make purchases in fast food restaurants. Increasingly, computer technology is used to deliver conversational skills training to clients with clinical conditions including schizophrenia (e.g. Ku et al. 2007) and intellectual disability (e.g. Mechling et al. 2005). Clinicians are also using conversational skills training in the management of aphasia. However, in this case, it is the conversational partners of clients with aphasia who receive training. The aim is to improve the social communication skills of these clients by making partners aware of how their own conversational behaviours may be an obstruction to effective communication with people with aphasia. For further discussion of this use of conversational skills training, the reader is referred to Whitworth et al. (2014).

Finally, some social communication interventions proceed by training clients in the use of social cognitive skills such as theory of mind and emotion recognition. The rationale of these interventions is that by enhancing social cognitive skills, it will be possible to alleviate clients' social communication problems—social cognition is, after all, a key domain of social communication. The techniques used to train these social cognitive skills are many and varied. Most commonly, they are implemented in children and adults with autism spectrum disorder, although social cognition training is also undertaken in other clinical populations. Williams et al. (2012) used the Transporters programme to train emotion recognition in 55 young children with autism and a range of intellectual ability. This programme features the adventures of eight animated mechanical vehicles with human faces which express 15 emotions. Kandalaft et al. (2013) used a virtual reality platform to train theory of mind and emotion recognition in eight young adults diagnosed with high-functioning autism. Silver et al. (2004) adopted a computerized emotion training program, which was originally developed for use with children with autism, to train the recognition of facial emotions in male patients with chronic schizophrenia. Bornhofen and McDonald (2008) used two strategies—errorless learning and self-instruction training—to remediate emotion perception deficits in 18 adult outpatients with severe TBI who were at least 6 months post-injury.

Two of the most widely employed techniques in social cognition training in autism are comic strip conversations (Gray 1994) and social stories (Gray 1995). That social cognition, and particularly theory of mind, is at the centre of these approaches is evident from the following remarks of Gray (1994, p. 2) in her explanation of the rationale of comic strip conversations: 'Students with autism have difficulty identifying the beliefs and motivations of others [...] Comic Strip Conversations regard the thoughts and feelings of others as holding equal importance to spoken words and actions in an interaction. Students are taught to use colors to identify the feelings behind thoughts and spoken words'.

Social stories have been variously employed in clinical interventions in clients with autism. These stories have been used to increase social communicative behaviours such as verbal greeting initiations (Reichow and Sabornie 2009). Thiemann and Goldstein (2001) used social stories to target four social communicative behaviours—securing attention, initiating comments, initiating requests and contingent responses—in an intervention with five students with autism. Social stories interventions have also been used to improve the social skills of children with autism during game play (Quirmbach et al. 2009), to increase prosocial behaviours (Crozier and Tincani 2007) and to decrease disruptive behaviours (Scattone et al. 2002; Ozdemir 2008). Social stories have been used in individual therapy (Bock et al. 2001) and in inclusive classroom settings (Chan and O'Reilly 2008), and have also been musically adapted (Brownell 2002). Hutchins and Prelock (2006) describe a family-centered collaborative approach to developing social stories and comic strip conversations.

Increasingly, clinicians and researchers are required to demonstrate the effectiveness of social communication interventions. Findings of efficacy studies have been variable, to say the least. Reichow et al. (2012) conducted a review of the effectiveness of social skills groups for improving social communication and social competence in 196 clients with ASD aged 6–21 years. There was some evidence that social skills groups improved social competence and friendship quality in these clients. However, there were no differences between treatment and control subjects in relation to emotion recognition and social communication. In a systematic review of treatments for pragmatic language disorders, Gerber et al. (2012) found preliminary support for the efficacy of treatment procedures that address social communication behaviours, with significant gains reported in topic management skills, narrative production and repairs of inadequate or ambiguous comments. In a randomized controlled trial, Begeer et al. (2011) failed to find strong evidence for the effectiveness of a 16-week theory of mind treatment in children with ASD aged 8–13 years. Williams et al. (2012) reported limited efficacy of the Transporters programme in teaching emotion recognition skills to young children with autism who had a lower range of cognitive ability. Significant treatment gains have been reported from the virtual reality application of social cognition and social skills training (Park et al. 2011; Kandalaft et al. 2013) and from conversation skills training (Chien et al. 2003).

Several literature reviews and research studies have examined the effectiveness of interventions based on the use of social stories. As with other social communication interventions, the effects of social stories interventions appear to be highly variable (Reynhout and Carter 2006), with findings of positive outcomes and negligible benefits reported by investigators. In a systematic review of the literature, Karkhaneh et al. (2010) found statistically significant benefits for outcomes related to social interaction in five of six trials that employed social stories. However, Kokina and Kern (2010) reported low to questionable overall effectiveness of social stories in a meta-analysis of single-subject research. Social stories have been found to be less effective than a teaching interaction procedure in developing social skills in children and adolescents with ASD (Leaf et al. 2012). In a review of the literature on social stories, Rust and Smith (2006) reported considerable variability in the quality of research methodology employed in intervention studies, and considered factors that should be addressed when testing the effectiveness of interventions based on social stories. Clearly, it will only be possible to make an accurate assessment of the effectiveness of social stories as a social communication intervention when rigorous research methodologies are consistently applied across studies.

As a final point, it should be noted that the various social communication interventions discussed in this section target clients who are verbal communicators.

However, interventions have also been found to produce social communication gains in non-verbal clients. In this way, Lerna et al. (2012) examined the effects of two interventions—a conventional language therapy and the Picture Exchange Communication System (PECS)—on the social communication skills of 18 non-verbal, preschool children with autism. Although there was no difference in the pre-treatment social communication skills of the children assigned to these two treatment conditions, only children who received PECS intervention showed a significant improvement on several social communication measures after a 6-month period of treatment. A strictly verbal conception of social communication neglects the social communication achievements of these children and other non-verbal communicators and should be avoided in a clinical context.

7.5   Future Research into Social Communication

It will not have escaped the reader's attention that many of the clinical studies examined in Sect. 7.3 treat social communication in rather vague and inexplicit ways. Some studies use measures that subsume social communication within subscales examining non-communicative social behaviours (e.g. social relationships). Other studies employ rating scales in which social communicative items appear in several different subscales. Still other studies straightforwardly identify social communication with pragmatics, rather than viewing pragmatics as one sub-domain within social communication. In fact, few clinical studies treat social communication as a distinctive social construct that warrants the type of systematic examination which is routinely afforded to other social behaviours. It behoves us to ask how this unsatisfactory situation has come about, and identify ways in which future investigators might improve research into social communication and its disorders.

The question of why so many clinical studies fail to give a good account of social communication is complex and can at best be answered only tentatively. One part of that answer lies in the disciplinary backgrounds of the investigators who undertake these studies. Psychiatrists and psychologists often lack the linguistic expertise to identify and characterize social communicative behaviours. Even speech-language pathologists, who do have the requisite expertise in language, often conflate social communication with the pragmatic language skills that form one of its component domains. Another part of the answer concerns the lack of clinical instruments to measure social communicative behaviours. Dedicated social communicative assessments such as the Children's Communication Checklist (Bishop 2003) are still underrepresented in the clinical disciplines that assess and treat children and adults with social communication disorders. In the absence of these instruments, clinicians and researchers must look to pre-existing social measures which either neglect or misrepresent social communication. And, finally, probably the most significant part of an answer to the question of why so many studies do not adequately address social communication is that clinicians and researchers are generally ignorant of the specific social behaviours that this construct may be taken to represent. This lack of knowledge is not a failing of individual investigators, but reflects the fact that there has been little serious effort made to characterize social communication in a rigorous way. The combined influence of these factors has served to undermine many clinical studies of social communication which have been conducted to date.

In this section, I will identify and examine three ways in which future research into social communication in a clinical context can move beyond the significant weaknesses of former studies. The first of these ways addresses the need for much greater clarity about the nature and extent of social communication. This will largely be a conceptual exercise which will reflect on the 'essence' or core attributes of social communication and the relationship of social communication to other behaviours in the social domain. The second way in which future research can address the weaknesses of former studies is to establish the clinical validity of the behaviours that constitute the essence of social communication. To the extent that these behaviours are the manifestation of a specific social competence, they must display predictable patterns of impairment in clients with social dysfunction—it is difficult to argue that these behaviours emanate from a specific social competence if certain behaviours are intact while others are impaired in an individual with social dysfunction. These behaviours must also fractionate from non-communicative social behaviours in subjects with and without social impairment. Needless to say, this is a huge research program which will not be completed in the short term. An equally large program, which will be the third way in which future research can address the weaknesses of former studies, is the development of reliable and sensitive clinical measures of social communication. It is only when these measures have been developed and are put to clinical use that investigators can begin to characterize with hitherto unseen accuracy the social communication impairments of a range of clients.

Although conceptual work may appear out of place in a clinical context, it must play a role in future research into social communication. It is only when clinicians and researchers are clear about the true nature and extent of social communication that we can expect to see a reduction of inaccurate characterizations of this notion in clinical studies. At the heart of this conceptual work must be a new view of social communication, one in which social communication is seen to emerge from the interaction of several key competences, namely, social perception, theory of mind (social cognition) and pragmatics. The speaker who can develop a topic of conversation is still not a competent social communicator if he develops that conversation in ways which are not of interest to the hearer. Pragmatic language skills must combine with ToM skills if a speaker is to extend a topic of conversation along lines that appeal to the interests, beliefs and emotional states of a hearer.

By the same token, a hearer may be able to establish that a speaker has flouted a maxim of conversation (e.g. relation) with a view to achieving some communicative effect. But if that hearer fails to ascertain the significance of a particular facial expression or lapse in eye gaze for the interpretation of the speaker's 'irrelevant' utterance, then there is a clear sense in which the hearer is not a competent social communicator. In this case, social perceptual skills must come into play alongside pragmatic language skills in order for social communication to be achieved. These interconnections between pragmatics, social perception and theory of mind lie at the very heart of what it means to engage in social communication. It is from these interconnections that serious conceptual work on the notion of social communication must now proceed.

Conceptual work, even rigorous conceptual work, can lead investigators on occasion down unproductive and erroneous routes of enquiry. When a list of the core social communicative behaviours is eventually determined, investigators must establish the clinical validity of those behaviours. Investigators must satisfy themselves that the behaviours they have identified as belonging to the domain of social communication not only 'sit well' alongside each other, but that they also achieve sufficient discrimination between this domain and a range of other social domains (e.g. social relationships). Social behaviours which reflect a shared, underlying competence can be expected to be intact or impaired alongside each other. Even behaviours which appear essentially related on conceptual grounds can begin to look quite disparate when one is consistently impaired and the other is intact in individual clients with social communication disorders. Also, it may be discovered that a certain communicative behaviour, for example, the initiation of conversation, displays as close an affinity with social relationships as it does with social communication. In such a case, there may be grounds for claiming that this communicative behaviour lacks the level of discrimination needed to be a core behaviour within the social communication domain. A key part of any future research effort must be expended towards establishing the clinical validity of the behaviours which are identified on conceptual grounds as integral to social communication.

Finally, when investigators are assured that the behaviours they have identified are truly reflective of the social communication domain, they must proceed to operationalize those behaviours within robust clinical measures. The development of any clinical rating scale is an arduous process. Investigators must establish, for example, that the items included in the scale are sufficiently sensitive to the domain under investigation. They must also be convinced that different clinicians using the same scale will arrive at the same ratings of a client's behaviours (interrater reliability). If there are pre-existing rating scales with good psychometric properties, investigators will also want to convince themselves that any new scale produces scores which are consistent with scores obtained on these other scales. Each of these tasks involves a significant commitment of research effort and resources over an extended period of time. Yet, this is an investment which clinicians and researchers must make if they are to obtain robust tools to measure social communication. With properly validated clinical measures in place, investigators can begin to make real progress on characterizing the social communication disorders of different clinical groups. They can also begin to explore, for the first time and with accuracy, the interrelationships between the component competences of social communication as well as the contribution of each of these competences to clients' social communication skills. It is only when studies of this type are undertaken that we can be said to have rectified the weaknesses of earlier clinical research into social communication.

7.6 Summary

There can be few aspects of social behaviour so frequently discussed, and yet so poorly characterized, as social communication. This chapter attempts to address the rather unsystematic efforts of clinical investigators to date to characterize this social construct by placing social communication at the centre of a discussion of pragmatic disorders. Social communication is characterized as a behaviour which draws on competences in several cognitive and linguistic domains, including pragmatics, theory of mind (social cognition) and social perception. Each of these domains is described on its own terms and then examined for the contribution it makes to social communication. The relationship between pragmatics and social communication is investigated across several clinical conditions in which there are marked pragmatic disorders, including autism spectrum disorder, schizophrenia and dementia. Clinical tools and techniques used to assess and treat social communication disorders in children and adults are examined, and directions for future research into social communication are explored.

Notes

1. Of course, a range of skills beyond the three domains listed are also necessary for social communication. A speaker must be able to decode language, attend to and perceive auditory and visual stimuli, and retrieve information from memory in order to engage in social communication. However, these skills are not in any way unique to social communication—they are fundamental to a number of behaviours—and so will not be discussed further in this context.
2. This tendency is exemplified by Russell (2007) who states that '[s]ocial communication or pragmatic impairments are characterized [...] as involving inappropriate or ineffective use of language and gesture in social contexts' (483).
3. Consensus on a definition of social cognition is hard to find. But there is general agreement that theory of mind is a central topic of social cognitive research. For a brief overview of social cognition, and its relation to pragmatics, the reader is referred to Scott-Phillips (2010).
4. Social models of disability and functioning are now integral to internationally recognized classification systems such as the International Classification of Functioning, Disability and Health (ICF) (World Health Organization 2001). The ICF uses a biopsychosocial model of disability which is an integration of medical and social models of disability.
5. A diagnosis of social communication disorder specifically excludes individuals with autism spectrum disorder (ASD). This is because children with social communication disorder lack the additional difficulties seen in ASD (e.g. repetitive behaviours and restricted interests).

6. The assumption of most clinical studies is that ToM deficits play a causal role in the social communication difficulties of patients. However, some investigations have considered a different relationship between ToM and social communication. Milders et al. (2006) ask if more limited opportunities for social communication following TBI might not lead to a deterioration in ToM skill: 'changes in patients' social interactions and reduced social communication might affect ToM ability, and ToM deficits occurring shortly after injury may further deteriorate as a result of the patients' impoverished social environment' (2006, p. 400). Milders et al. did find ToM impairments in their patients with TBI both shortly after injury and at 1-year follow-up. However, ToM skills did not deteriorate during this time, leading these investigators to conclude that the ToM impairments of these patients were a direct consequence of brain damage, and not the result of any changes in the social environment during the year to follow-up.

7. In describing their motivation for using the SDI, Hooker and Park (2002) capture a problem of most clinical measures which assess social functioning—their failure to assess communication as an independent aspect of social functioning. Hooker and Park (2002, p. 43) state that 'whereas previous measures have embedded communication problems into other measures of functioning—such as relationship problems—this measure [the SDI] has a specific communication subscale'.

8. Solomon et al. (2011) found that individuals (aged 11–18 years) at clinical high risk for psychosis and individuals (aged 14–20 years) with first episode psychosis displayed significantly poorer scores than typically developing individuals on the Communication subscale of the Social Responsiveness Scale (Constantino 2002). However, the pragmatic language skills of clinical subjects, as measured on the Scripted Language, Context and Non-Verbal Communication subscales of the CCC-2 (Bishop 2003), were comparable to those of typically developing individuals.

9. It is worth remarking that the number of studies which examine this relationship in adults is very small indeed. Typically, adult studies neglect social communication in favour of social integration and social functioning, with pragmatic language skills related to the latter social constructs rather than to the former one. Social integration is often investigated in adults with TBI. In this way, Galski et al. (1998) reported that discourse and pragmatic behaviours correlated with social integration in 30 patients with TBI more strongly than age, gender, education and other conventional psychosocial factors. Also, Struchen et al. (2011) reported that two social communication measures contributed significantly to social integration in 184 adults with TBI.

10. The reader is referred to Chap. 3, this volume and to Chap. 5 in Cummings (2009) for discussion of the cognitive substrates of pragmatic disorders.

11. Given the widespread clinical use of functional communication measures, a question of some interest is the exact relationship between functional communication and social communication. Although there is no definitive answer to this question—and the author is not aware of any research that has addressed

this relationship—it is clear that both notions are taken to include similar behaviours. The National Joint Committee for the Communication Needs of Persons with Severe Disabilities defines functional communication skills as 'forms of behavior that express needs, wants, feelings, and preferences that others can understand [...] Functional communication skills vary in their form and may include personalized movements, gestures, verbalizations, signs, pictures, words, and augmentative and alternative communication devices.

12. Few studies have attempted to establish the prevalence of social communication disorders in the general population. One exception is Skuse et al. (2009) who estimated the prevalence of social communication disorders in a general population of 8,094 children (4,167 boys and 3,927 girls) who were part of the Avon Longitudinal Study of Parents and Children (Golding et al. 2001). Social communication disorders were assessed on the Social Communication Disorders Checklist (SCDC) (Skuse et al. 2005). The 12 individual symptoms rated by parents on the SCDC revealed that these symptoms were 'very or often true' in 0.7–3.9 % of girls, and in 2.3–6.2 % of boys. Boys had mean scores on the SCDC which were 30 % higher than those of girls. There was a large and significant association between SCDC scores and the pragmatic competence score on the Children's Communication Checklist (Bishop 1998). Social communication deficits correlated positively with peer relationship problems for both boys and girls, with SCDC scores contributing 4.4 % of the variance for boys and 1.9 % of the variance for girls.

13. For reviews of social communication assessments and treatments in children, the reader is referred to Landa (2005) and Gerber et al. (2012), respectively.

14. The issue of the reliability of carers and parents as informants has been examined by comparing their ratings of clients' social communication skills with those of professionals, typically speech and language therapists and teachers. Bishop et al. (2006) examined inter-rater reliability between parent and teacher ratings on the Children's Communication Checklist. Inter-rater reliability was generally weak with correlations exceeding 0.5 on only the speech, syntax and coherence scales and on the General Communication Composite of the checklist. Bishop and Baird (2001) found that correlations between ratings for parents and professionals on the individual pragmatic scales of the checklist ranged from 0.30 to 0.58, with a correlation of 0.46 for the pragmatic composite. When the checklist was completed by teachers and speech and language therapists, Bishop (1998) reported inter-rater reliability and internal consistency of around 0.80 on the five pragmatic subscales. These findings clearly indicate that clinicians need to be somewhat circumspect about the judgements and reports of informants in matters relating to social communication.

15. The adult version of the CCC—the Communication Checklist-Adult (CC-A) (Whitehouse and Bishop 2009)—is a 70-item questionnaire which is completed by a respondent who has regular contact with the individual undergoing assessment. It is suitable for use with adults who have a developmental disorder such as specific language impairment, ASD, Down's syndrome, fragile

X syndrome, and learning difficulties, but may also be used with adults who have an acquired disorder such as a head injury.

16. That Andreasen (1986) intended the TLC to represent a shift away from viewing linguistic abnormalities in schizophrenia as the manifestation of thought disorder towards viewing them as a communication disorder is evident in the following comments: 'The various disorders which comprised the concept of "formal thought disorder" can be better conceptualized as "disorders of thought, language, and communication". If viewed from an empirical perspective, most of them are in fact disorders of communication, and the notion of thought need only be invoked to explain a few of them' (473).

17. Adams (2005, p. 181) defines social communication as 'the interdependence of social interaction, social cognition, pragmatics and language processing'.

18. Kopelowicz et al. (2006) convey something of this breadth when they state that social skills comprise 'the full range of human social performance' (S12). Their list of these skills is particularly comprehensive and covers many of the same behaviours (e.g. social perception) that are integral to social communication: 'verbal, nonverbal, and paralinguistic behaviors; accurate social perception; effective processing of social information to make decisions and responses that conform to the normative, reasonable expectations of situations, and rules of society; assertiveness; conversational skills; skills related to management and stabilization of one's mental disorder and expressions of empathy, affection, sadness, and other emotions that are appropriate to the context and expectations of others' (S12).

Bibliography

Aarsen, F. K., Van Dongen, H. R., Paquier, P. F., Van Mourik, M., & Catsman-Berrevoets, C. E. (2004). Long-term sequelae in children after cerebellar astrocytoma surgery. *Neurology, 62,* 1311–1316.

Abbeduto, L., Pavetto, M., Kesin, E., Weissman, M. D., Karadottir, S., O'Brien, A., et al. (2001). The linguistic and cognitive profile of Down syndrome: Evidence from a comparison with fragile X syndrome. *Down's Syndrome Research and Practice, 7,* 9–15.

Aboulafia-Brakha, T., Christe, B., Martory, M. D., & Annoni, J. M. (2011). Theory of mind tasks and executive functions: A systematic review of group studies in neurology. *Journal of Neuropsychology, 5,* 39–55.

Abu-Akel, A., & Abushua'leh, K. (2004). 'Theory of mind' in violent and nonviolent patients with paranoid schizophrenia. *Schizophrenia Research, 69,* 45–53.

Adair, J. C., Cooke, N., & Jankovic, J. (2007). Alexia without agraphia in Creutzfeldt-Jakob disease. *Journal of the Neurological Sciences, 263,* 208–210.

Adams, C. (2005). Social communication intervention for school-age children: Rationale and description. *Seminars in Speech and Language, 26,* 181–188.

Adams, C., Clarke, E., & Haynes, R. (2009). Inference and sentence comprehension in children with specific or pragmatic language impairment. *International Journal of Language and Communication Disorders, 44,* 301–318.

Adams, C., Green, J., Gilchrist, A., & Cox, A. (2002). Conversational behaviour of children with Asperger syndrome and conduct disorder. *Journal of Child Psychology and Psychiatry, 43,* 679–690.

Adams, C., Lloyd, J., Aldred, C., & Baxendale, J. (2006). Exploring the effects of communication intervention for developmental pragmatic language impairments: A signal-generation study. *International Journal of Language & Communication Disorders, 41,* 41–65.

Adams, C., Lockton, E., Freed, J., Gaile, J., Earl, G., McBean, K., et al. (2012a). The Social Communication Intervention Project: A randomized controlled trial of the effectiveness of speech and language therapy for school-age children who have pragmatic and social communication problems with or without autism spectrum disorder. *International Journal of Language & Communication Disorders, 47,* 233–244.

Adams, C., Lockton, E., Gaile, J., Earl, G., & Freed, J. (2012b). Implementation of a manualized communication intervention for school-aged children with pragmatic and social communication needs in a randomized controlled trial: The social communication intervention project. *International Journal of Language & Communication Disorders, 47,* 245–256.

Alarcon, N. B., & Rogers, M. A. (2007). *Supported communication intervention for aphasia.* Rockville: American Speech-Language-Hearing Association.

Alderman, N. (2007). Prevalence, characteristics and causes of aggressive behaviour observed within a neurobehavioural rehabilitation service: Predictors and implications for management. *Brain Injury, 21,* 891–911.

Alderman, N., Knight, C., & Henman, C. (2002). Aggressive behaviour observed within a neu-robehavioural rehabilitation service: Utility of the OAS-MNR in clinical audit and applied research. *Brain Injury, 16*, 469–489.

Allen, M. L., Haywood, S., Rajendran, G., & Branigan, H. (2011). Evidence for syntactic align-ment in children with autism. *Developmental Science, 14*, 540–548.

Amanzio, M., Geminiani, G., Leotta, D., & Cappa, S. (2008). Metaphor comprehension in Alzheimer's disease: Novelty matters. *Brain and Language, 107*, 1–10.

American Psychiatric Association. (2013). *Diagnostic and statistical manual of mental disorders* (5th ed.). Washington, DC: American Psychiatric Association.

Anastassiou-Hadjicharalambous, X., & Warden, D. (2008). Cognitive and affective perspective-taking in conduct-disordered children high and low on callous-unemotional traits. *Child and Adolescent Psychiatry and Mental Health, 2*, 16.

Andelic, N., Anke, A., Skandsen, T., Sigurdardottir, S., Sandhaug, M., Ader, T., et al. (2012). Incidence of hospital-admitted severe traumatic brain injury and in-hospital fatality in Norway: A national cohort study. *Neuroepidemiology, 38*, 259–267.

Anderson, P. J. (2008). Towards a developmental model of executive function. In V. Anderson, R. Jacobs, & P. J. Anderson (Eds.), *Executive functions and the frontal lobes: A lifespan per-spective* (pp. 3–22). London: Taylor & Francis.

Anderson, V. A., Morse, S. A., Catroppa, C., Haritou, F., & Rosenfeld, J. V. (2004). Thirty month outcome from early childhood head injury: A prospective analysis of neurobehavioural recov-ery. *Brain, 127*, 2608–2620.

Andersson, C. B., & Thomsen, P. H. (1998). Electively mute children: An analysis of 37 Danish cases. *Nordic Journal of Psychiatry, 52*, 231–238.

Andreasen, N. C. (1986). Scale for the assessment of thought, language, and communication (TLC). *Schizophrenia Bulletin, 12*, 473–482.

Andreetta, S., Cantagallo, A., & Marini, A. (2012). Narrative discourse in anomic aphasia. *Neuropsychologia, 50*, 1787–1792.

Andreou, C., Bozikas, V. P., Papouliakos, I., Kosmidis, M. H., Garyfallos, G., Karavatos, A., et al. (2008). Factor structure of the Greek translation of the scale for the assessment of thought, language and communication. *Australian and New Zealand Journal of Psychiatry, 42*, 636–642.

Angeleri, R., Bosco, F. M., Gabbatore, I., Bara, B. G., & Sacco, K. (2012). Assessment battery for communication (ABaCo): Normative data. *Behavior Research Methods, 44*, 845–861.

Angeleri, R., Bosco, F. M., Zettin, M., Sacco, K., Colle, L., & Bara, B. G. (2008). Communicative impairment in traumatic brain injury: A complete pragmatic assessment. *Brain and Language, 107*, 229–245.

Arkkila, E., Räsänen, P., Roine, R. P., Sintonen, H., & Vilkman, E. (2008). Health-related quality of life of adults with childhood diagnosis of specific language impairment. *Folia Phoniatrica et Logopaedica, 60*, 233–240.

Armstrong, K., Kose, S., Williams, L., Woolard, A., & Heckers, S. (2012). Impaired associative inference in patients with schizophrenia. *Schizophrenia Bulletin, 38*, 622–629.

Arnett, P. A., Rao, S. M., Grafman, J., Bernardin, L., Luchetta, T., Binder, J. R., et al. (1997). Executive functions in multiple sclerosis: An analysis of temporal ordering, semantic encod-ing, and planning abilities. *Neuropsychology, 11*, 535–544.

Arnett, W. L., Chenery, H. J., Angwin, A. J., Murdoch, B. E., Silburn, P. A., & Copland, D. A. (2010). Decreased semantic competitive inhibition in Parkinson's disease: Evidence from an investigation of word search performance. *International Journal of Speech-Language Pathology, 12*, 437–445.

Arnott, W. L., Jordan, F. M., Murdoch, B. E., & Lethlean, J. B. (1997). Narrative discourse in multiple sclerosis: An investigation of conceptual structure. *Aphasiology, 11*, 969–991.

Arnott, W. L., Sali, L., & Copland, D. (2011). Impaired reading comprehension in schizophrenia: Evidence for underlying phonological processing deficits. *Psychiatry Research, 187*, 6–10.

Asberg, J. (2010). Patterns of language and discourse comprehension skills in school-aged chil-dren with autism spectrum disorders. *Scandinavian Journal of Psychology, 51*, 534–539.

Asberg, J., Kopp, S., Berg-Kelly, K., & Gillberg, C. (2010). Reading comprehension, word decoding and spelling in girls with autism spectrum disorders (ASD) or attention-deficit/hyperactivity disorder (AD/HD): Performance and predictors. *International Journal of Language & Communication Disorders, 45,* 61–71.

Ash, S., McMillan, C., Gross, R. G., Cook, P., Morgan, B., Boller, A., et al. (2011). The organization of narrative discourse in Lewy body spectrum disorder. *Brain and Language, 119,* 30–41.

Ash, S., McMillan, C., Gunawardena, D., Avants, B., Morgan, B., Khan, A., et al. (2010). Speech errors in progressive non-fluent aphasia. *Brain and Language, 113,* 13–20.

Ash, S., Moore, P., Antani, S., McCawley, G., Work, M., & Grossman, M. (2006). Trying to tell a tale: Discourse impairments in progressive aphasia and frontotemporal dementia. *Neurology, 66,* 1405–1413.

Austin, J. L. (1962). *How to do things with words.* Oxford: Clarendon Press.

Auther, A. M., Smith, C. W., & Cornblatt, B. A. (2006). *Global functioning: Social scale (GF: Social).* Glen Oaks: Zucker-Hillside Hospital.

Averback, B. B., Evans, S., Chouhan, V., Bristow, E., & Shergill, S. S. (2011). Probabilistic learning and inference in schizophrenia. *Schizophrenia Research, 127,* 115–122.

Babikian, T., Satz, P., Zaucha, K., Light, R., Lewis, R. S., & Asarnow, R. F. (2011). The UCLA longitudinal study of neurocognitive outcomes following mild pediatric traumatic brain injury. *Journal of the International Neuropsychological Society, 17,* 886–895.

Bach, K. (1994). Semantic slack: What is said and more. In S. L. Tsohatzidis (ed.), *Foundations of speech act theory: Philosophical and linguistic perspectives* (pp. 267–291). London: Routledge.

Bach, L. J., Happé, F., Fleminger, S., & David, A. S. (2006). Intact theory of mind in TBI with behavioural disturbance. *Brain and Cognition, 60,* 196–198.

Baddeley, A. D. (1986). *Working memory.* Oxford: Oxford University Press.

Baddeley, A. D. (1992). Working memory. *Science, 255,* 556–559.

Baddeley, A. D. (2002). Fractionating the central executive. In D. T. Stuss & R. T. Knight (Eds.), *Principles of frontal lobe function* (pp. 246–260). New York: Oxford University Press.

Baddeley, A. D., & Hitch, G. (1974). Working memory. In G. A. Bower (Ed.), *The psychology of learning and motivation* (pp. 47–89). New York: Academic Press.

Baillargeon, R., Scott, R. M., & He, Z. (2010). False-belief understanding in infants. *Trends in Cognitive Sciences, 14,* 110–118.

Bak, T. H., & Hodges, J. R. (2004). The effects of motor neurone disease on language: Further evidence. *Brain and Language, 89,* 354–361.

Ball, L. J., Beukelman, D. R., & Pattee, G. L. (2004). Communication effectiveness of individuals with amyotrophic lateral sclerosis. *Journal of Communication Disorders, 37,* 197–215.

Bara, B. G. (2010). *Cognitive pragmatics: The mental processes of communication.* Cambridge: MIT Press.

Bara, B. G. (2011). Cognitive pragmatics: The mental processes of communication. *Intercultural Pragmatics, 8,* 443–485.

Bara, B. G., Bosco, F. M., & Bucciarelli, M. (1999). Developmental pragmatics in normal and abnormal children. *Brain and Language, 68,* 507–528.

Bara, B. G., Bucciarelli, M., & Colle, L. (2001). Communicative abilities in autism: Evidence for attentional deficits. *Brain and Language, 77,* 216–240.

Bara, B. G., Bucciarelli, M., & Geminiani, G. C. (2000). Development and decay of extra-linguistic communication. *Brain and Cognition, 43,* 21–27.

Bara, B. G., & Tirassa, M. (2000). Neuropragmatics: Brain and communication. *Brain and Language, 71,* 10–14.

Bara, B. G., Tirassa, M., & Zettin, M. (1997). Neuropragmatics: Neuropsychological constraints on formal theories of dialogue. *Brain and Language, 59,* 7–49.

Barnes, M. A., & Dennis, M. (1998). Discourse after early-onset hydrocephalus: Core deficits in children of average intelligence. *Brain and Language, 61,* 309–334.

Barnes, M. A., Faulkner, H., Wilkinson, M., & Dennis, M. (2004). Meaning construction and integration in children with hydrocephalus. *Brain and Language, 89,* 47–56.

Baron-Cohen, S., Golan, O., & Ashwin, E. (2012). Teaching emotion recognition to children with autism spectrum conditions. *BJEP Monograph Series II, Number 8—Educational Neuroscience, 1*, 115–127.

Baron-Cohen, S., Leslie, A. M., & Frith, U. (1985). Does the autistic child have a "theory of mind"? *Cognition, 21*, 37–46.

Bastiaanse, R., & Prins, R. (2014). Aphasia. In L. Cummings (Ed.), *Cambridge handbook of communication disorders* (pp. 224–246). Cambridge: Cambridge University Press.

Bates, E. (1976). *Language and context: The acquisition of pragmatics*. New York: Academic Press.

Bayles, K. A., Tomoeda, C. K., & Trosset, M. W. (1992). Relation of linguistic communication abilities of Alzheimer's patients to stage of disease. *Brain and Language, 42*, 454–472.

Bazin, N., Lefrere, F., Passerieux, C., Sarfati, Y., & Hardy-Baylé, M. C. (2002). Formal thought disorders: French translation of the thought, language and communication assessment scale. *L'Encéphale, 28*, 109–119.

Bearden, C. E., Wu, K. N., Caplan, R., & Cannon, T. D. (2011). Thought disorder and communication deviance as predictors of outcome in youth at clinical high risk for psychosis. *Journal of the American Academy of Child and Adolescent Psychiatry, 50*, 669–680.

Beauchamp, M., Catroppa, C., Godfrey, C., Morse, S., Rosenfeld, J. V., & Anderson, V. (2011). Selective changes in executive functioning ten years after severe childhood traumatic brain injury. *Developmental Neuropsychology, 36*, 578–595.

Becchio, C., Adenzato, M., & Bara, B. G. (2006). How the brain understands intention: Different neural circuits identify the componential features of motor and prior intentions. *Consciousness and Cognition, 15*, 64–74.

Begeer, S., Gevers, C., Clifford, P., Verhoeve, M., Kat, K., Hoddenbach, E., et al. (2011). Theory of mind training in children with autism: A randomized controlled trial. *Journal of Autism and Developmental Disorders, 41*, 997–1006.

Behrns, I., Ahlsén, E., & Wengelin, Å. (2010). Aphasia and text writing. *International Journal of Language & Communication Disorders, 45*, 230–243.

Beitchman, J. H., Adlaf, E. M., Douglas, L., Atkinson, L., Young, A., Johnson, C. J., et al. (2001). Comorbidity of psychiatric and substance use disorders in late adolescence: A cluster analytic approach. *American Journal of Drug and Alcohol Abuse, 27*, 421–440.

Beitchman, J. H., Douglas, L., Wilson, B., Johnson, C., Young, A., Atkinson, L., et al. (1999). Adolescent substance use disorders: Findings from a 14-year follow-up of speech/language-impaired and control children. *Journal of Clinical Child Psychology, 28*, 312–321.

Béjot, Y., Aboa-Eboulé, C., Durier, J., Rouaud, O., Jacquin, A., Ponavoy, E., et al. (2011). Prevalence of early dementia after first-ever stroke: A 24-year-population-based study. *Stroke, 42*, 607–612.

Bellack, A. S., Brown, C. H., & Thomas-Lorhman, S. (2006). Psychometric characteristics of role-play assessments of social skill in schizophrenia. *Behavior Therapy, 37*, 339–352.

Bellani, M., Moretti, A., Perlini, C., & Brambilla, P. (2011). Language disturbances in ADHD. *Epidemiology and Psychiatric Sciences, 20*, 311–315.

Benner, G. J. (2005). Language skills of elementary-aged children with emotional and behavioural disorders. *Great Plains Research, 15*, 251–265.

Bennett, K. J., Stephen Brown, K., Boyle, M., Racine, Y., & Offord, D. (2003). Does low reading achievement at school entry cause conduct problems? *Social Science & Medicine, 56*, 2443–2448.

Benton, E., & Bryan, K. (1996). Right cerebral hemisphere damage: Incidence of language problems. *International Journal of Rehabilitation Research, 19*, 47–54.

Ben-Yizhak, N., Yirmiya, N., Seidman, I., Alon, R., Lord, C., & Sigman, M. (2011). Pragmatic language and school related linguistic abilities in siblings of children with autism. *Journal of Autism and Developmental Disorders, 41*, 750–760.

Berg, E., Björnram, C., Hartelius, L., Laakso, K., & Johnels, B. (2003). High-level language difficulties in Parkinson's disease. *Clinical Linguistics & Phonetics, 17*, 63–80.

Berthiaume, K. S., Lorch, E. P., & Milich, R. (2010). Getting clued in: Inferential processing and comprehension monitoring in boys with ADHD. *Journal of Attention Disorders, 14*, 31–42.

Best, J. R., & Miller, P. H. (2010). A developmental perspective on executive function. *Child Development, 81*, 1641–1660.

Best, W., Greenwood, A., Grassly, J., & Hickin, J. (2008). Bridging the gap: Can impairment-based therapy for anomia have an impact at the psycho-social level? *International Journal of Language & Communication Disorders, 43*, 390–407.

Biddle, K. R., McCabe, A., & Bliss, L. S. (1996). Narrative skills following traumatic brain injury in children and adults. *Journal of Communication Disorders, 29*, 447–469.

Biederman, J., & Faraone, S. V. (2006). The effects of attention-deficit/hyperactivity disorder on employment and household income. *Medscape General Medicine, 8*, 12.

Biederman, J., Mick, E., Faraone, S. V., Braaten, E., Doyle, A., Spencer, T., et al. (2002). Influence of gender on attention deficit hyperactivity disorder in children referred to a psychiatric clinic. *American Journal of Psychiatry, 159*, 36–42.

Bignell, S., & Cain, K. (2007). Pragmatic aspects of communication and language comprehension in groups of children differentiated by teacher ratings of inattention and hyperactivity. *British Journal of Developmental Psychology, 25*, 499–512.

Birchwood, M., Smith, J., Cochrane, R., Wetton, S., & Copestake, S. (1990). The Social Functioning Scale. The development and validation of a new scale of social adjustment for use in family intervention programmes with schizophrenic patients. *British Journal of Psychiatry, 157*, 853–859.

Birkett, P., Clegg, J., Bhaker, R., Lee, K.-H., Mysore, A., Parks, R., et al. (2011). Schizophrenia impairs phonological speech production: A preliminary report. *Cognitive Neuropsychiatry, 16*, 40–49.

Bishop, D. V. M. (1998). Development of the Children's Communication Checklist (CCC): A method for assessing qualitative aspects of communicative impairment in children. *Journal of Child Psychology and Psychiatry, 39*, 879–891.

Bishop, D. V. M. (2000). Pragmatic language impairment: A correlate of SLI, a distinct subgroup, or part of the autistic continuum? In D. V. M. Bishop & L. B. Leonard (Eds.), *Speech and language impairments in children: Causes, characteristics, intervention and outcome* (pp. 99–113). Hove: Psychology Press Ltd.

Bishop, D. V. M. (2003). *Children's communication checklist—revised* (2nd ed.). London: Psychological Corporation.

Bishop, D. V. M. (2009). Genes, cognition, and communication: Insights from neurodevelopmental disorders. *Annals of the New York Academy of Sciences, 156*, 1–18.

Bishop, D. V. M., & Baird, G. (2001). Parent and teacher report of pragmatic aspects of communication: Use of the children's communication checklist in a clinical setting. *Developmental Medicine & Child Neurology, 43*, 809–818.

Bishop, D. V. M., Chan, J., Adams, C., Hartley, J., & Weir, F. (2000). Conversational responsiveness in specific language impairment: Evidence of disproportionate pragmatic difficulties in a subset of children. *Development and Psychopathology, 12*, 177–199.

Bishop, D. V. M., Laws, G., Adams, C., & Norbury, C. F. (2006). High heritability of speech and language impairments in 6-year-old twins demonstrated using parent and teacher report. *Behavior Genetics, 36*, 173–184.

Bishop, D. V. M., & Norbury, C. F. (2002). Exploring the borderlands of autistic disorder and specific language impairment: A study using standardised diagnostic instruments. *Journal of Child Psychology and Psychiatry, 43*, 917–929.

Bishop, D. V. M., & Norbury, C. F. (2005). Executive functions in children with communication impairments in relation to autistic symptomatology. I: Generativity. *Autism, 9*, 7–27.

Blake, L., & Margaret, T. (2003). Affective language and humor appreciation after right hemisphere brain damage. *Seminars in Speech and Language, 24*, 107–119.

Blake, L., & Margaret, T. (2006). Clinical relevance of discourse characteristics after right hemisphere brain damage. *American Journal of Speech-Language Pathology, 15*, 255–267.

Blanchard, L. T., Gurka, M. J., & Blackman, J. A. (2006). Emotional, developmental, and behavioral health of American children and their families: A report from the 2003 National Survey of Children's Health. *Pediatrics, 117*, e1202–e1212.

Blood, G. W., Blood, I. M., Michael Tramontana, G., Sylvia, A. J., Boyle, M. P., & Motzko, G. R. (2011). Self-reported experience of bullying of students who stutter: Relations with life satisfaction, life orientation, and self-esteem. *Perceptual and Motor Skills, 113*, 353–364.

Bloom, B., Cohen, R. A., & Freeman, G. (2011). Summary health statistics for U.S. children: National Health Interview Survey, 2010. *Vital and Health Statistics, 250*, 1–80.

Bo, S., Abu-Akel, A., Kongerslev, M., Haahr, U. H., & Simonsen, E. (2011). Risk factors for violence among patients with schizophrenia. *Clinical Psychology Review, 31*, 711–726.

Bock, M., Rogers, M. F., & Myles, B. S. (2001). Using social stories and comic strip conversations to interpret social situations for an adolescent with Asperger syndrome. *Intervention in School and Clinic, 36*, 310–313.

Bodden, M. E., Mollenhauer, B., Trenkwalder, C., Cabanel, N., Eggert, K. M., Unger, M. M., et al. (2010). Affective and cognitive theory of mind in patients with Parkinson's disease. *Parkinsonism & Related Disorders, 16*, 466–470.

Body, R., & Parker, M. (2005). Topic repetitiveness after traumatic brain injury: An emergent, jointly managed behaviour. *Clinical Linguistics & Phonetics, 19*, 379–392.

Body, R., Perkins, M., & McDonald, S. (1999). Pragmatics, cognition, and communication in traumatic brain injury. In S. McDonald, L. Togher, & C. Code (eds.), *Communication disorders following traumatic brain injury* (pp. 81–112). Hove: Psychology Press.

Bogart, E., Togher, L., Power, E., & Docking, K. (2012). Casual conversations between individuals with traumatic brain injury and their friends. *Brain Injury, 26*, 221–233.

Bora, E., Eryavuz, A., Kayahan, B., Sungu, G., & Veznedaroglu, B. (2006). Social functioning, theory of mind and neurocognition in outpatients with schizophrenia; mental state decoding may be a better predictor of social functioning than mental state reasoning. *Psychiatry Research, 145*, 95–103.

Bornhofen, C., & McDonald, S. (2008). Comparing strategies for treating emotion perception deficits in traumatic brain injury. *Journal of Head Trauma Rehabilitation, 23*, 103–115.

Bosco, F. M., Angeleri, R., Zuffranieri, M., Bara, B. G., & Sacco, K. (2012a). Assessment battery for communication: development of two equivalent forms. *Journal of Communication Disorders, 45*, 290–303.

Bosco, F. M., Bono, A., & Bara, B. G. (2012b). Recognition and repair of communicative failures: The interaction between theory of mind and cognitive complexity in schizophrenic patients. *Journal of Communication Disorders, 45*, 181–197.

Bosco, F. M., Bucciarelli, M., & Bara, B. G. (2006a). Recognition and repair of communicative failures: A developmental perspective. *Journal of Pragmatics, 38*, 1398–1429.

Bosco, F. M., Friedman, O., & Leslie, A. M. (2006b). Recognition of pretend and real actions in play by 1- and 2-year-olds: Early success and why they fail. *Cognitive Development, 21*, 3–10.

Botting, N., & Adams, C. (2005). Semantic and inferencing abilities in children with communication disorders. *International Journal of Language & Communication Disorders, 40*, 49–66.

Botting, N., & Conti-Ramsden, G. (2000). Social and behavioural difficulties in children with language impairment. *Child Language Teaching and Therapy, 16*, 105–120.

Boucher, J. (2012). Research review: Structural language in autistic spectrum disorder—characteristics and causes. *Journal of Child Psychology and Psychiatry, and Allied Disciplines, 53*, 219–233.

Bowie, C. R., & Harvey, P. D. (2008). Communication abnormalities predict functional outcomes in chronic schizophrenia: Differential associations with social and adaptive functions. *Schizophrenia Research, 103*, 240–247.

Boyle, C. A., Boulet, S., Schieve, L. A., Cohen, R. A., Blumberg, S. J., Yeargin-Allsopp, M., et al. (2011). Trends in the prevalence of developmental disabilities in US children, 1997–2008. *Pediatrics, 127*, 1034–1042.

Bozikas, V. P., Giannakou, M., Kosmidis, M. H., Kargopoulos, P., Kioseoglou, G., Liolios, D., et al. (2011). Insights into theory of mind in schizophrenia: The impact of cognitive impairment. *Schizophrenia Research, 130*, 130–136.

Braden, C., Hawley, L., Newman, J., Morey, C., Gerber, D., & Harrison-Felix, C. (2010). Social communication skills group treatment: A feasibility study for persons with traumatic brain injury and comorbid conditions. *Brain Injury, 24*, 1298–1310.

Brauner, C. B., & Stephens, C. B. (2006). Estimating the prevalence of early childhood serious emotional/behavioral disorders: Challenges and recommendations. *Public Health Reports, 121*, 303–310.

Brito e Silva, E. T., B., Caixeta, L. F., Dias Soares, V. L., & Fonseca Sagawa, G. R. (2011). HIV-associated dementia in older adults: Clinical and tomographic aspects. *International Psychogeriatrics, 23*, 1061–1069.

Brock, J. (2007). Language abilities in Williams syndrome: A critical review. *Development and Psychopathology, 19*, 97–127.

Brookshire, B. L., Chapman, S. B., Song, J., & Levin, H. S. (2000). Cognitive and linguistic correlates of children's discourse after closed head injury: A three-year follow-up. *Journal of the International Neuropsychological Society, 6*, 741–751.

Brown, T. E. (2006). Executive functions and attention deficit hyperactivity disorder: Implications of two conflicting views. *International Journal of Disability, Development and Education, 53*, 35–46.

Brownell, M. D. (2002). Musically adapted social stories to modify behaviors in students with autism: Four case studies. *Journal of Music Therapy, 39*, 117–144.

Brownlie, E. B., Beitchman, J. H., Escobar, M., Young, A., Atkinson, L., Johnson, C., et al. (2004). Early language impairment and young adult delinquent and aggressive behaviour. *Journal of Abnormal Child Psychology, 32*, 453–467.

Bruce, B., Thernlund, G., & Nettelbladt, U. (2006). ADHD and language impairment: A study of the parent questionnaire FTF (Five to Fifteen). *European Child & Adolescent Psychiatry, 15*, 52–60.

Brundage, S. B., Graap, K., Gibbons, K. F., Ferrer, M., & Brooks, J. (2006). Frequency of stuttering during challenging and supportive virtual reality job interviews. *Journal of Fluency Disorders, 31*, 325–339.

Brüne, M., Blank, K., Witthaus, H., & Saft, C. (2011). "Theory of mind" is impaired in Huntington's disease. *Movement Disorders, 26*, 671–678.

Brüne, M., & Bodenstein, L. (2005). Proverb comprehension reconsidered—"theory of mind" and the pragmatic use of language in schizophrenia. *Schizophrenia Research, 75*, 233–239.

Bryan, K. L. (1989). *The right hemisphere language battery*. Leicester: Far Communications.

Bryan, K. (2004). Preliminary study of the prevalence of speech and language difficulties in young offenders. *International Journal of Language & Communication Disorders, 39*, 391–400.

Bryan, K., Freer, J., & Furlong, C. (2007). Language and communication difficulties in juvenile offenders. *International Journal of Language & Communication Disorders, 42*, 505–520.

Bucciarelli, M., Colle, L., & Bara, B. G. (2003). How children comprehend speech acts and communicative gestures. *Journal of Pragmatics, 35*, 207–241.

Buchanan, R. J., Martin, R. A., Moore, L., Wang, S., & Ju, H. (2005). Nursing home residents with multiple sclerosis and dementia compared to other multiple sclerosis residents. *Multiple Sclerosis, 11*, 610–616.

Budd, M. A., Kortte, K., Cloutman, L., Newhart, M., Gottesman, R. F., Davis, C., et al. (2010). The nature of naming errors in primary progressive aphasia versus acute post-stroke aphasia. *Neuropsychology, 24*, 581–589.

Buitelaar, J. K., van der Wees, M., Swaab-Barneveld, H., & van der Gaag, R. J. (1999). Theory of mind and emotion-recognition functioning in autistic spectrum disorders and in psychiatric control and normal children. *Development and Psychopathology, 11*, 39–58.

Burdon, L., & Dickens, G. (2009). Asperger syndrome and offending behaviour. *Learning Disability Practice, 12*, 14–20.

Byrne, M. E., Crowe, T. A., & Griffin, P. S. (1998). Pragmatic language behaviors of adults diagnosed with chronic schizophrenia. *Psychological Reports, 83*, 835–846.

Bögels, S. M., Alden, L., Beidel, D. C., Clark, L. A., Pine, D. S., Stein, M. B., et al. (2010). Social anxiety disorder: Questions and answers for the DSM-V. *Depression and Anxiety, 27*, 168–189.

Caglayan, A. O. (2010). Genetic causes of syndromic and non-syndromic autism. *Developmental Medicine and Child Neurology, 52*, 130–138.

Carbone, D., Schmidt, L. A., Cunningham, C. C., McHolm, A. E., Edison, S., St. Pierre, J., & Boyle, M. H. (2010). Behavioral and socio-emotional functioning in children with selective mutism: A comparison with anxious and typically developing children across multiple informants. *Journal of Abnormal Child Psychology, 38*, 1057–1067

Cardy, J. E., Cardy, O., Tannock, R., Johnson, A. M., & Johnson, C. J. (2010). The contribution of processing impairments to SLI: Insights from attention-deficit/hyperactivity disorder. *Journal of Communication Disorders, 43*, 77–91.

Carlomagno, S., Giannotti, S., Vorano, L., & Marini, A. (2011). Discourse information content in non-aphasic adults with brain injury: A pilot study. *Brain Injury, 25*, 1010–1018.

Carlomagno, S., Santoro, A., Menditti, A., Pandolfi, M., & Marini, A. (2005). Referential communication in Alzheimer's type dementia. *Cortex, 41*, 520–534.

Carota, A., & Bogousslavsky, J. (2012). Mood disorders after stroke. *Frontiers of Neurology and Neuroscience, 30*, 70–74.

Carretti, B., Cornoldi, C., De Beni, R., & Romanò, M. (2005). Updating in working memory: A comparison of good and poor comprehenders. *Journal of Experimental Child Psychology, 91*, 45–66.

Carroll, J. M., Maughan, B., Goodman, R., & Meltzer, H. (2005). Literacy difficulties and psychiatric disorders: Evidence for comorbidity. *Journal of Child Psychology and Psychiatry, 46*, 524–532.

Carrow-Woolfolk, E. (1999). *Comprehensive assessment of spoken language*. Circle Pines: American Guidance Service.

Carruthers, P., & Smith, P. K. (1996). Introduction. In P. Carruthers & P. K. Smith (Eds.), *Theories of theories of mind* (pp. 1–10). Cambridge: Cambridge University Press.

Cashin, A., & Newman, C. (2009). Autism in the criminal justice detention system: A review of the literature. *Journal of Forensic Nursing, 5*, 70–75.

Castelli, I., Pini, A., Alberoni, M., Liverta-Sempio, O., Baglio, F., Massaro, D., et al. (2011). Mapping levels of theory of mind in Alzheimer's disease: A preliminary study. *Aging & Mental Health, 15*, 157–168.

Cavallo, M., Adenzato, M., Macpherson, S. E., Karwig, G., Enrici, I., & Abrahams, S. (2011). Evidence of social understanding impairment in patients with amyotrophic lateral sclerosis. *PLoS One, 6*, e25948.

Centers for Disease Control and Prevention. (2012a). *What are developmental disabilities?* Retrieved from www.cdc.gov/ncbddd/dd/default.htm

Centers for Disease Control and Prevention. (2012b). Prevalence of autism spectrum disorders—autism and developmental disabilities monitoring network, 14 sites, United States, 2008. *Morbidity and Mortality Weekly Report. Surveillance Summaries, 61*, 1–19.

Champagne-Lavau, M., Fossard, M., Martel, G., Chapdelaine, C., Blouin, G., Rodriguez, J.-P., et al. (2009). Do patients with schizophrenia attribute mental states in a referential communication task? *Cognitive Neuropsychiatry, 14*, 217–239.

Chan, J. M., & O'Reilly, M. F. (2008). A Social stories™ intervention package for students with autism in inclusive classroom settings. *Journal of Applied Behavior Analysis, 41*, 405–409.

Channon, S., & Watts, M. (2003). Pragmatic language interpretation after closed head injury: Relationship to executive functioning. *Cognitive Neuropsychiatry, 8*, 243–260.

Chapman, S. B., Gamino, J. F., Cook, L. G., Hanten, G., Li, X., & Levin, H. S. (2006). Impaired discourse gist and working memory in children after brain injury. *Brain and Language, 97*, 178–188.

Chapman, S. B., Highley, A. P., & Thompson, J. L. (1998). Discourse in fluent aphasia and Alzheimer's disease: Linguistic and pragmatic considerations. *Journal of Neurolinguistics, 11*, 55–78.

Chapman, S. B., Sparks, G., Levin, H. S., Dennis, M., Roncadin, C., Zhang, L., et al. (2004). Discourse macrolevel processing after severe pediatric traumatic brain injury. *Developmental Neuropsychology, 25*, 37–60.

Chapman, S. B., Ulatowska, H. K., Franklin, L. R., Shobe, A. E., Thompson, J. L., & McIntire, D. D. (1997). Proverb interpretation in fluent aphasia and Alzheimer's disease: Implications beyond abstract thinking. *Aphasiology, 11*, 337–350.

Charman, T., Baron-Cohen, S., Swettenham, J., Baird, G., Cox, A., & Drew, A. (2000). Testing joint attention, imitation, and play as infancy precursors to language and theory of mind. *Cognitive Development, 15*, 481–498.

Cheang, H. S., & Pell, M. D. (2006). A study of humour and communicative intention following right hemisphere stroke. *Clinical Linguistics & Phonetics, 20*, 447–462.

Chenery, H. J., Copland, D. A., & Murdoch, B. E. (2002). Complex language functions and sub-cortical mechanisms: Evidence from Huntington's disease and patients with non-thalamic subcortical lesions. *International Journal of Language & Communication Disorders, 37*, 459–474.

Chevallier, C., Wilson, D., Happé, F., & Noveck, I. (2010). Scalar inferences in autism spectrum disorders. *Journal of Autism and Developmental Disorders, 40*, 1104–1117.

Chevallier, C., Kohls, G., Troiani, V., Brodkin, E. S., & Schultz, R. T. (2012). The social motivation theory of autism. *Trends in Cognitive Sciences, 16*, 231–239.

Chien, H.-C., Ku, C.-H., Lu, R.-B., Chu, H., Tao, Y.-H., & Chou, Kuei.-Ru. (2003). Effects of social skills training on improving social skills of patients with schizophrenia. *Archives of Psychiatric Nursing, 17*, 228–236.

Chin, H. Y., & Bernard-Opitz, V. (2000). Teaching conversational skills to children with autism: Effect on the development of a theory of mind. *Journal of Autism and Developmental Disorders, 30*, 569–583.

Ciaramidaro, A., Adenzato, M., Enrici, I., Erk, S., Pia, L., Bara, B. G., et al. (2007). The intentional network: How the brain reads varieties of intentions. *Neuropsychologia, 45*, 3105–3113.

Clark, H. H. (1992). *Arenas of language use*. Chicago: The University of Chicago Press.

Clegg, J., Hollis, C., Mawhood, L., & Rutter, M. (2005). Developmental language disorders—a follow-up in later adult life. Cognitive, language and psychosocial outcomes. *Journal of Child Psychology and Psychiatry, 46*, 128–149.

Cleland, J., Gibbon, F., Peppé, S., O'Hare, A., & Rutherford, M. (2010). Phonetic and phonological errors in children with high functioning autism and Asperger syndrome. *International Journal of Speech-Language Pathology, 12*, 69–76.

Cocoran, R. (2003). Inductive reasoning and the understanding of intention in schizophrenia. *Cognitive Neuropsychiatry, 8*, 223–235.

Coelho, C. A., & Flewellyn, L. (2003). Longitudinal assessment of coherence in an adult with fluent aphasia. *Aphasiology, 17*, 173–182.

Coelho, C. A., Grela, B., Corso, M., Gamble, A., & Feinn, R. (2005a). Microlinguistic deficits in the narrative discourse of adults with traumatic brain injury. *Brain Injury, 19*, 1139–1145.

Coelho, C., Ylvisaker, M., & Turkstra, L. S. (2005b). Nonstandardized assessment approaches for individuals with traumatic brain injuries. *Seminars in Speech and Language, 26*, 223–241.

Cohan, S. L., Chavira, D. A., Shipon-Blum, E., Hitchcock, C., Roesch, S. C., & Stein, M. B. (2008). Refining the classification of children with selective mutism: A latent profile analysis. *Journal of Clinical Child and Adolescent Psychiatry, 37*, 770–784.

Cohen, N. J., Vallance, D. D., Barwick, M., Im, N., Menna, R., Horodezky, N. B., et al. (2000). The interface between ADHD and language impairment: An examination of language, achievement, and cognitive processing. *Journal of Child Psychology and Psychiatry, 41*, 353–362.

Colle, L., Baron-Cohen, S., Wheelwright, S., & van der Lely, H. K. (2008). Narrative discourse in adults with high-functioning autism or Asperger syndrome. *Journal of Autism and Developmental Disorders, 38*, 28–40.

Colvert, E., Rutter, M., Kreppner, J., Beckett, C., Castle, J., Groothues, C., et al. (2008). Do theory of mind and executive function deficits underlie the adverse outcomes associated with profound early deprivation?: Findings from the English and Romanian adoptees study. *Journal of Abnormal Child Psychology, 36*, 1057–1068.

Comblain, A., & Elbouz, M. (2002). The fragile-X syndrome: What about the deficit in the pragmatic component of language? *Journal of Cognitive Education and Psychology, 2,* 244–265.

Condray, R., Steinhauer, S. R., van Kammen, D. P., & Kasparek, A. (2002). The language system in schizophrenia: Effects of capacity and linguistic structure. *Schizophrenia Bulletin, 28,*
475–490.

Confavreux, C., & Vukusic, S. (2006). Natural history of multiple sclerosis: A unifying concept.
Brain, 129, 606–616.

Constantino, J. N. (2002). *Social responsiveness scale.* Los Angeles: Western Psychological
Services.

Constantino, J. N., & Gruber, C. P. (2005). *Social responsiveness scale (SRS).* Los Angeles:
Western Psychological Services.

Conti-Ramsden, G., & Botting, N. (2004). Social difficulties and victimization in children with
SLI at 11 years of age. *Journal of Speech, Language, and Hearing Research, 47,* 145–161.

Conti-Ramsden, G., Durkin, K., Simkin, Z., & Knox, E. (2009). Specific language impairment
and school outcomes. I: Identifying and explaining variability at the end of compulsory education. *International Journal of Language & Communication Disorders, 44,* 15–35.

Coplan, R. J., & Weeks, M. (2009). Shy and soft-spoken: Shyness, pragmatic language, and
socio-emotional adjustment in early childhood. *Infant and Child Development, 18,* 238–254.

Cordery, R. J., Alner, K., Cipolotti, L., Ron, M., Kennedy, A., Collinge, J., et al. (2005). The neuropsychology of variant CJD: A comparative study with inherited and sporadic forms of prion
disease. *Journal of Neurology, Neurosurgery, and Psychiatry, 76,* 330–336.

Cornish, K., Burack, J. A., Rahman, A., Munir, F., Russo, N., & Grant, C. (2005). Theory of
mind deficits in children with fragile X syndrome. *Journal of Intellectual Disability Research,
49,* 372–378.

Cornwell, P. L., Murdoch, B. E., Ward, E. C., & Kellie, S. (2003). Perceptual evaluation of
motor speech following treatment for childhood cerebellar tumour. *Clinical Linguistics &
Phonetics, 17,* 597–615.

Coster, F. W., Goorhuis-Brouwer, S. M., Nakken, H., & Lutje Spelberg, H. C. (1999). Specific
language impairments and behavioural problems. *Folia Phoniatrica et Logopaedica, 51,*
99–107.

Côté, H., Payer, M., Giroux, F., & Joanette, Y. (2007). Towards a description of clinical communication impairment profiles following right-hemisphere damage. *Aphasiology, 21,* 739–749.

Covey, T. J., Zivadinov, R., Shucard, J. L., & Shucard, D. W. (2011). Information process-
ing speed, neural inefficiency, and working memory performance in multiple sclerosis:
Differential relationships with structural magnetic resonance imaging. *Journal of Clinical and
Experimental Neuropsychology, 33,* 1129–1145.

Covington, M. A., He, C., Brown, C., Naçi, L., McClain, J. T., Fjordbak, B. S., et al. (2005).
Schizophrenia and the structure of language: The linguist's view. *Schizophrenia Research, 77,*
85–98.

Cram, D., & Hedley, P. (2005). Pronouns and procedural meaning: The relevance of spaghetti
code and paranoid delusion. *Oxford Working Papers in Linguistics, Philology and Phonetics,
10,* 187–210.

Crone, E. A., Somsen, R. J., Zanolie, K., & van der Molen, M. W. (2006). A heart rate analysis of
developmental change in feedback processing and rule shifting from childhood to early adulthood. *Journal of Experimental Child Psychology, 95,* 99–116.

Crozier, S., & Tincani, M. (2007). Effects of social stories on prosocial behaviour of preschool
children with autism spectrum disorders. *Journal of Autism and Developmental Disorders,
37,* 1803–1814.

Crystal, D., & Varley, R. (1998). *Introduction to language pathology.* London: Whurr.

Cuerva, A. G., Sabe, L., Kuzis, G., Tiberti, C., Dorrego, F., & Starkstein, S. E. (2001). Theory of
mind and pragmatic abilities in dementia. *Neuropsychiatry, Neuropsychology, and Behavioral
Neurology, 14,* 153–158.

Cuetos, F., Herrera, E., & Ellis, A. W. (2010). Impaired word recognition in Alzheimer's disease:
The role of age of acquisition. *Neuropsychologia, 48,* 3329–3334.

Cullen, B., Samuels, J., Grados, M., Landa, R., Joseph Bienvenu, O., Liang, K.-Y., et al. (2008). Social and communication difficulties and obsessive-compulsive disorder. *Psychopathology, 41*, 194–200.

Cummings, L. (2002). Why we need to avoid theorising about rationality: A Putnamian criticism of Habermas's epistemology. *Social Epistemology, 16*, 117–131.

Cummings, L. (2005). *Pragmatics: A multidisciplinary perspective.* Edinburgh: Edinburgh University Press.

Cummings, L. (2007a). Pragmatics and adult language disorders: Past achievements and future directions. *Seminars in Speech and Language, 28*, 98–112.

Cummings, L. (2007b). Clinical pragmatics: A field in search of phenomena? *Language & Communication, 27*, 396–432.

Cummings, L. (2008). *Clinical linguistics.* Edinburgh: Edinburgh University Press.

Cummings, L. (2009). *Clinical pragmatics.* Cambridge: Cambridge University Press.

Cummings, L. (2010a). Clinical pragmatics. In L. Cummings (Ed.), *The Routledge pragmatics encyclopedia* (pp. 40–43). London: Routledge.

Cummings, L. (2010b). Neuropragmatics. In L. Cummings (ed.), *The Routledge pragmatics encyclopedia* (pp. 292–294). London: Routledge.

Cummings, L. (2011). Pragmatic disorders and their social impact. *Pragmatics and Society, 2*, 17–36.

Cummings, L. (2012a). Pragmatic disorders. In H.-J. Schmid (ed.), *Cognitive pragmatics* (Vol. 4, pp. 291–315). Handbook of Pragmatics. Berlin: De Gruyter.

Cummings, L. (2012b). Establishing diagnostic criteria: The role of clinical pragmatics. *Lodz Papers in Pragmatics, 8*, 61–84.

Cummings, L. (2012c). Theorising context: The case of clinical pragmatics. In R. Finkbeiner, J. Meibauer, & P. Schumacher (eds.), *What is context? Theoretical and experimental evidence* (pp. 55–80). Amsterdam: John Benjamins.

Cummings, L. (2012d). Theorising in pragmatics: Commentary on Bara's cognitive pragmatics: The mental processes of communication (MIT Press, 2010). *Intercultural Pragmatics, 9*, 113–120.

Cummings, L. (2013a). Clinical pragmatics and theory of mind. In A. Capone, F. Lo Piparo, & M. Carapezza (eds.), *Perspectives on linguistic pragmatics* (Vol. 2, pp. 23–56). Series: Perspectives in pragmatics, philosophy & psychology. Dordrecht: Springer.

Cummings, L. (2013b). Clinical linguistics: A primer. *International Journal of Language Studies, 7*, 1–30.

Cummings, L. (2013c). Clinical linguistics: State of the art. *International Journal of Language Studies, 7*, 1–32

Cummings, L. (2014a). *Communication disorders.* Houndmills: Palgrave Macmillan.

Cummings, L. (2014b). Pragmatic disorders and theory of mind. In L. Cummings (ed.), *Cambridge handbook of communication disorders* (pp. 559–577). Cambridge: Cambridge University Press.

Cummings, L. (2014c). Pragmatics. In N. Whitworth & R.-A. Knight (Eds.), *Methods in teaching clinical phonetics and linguistics.* Guildford: J&R Press.

Cummings, L. (2014d). Clinical pragmatics. In Y. Huang (ed.), *Oxford handbook of pragmatics.* Oxford: Oxford University Press.

Cutica, I., Bucciarelli, M., & Bara, B. (2006). Neuropragmatics: Extralinguistic pragmatic ability is better preserved in left-hemisphere-damaged patients than in right-hemisphere-damaged patients. *Brain and Language, 98*, 12–25.

Dahlberg, C. A., Cusick, C. P., Hawley, L. A., Newman, J. K., Morey, C. E., Harrison-Felix, C. L., et al. (2007). Treatment efficacy of social communication skills training after traumatic brain injury: A randomized treatment and deferred treatment controlled trial. *Archives of Physical Medicine and Rehabilitation, 88*, 1561–1573.

Daily, D. K., Ardinger, H. H., & Holmes, G. E. (2000). Identification and evaluation of mental retardation. *American Family Physician, 61*, 1059–1067.

Damico, J. S. (1985). Clinical discourse analysis: A functional approach to language assessment. In C. S. Simon (Ed.), *Communication skills and classroom success* (pp. 165–203). London: Taylor & Francis.

Damico, J. S. (1991). Clinical discourse analysis: A functional approach to language assessment. Assessment and therapy methodologies for language and learning disabled students. In

C. S. Simon (ed.), Communication skills and classroom success (pp. 125–150). Eau Claire: Thinking Publications.

DaParma, A., Geffner, D., & Martin, N. (2011). Prevalence and nature of language impairment in children with attention deficit/hyperactivity disorder. *Contemporary Issues in Communication Science and Disorders, 38*, 119–125.

Dardier, V., Bernicot, J., Delanoë, A., Vanberten, M., Fayada, C., Chevignard, M., et al. (2011). Severe traumatic brain injury, frontal lesions, and social aspects of language use: A study of French-speaking adults. *Journal of Communication Disorders, 44*, 359–378.

David, N., Aumann, C., Bewernick, B. H., Santos, N. S., Lehnhardt, F. G., & Vogeley, K. (2010). Investigation of mentalizing and visuospatial perspective taking for self and other in Asperger syndrome. *Journal of Autism and Developmental Disorders, 40*, 290–299.

Davidson, B., Worrall, L., & Hickson, L. (2006). Social communication in older age: Lessons from people with aphasia. *Topics in Stroke Rehabilitation, 13*, 1–13.

Davidson, P. S. R., Gao, F. Q., Mason, W. P., Winocur, G., & Anderson, N. D. (2008). Verbal fluency, trail making, and Wisconsin card sorting test performance following right frontal lobe tumor resection. *Journal of Clinical and Experimental Neuropsychology, 30*, 18–32.

Davis, M. H. (1983). Measuring individual differences in empathy: Evidence for a multidimensional approach. *Journal of Personality and Social Psychology, 44*, 113–126.

Dawes, S., Suarez, P., Casey, C. Y., Cherner, M., Marcotte, T. D., Letendre, S., Grant, I., Heaton, R. K., & HNRC Group. (2008). Variable patterns of neuropsychological performance in HIV-1 infection. *Journal of Clinical and Experimental Neuropsychology, 30*, 613–626.

De Carvalho, I. A. M., Bahia, V. S. & Mansur, L. L. (2008). Functional communication ability in frontotemporal lobar degeneration and Alzheimer's disease. *Dementia & Neuropsychologia, 2*, 31–36.

De Neys, W., & Schaeken, W. (2007). When people are more logical under cognitive load: Dual task impact on scalar implicature. Experimental Psychology 54:128-133

De Rijk, M. C., Breteler, M. M., Graveland, G. A., Ott, A., Grobbee, D. E., van de Meché, F. G., et al. (1995). Prevalence of Parkinson's disease in the elderly: The Rotterdam study. *Neurology, 45*, 2143–2146.

De Smet, H. J., Baillieux, H., Wackenier, P., De Praeter, M., Engelborghs, S., Paquier, P. F, et al. (2009). Long-term cognitive deficits following posterior fossa tumor resection: a neuropsychological and functional neuroimaging follow-up study. *Neuropsychology, 23*, 694–704

Demir, S. Ö., Görgülü, G., & Köseoğlu, F. (2006). Comparison of rehabilitation outcome in patients with aphasic and non-aphasic traumatic brain injury. *Journal of Rehabilitation Medicine, 38*, 68–71.

Dennis, M., & Barnes, M. A. (1993). Oral discourse after early-onset hydrocephalus: Linguistic ambiguity, figurative language, speech acts, and script-based inferences. *Journal of Pediatric Psychology, 18*, 639–652.

Dennis, M., & Barnes, M. (2001). Comprehension of literal, inferential, and intentional text comprehension in children with mild or severe closed-head injury. *Journal of Head Trauma Rehabilitation, 16*, 456–468.

Dennis, M., Lazenby, A. L., & Lockyer, L. (2001a). Inferential language in high-function children with autism. *Journal of Autism and Developmental Disorders, 31*, 47–54.

Dennis, M., Purvis, K., Barnes, M. A., Wilkinson, M., & Winner, E. (2001b). Understanding of literal truth, ironic criticism, and deceptive praise following childhood head injury. *Brain and Language, 78*, 1–16.

Department for Education and Employment. (1994). *Code of practice for the identification and assessment of special educational needs.* London: DfEE.

Déry, M., Toupin, J., Pauzé, R., Mercier, H., & Fortin, L. (1999). Neuropsychological characteristics of adolescents with conduct disorder: Association with attention-deficit-hyperactivity and aggression. *Journal of Abnormal Child Psychology, 27*, 225–236.

Dewart, H., & Summers, S. [1988] (1995). *The pragmatics profile of early communication skills.* Windsor: NFER-NELSON

Di Legge, S., Saposnik, G., Nilanont, Y., & Hachinski, V. (2006). Neglecting the difference: Does right or left matter in stroke outcome after thrombolysis? *Stroke, 37*, 2066–2069.

Di Rocco, C., Chieffo, D., Frassanito, P., Caldarelli, M., Massimi, L., & Tamburrini, G. (2011). Heralding cerebellar mutism: evidence for pre-surgical language impairment as primary risk factor in posterior fossa surgery. *Cerebellum, 10*, 551–562.

Di Rocco, C., Chieffo, D., Pettorini, B. L., Massimi, L., Caldarelli, M., & Tamburrini, G. (2010). Preoperative and postoperative neurological, neuropsychological and behavioral impairment in children with posterior cranial fossa astrocytomas and medulloblastomas: The role of the tumor and the impact of the surgical treatment. *Child's Nervous System, 26*, 1173–1188.

Diamond, A., Kirkham, N., & Amso, D. (2002). Conditions under which young children can hold two rules in mind and inhibit a prepotent response. *Developmental Psychology, 38*, 352–362.

Dickerson, F. B., Boronow, J. J., Stallings, C. R., Origoni, A. E., Cole, S., & Yolken, R. H. (2004). Association between cognitive functioning and employment status of persons with bipolar disorder. *Psychiatric Services, 55*, 54–58.

Dickey, C. C., Panych, L. P., Voglmaier, M. M., Niznikiewicz, M. A., Terry, D. P., Murphy, C., et al. (2011). Facial emotion recognition and facial affect display in schizotypal personality disorder. *Schizophrenia Research, 131*, 242–249.

Dickey, L., Kagan, A., Patrice Lindsay, M., Fang, J., Rowland, A., & Black, S. (2010). Incidence and profile of inpatient stroke-induced aphasia in Ontario, Canada. *Archives of Physical Medicine and Rehabilitation, 91*, 196–202.

Dickinson, D., Bellack, A. S., & Gold, J. M. (2007). Social/communication skills, cognition, and vocational functioning in schizophrenia. *Schizophrenia Bulletin, 33*, 1213–20.

Diesfeldt, H. F. (2011). The phonological variant of primary progressive aphasia, a single case study. *Tijdschrift voor Gerontologie en Geriatrie, 42*, 79–90.

Dipper, L. T., Bryan, K. L., & Tyson, J. (1997). Bridging inference and relevance theory: An account of right hemisphere damage. *Clinical Linguistics & Phonetics, 11*, 213–228.

Dirnberger, G., Frith, C. D., & Jahanshahi, M. (2005). Executive dysfunction in Parkinson's disease is associated with altered pallidal-frontal processing. *Neuroimage, 25*, 588–599.

Docking, K. M., Murdoch, B. E., & Suppiah, R. (2007). The impact of a cerebellar tumour on language function in childhood. *Folia Phoniatrica et Logopaedica, 59*, 190–200.

Docking, K. M., Ward, E. C., & Murdoch, B. E. (2005). Language outcomes subsequent to treatment of brainstem tumour in childhood. *NeuroRehabilitation, 20*, 107–124.

Dolan, M., & Fullam, R. (2004). Theory of mind and mentalizing ability in antisocial personality disorders with and without psychopathy. *Psychological Medicine, 34*, 1093–1102.

Donno, R., Parker, G., Gilmour, J., & Skuse, D. H. (2010). Social communication deficits in disruptive primary-school children. *British Journal of Psychiatry, 196*, 282–289.

Douglas, J. M. (2010a). Relation of executive functioning to pragmatic outcome following severe traumatic brain injury. *Journal of Speech, Language, and Hearing Research, 53*, 365–382.

Douglas, J. M. (2010b). Using the La Trobe Communication Questionnaire to measure perceived social communication ability in adolescents with traumatic brain injury. *Brain Impairment, 11*, 171–182.

Douglas, J. M., Bracy, C. A., & Snow, P. C. (2007). Measuring perceived communicative ability after traumatic brain injury: Reliability and validity of the La Trobe Communication Questionnaire. *Journal of Head Trauma Rehabilitation, 22*, 31–38.

Douglas, J. M., O'Flaherty, C. A., & Snow, P. C. (2000). Measuring perception of communicative ability: The development and evaluation of the La Trobe Communication Questionnaire. *Aphasiology, 14*, 251–268.

Dreessen, L., Arntz, A., Hendriks, T., Keune, N., & van den Hout, M. (1999). Avoidant personality disorder and implicit schema-congruent information processing bias: A pilot study with a pragmatic inference task. *Behaviour Research and Therapy, 37*, 619–632.

Drew, A., Baird, G., Taylor, E., Milne, E., & Charman, T. (2007). The Social Communication Assessment for Toddlers with Autism (SCATA): An instrument to measure the frequency, form and function of communication in toddlers with autism spectrum disorder. *Journal of Autism and Developmental Disorders, 37*, 648–666.

Duchan, J. F. (1984). Language assessment: The pragmatics revolution. In R. C. Naremore (Ed.), *Language science: Recent advances* (pp. 147–180). San Diego: College-Hill Press.

Duchan, J. F. (2011). A history of speech-language pathology: The pragmatics revolution 1975–2000. Retrieved from www.acsu.buffalo.edu/~duchan/1975-2000.html

Dumontheil, I., Apperly, I. A., & Blakemore, S.-J. (2010). Online usage of theory of mind continues to develop in late adolescence. *Developmental Science, 13*, 331–338.

Dunn, L. M., Dunn, L. M., Whetton, C., & Burley, J. (1997). The British picture vocabulary scale (2nd ed.). National Foundation for Educational Research, NFER-Nelson.

Durkin, K., Fraser, J., & Conti-Ramsden, G. (2012). School-age prework experiences of young people with a history of specific language impairment. *Journal of Special Education, 45*, 242–255.

Eales, M. J. (1993). Pragmatic impairments in adults with childhood diagnoses of autism or developmental receptive language disorder. *Journal of Autism and Developmental Disorders, 23*, 593–617.

Ecker, U. K., Lewandowsky, S., Oberauer, K., & Chee, A. E. (2010). The components of working memory updating: An experimental decomposition and individual differences. *Journal of Experimental Psychology. Learning, Memory, and Cognition, 36*, 170–189.

Eddy, C. M., Mitchell, I. J., Beck, S. R., Cavanna, A. E., & Rickards, H. E. (2010). Impaired comprehension of nonliteral language in Tourette syndrome. *Cognitive and Behavioral Neurology, 23*, 178–184.

El Hachioui, H., van de Sandt-Koenderman, M. V., Dippel, D. W., Koudstaal, P. J., & Visch-Brink, E. G. (2011). A 3-year evolution of linguistic disorders in aphasia after stroke. *International Journal of Rehabilitation Research, 34*, 215–221.

El Hachioui, H., Sandt-Koenderman, M. W., Dippel, D. W., Koudstaal, P. J., & Visch-Brink, E. G. (2012). The ScreeLing: Occurrence of linguistic deficits in acute aphasia post-stroke. *Journal of Rehabilitation Medicine, 44*, 429–435.

Elbro, C., Dalby, M., & Maarbjerg, S. (2011). Language-learning impairments: A 30-year follow-up of language-impaired children with and without psychiatric, neurological and cognitive difficulties. *International Journal of Language & Communication Disorders, 46*, 437–448.

Elliott, R. (2003). Executive functions and their disorders. *British Medical Bulletin, 65*, 49–59.

Ellis, C., & Peach, R. K. (2009). Sentence planning following traumatic brain injury. *NeuroRehabilitation, 24*, 255–266.

Ellis, C., Rosenbek, J. C., Rittman, M. R., & Boylstein, C. A. (2005). Recovery of cohesion in narrative discourse after left-hemisphere stroke. *Journal of Rehabilitation Research & Development, 42*, 737–746.

Elman, R. J. (2005). Social and life participation approaches to aphasia intervention. In L. L. LaPointe (Ed.), *Aphasia and related neurogenic language disorders* (pp. 39–50). New York: Thieme.

Elsegood, K. J., & Duff, S. C. (2010). Theory of mind in men who have sexually offended against children: A UK comparison study between child sex offenders and nonoffender controls. *Sexual Abuse, 22*, 112–131.

Emery, V. O. (2000). Language impairment in dementia of the Alzheimer type: A hierarchical decline? *International Journal of Psychiatry in Medicine, 30*, 145–164.

Emre, M., Aarsland, D., Brown, R., Burn, D. J., Duyckaerts, C., Mizuno, Y., et al. (2007). Clinical diagnostic criteria for dementia associated with Parkinson's disease. *Movement Disorders, 22*, 1689–1707.

Engelhardt, P. E., Ferreira, F., & Nigg, J. T. (2009). Priming sentence production in adolescents and adults with attention-deficit/hyperactivity disorder. *Journal of Abnormal Child Psychology, 37*, 995–1006.

Erez, A. B.-H., Rothschild, E., Katz, N., Tuchner, M., & Hartman-Maeir, A. (2009). Executive functioning, awareness, and participation in daily life after mild traumatic brain injury: A preliminary study. *American Journal of Occupational Therapy, 63*, 634–640.

Estigarribia, B., Martin, G. E., Roberts, J. E., Spencer, A., Gucwa, A., & Sideris, J. (2011). Narrative skill in boys with fragile X syndrome with and without autism spectrum disorder. *Applied Psycholinguistics, 32*, 359–388.

Ewing-Cobbs, L., & Barnes, M. (2002). Linguistic outcomes following traumatic brain injury in children. *Seminars in Pediatric Neurology, 9*, 209–217.

Farmer, M., & Oliver, A. (2005). Assessment of pragmatic difficulties and socio-emotional adjustment in practice. *International Journal of Language & Communication Disorders, 40*, 403–429.

Farrant, B. M., Fletcher, J., & Maybery, M. T. (2006). Specific language impairment, theory of mind, and visual perspective taking: Evidence for simulation theory and the developmental role of language. *Child Development, 77*, 1842–1853.

Fay, W. H. (1979). Personal pronouns and the autistic child. *Journal of Autism and Developmental Disorders, 9*, 247–260.

Feeney, R., Desha, L., Ziviani, J., & Nicholson, J. M. (2012). Health-related quality-of-life of children with speech and language difficulties: A review of the literature. *International Journal of Speech-Language Pathology, 14*, 59–72.

Fernandez-Duque, D., Baird, J. A., & Black, S. E. (2009). False-belief understanding in frontotemporal dementia and Alzheimer's disease. *Journal of Clinical and Experimental Neuropsychology, 31*, 489–497.

Fernandez-Duque, D., & Black, S. (2005). Impaired recognition of negative facial emotions in patients with frontotemporal dementia. *Neuropsychologia, 43*, 1673–1687.

Fiddick, L., Cosmides, L., & Tooby, J. (2000). No interpretation without representation: The role of domain-specific representations and inferences in the Wason selection task. *Cognition, 77*, 1–79.

Fodor, J. A. (1983). *The modularity of mind: An essay on faculty psychology.* Cambridge: MIT Press.

Fong, G. C., Cheng, T. S., Lam, K., Cheng, W. K., Mok, K. Y., Cheung, C. M., et al. (2005). An epidemiological study of motor neuron disease in Hong Kong. *Amyotrophic Lateral Sclerosis and Other Motor Neuron Disorders, 6*, 164–168.

Fontenot, J. L., Hayes, S. L., & Frilot, C. (2011). Language deficits and behavior problems in children placed in alternate education settings. *Contemporary Issues in Communication Science and Disorders, 38*, 36–40.

Forman, H., Mäntylä, T., & Carelli, M. G. (2011). Time keeping and working memory development in early adolescence: A 4-year follow-up. *Journal of Experimental Child Psychology, 108*, 170–179.

Foster-Cohen, S. H. (1994). Exploring the boundary between syntax and pragmatics: Relevance and the binding of pronouns. *Journal of Child Language, 21*, 237–255.

Frank, B., Schoch, B., Hein-Kropp, C., Dimitrova, A., Hövel, M., Ziegler, W., et al. (2007). Verb generation in children and adolescents with acute cerebellar lesions. *Neuropsychologia, 45*, 977–988.

Frank, B., Schoch, B., Hein-Kropp, C., Hövel, M., Gizewski, E. R., Karnath, H.-O., et al. (2008). Aphasia, neglect and extinction are no prominent clinical signs in children and adolescents with acute surgical cerebellar lesions. *Experimental Brain Research, 184*, 511–519.

Frank, E. M., McDade, H. L., & Scott, W. K. (1996). Naming in dementia secondary to Parkinson's, Huntington's, and Alzheimer's diseases. *Journal of Communication Disorders, 29*, 183–197.

Frattali, C. M., Thompson, C. M., Holland, A. L., Wohl, C. B., & Ferketic, M. M. (1995). *ASHA functional assessment of communication skills (FACS).* Rockville: American Speech-Language-Hearing Association.

Freed, J., Adams, C., & Lockton, E. (2011). Literacy skills in primary school-aged children with pragmatic language impairment: A comparison with children with specific language impairment. *International Journal of Language & Communication Disorders, 46*, 334–347.

Friedman, N. P., Haberstick, B. C., Willcutt, E. G., Miyake, A., Young, S. E., Corley, R. P., et al. (2007). Greater attention problems during childhood predict poorer executive functioning in late adolescence. *Psychological Science, 18*, 893–900.

Gagnon, L., Goulet, P., Giroux, F., & Joanette, Y. (2003). Processing of metaphoric and non-metaphoric alternative meanings of words after right- and left-hemispheric lesion. *Brain and Language, 87*, 217–226.

Gallagher, T. M., & Darnton, B. A. (1978). Conversational aspects of the speech of language-dis-ordered children: Revision behaviors. *Journal of Speech and Hearing Research, 21,* 118–135.

Galski, T., Tompkins, C., & Johnston, M. V. (1998). Competence in discourse as a measure of social integration and quality of life in persons with traumatic brain injury. *Brain Injury, 12,* 769–782.

Ganesalingam, K., Yeates, K. O., Taylor, H. G., Walz, N. C., Stancin, T., & Wade, S. (2011). Executive functions and social competence in young children 6 months following traumatic brain injury. *Neuropsychology, 25,* 466–476.

Gantman, A., Kapp, S. K., Orenski, K., & Laugeson, E. A. (2012). Social skills training for young adults with high-functioning autism spectrum disorders: A randomized controlled pilot study. *Journal of Autism and Developmental Disorders, 42,* 1094–1103.

Gao, C., Shi, Q., Tian, C., Chen, C., Han, J., Zhou, W., et al. (2011). The epidemiological, clinical, and laboratory features of sporadic Creutzfeldt-Jakob disease patients in China: Surveillance data from 2006 to 2010. *PloS One, 6,* e24231.

Gardner, H., & Brownell, H. H. (1986). *Right hemisphere communication battery.* Boston: Psychology Service, Veterans Administration Medical Center.

Garrett, M., & Harnish, R. M. (2007). Experimental pragmatics. In L. de Saussure, P. J. Schulz (eds.), *Pragmatic interfaces* (pp. 65–90). Amsterdam: John Benjamins.

Gasser-Moritz, S., Herbet, G., Maldonado, I. L., & Duffau, H. (2012). Lexical access speed is significantly correlated with the return to professional activities after awake surgery for low-grade gliomas. *Journal of Neuro-Oncology, 107,* 633–641.

Gerber, S., Brice, A., Capone, N., Fujiki, M., & Timler, G. (2012). Language use in social inter-actions of school-age children with language impairments: An evidence-based systematic review of treatment. *Language, Speech, and Hearing Services in Schools, 43,* 235–249.

Geurts, H. M., Verte, S., Oosterlaan, J., Roeyers, H., & Sergeant, J. A. (2004). How specific are executive functioning deficits in attention deficit hyperactivity disorder and autism. *Journal of Child Psychology and Psychiatry, 45,* 836–854.

Giancola, P. R., & Mezzich, A. C. (2000). Neuropsychological deficits in female adolescents with a substance use disorder: Better accounted for by conduct disorder? *Journal of Studies on Alcohol, 61,* 809–817.

Gibbons, Z. C., Snowden, J. S., Thompson, J. C., Happé, F., Richardson, A., & Neary, D. (2007). Inferring thought and action in motor neurone disease. *Neuropsychologia, 45,* 1196–1207.

Gibbs, R. W. (2010). Idiom. In L. Cummings (Ed.), *The Routledge pragmatics encyclopedia* (pp. 204–205). London: Routledge.

Gibbs, R. W., & Moise, J. F. (1997). Pragmatics in understanding what is said. *Cognition, 62,* 51–74.

Gil, M., Cohen, M., Korn, C., & Groswasser, Z. (1996). Vocational outcome of aphasic patients following severe traumatic brain injury. *Brain Injury, 10,* 39–45.

Gilmour, J., Hill, B., Place, M., & Skuse, D. H. (2004). Social communication deficits in conduct disorder: A clinical and community survey. *Journal of Child Psychology and Psychiatry, 45,* 967–978.

Ginsberg, Y., Hirvikoski, T., & Lindefors, N. (2010). Attention deficit hyperactivity disorder (ADHD) among longer-term prison inmates is a prevalent, persistent and disabling disorder. *BMC Psychiatry, 10,* 112.

Giora, R., Zaidel, E., Soroker, N., Batori, G., & Kasher, A. (2000). Differential effects of right- and left-hemisphere damage on understanding sarcasm and metaphor. *Metaphor and Symbol, 15,* 63–83.

Girardi, A., Macpherson, S. E., & Abrahams, S. (2011). Deficits in emotional and social cogni-tion in amyotrophic lateral sclerosis. *Neuropsychology, 25,* 53–65.

Girotto, V., Kemmelmeier, M., Sperber, D., & van der Henst, J.-B. (2001). Inept reasoners or pragmatic virtuosos? Relevance and the deontic selection task. *Cognition, 81,* 69–76.

Golan, O., Baron-Cohen, S., & Golan, Y. (2008). The 'Reading the Mind in Films' task [child version]: Complex emotion and mental state recognition in children with and without autism spectrum conditions. *Journal of Autism and Developmental Disorders, 38,* 1534–1541.

Golan, O., Baron-Cohen, S., & Hill, J. (2006). The Cambridge Mindreading (CAM) Face-Voice Battery: Testing complex emotion recognition in adults with and without Asperger syndrome. *Journal of Autism and Developmental Disorders, 36*, 169–183.

Golding, J., Pembrey, M., Jones, R., & The ALSPAC Study Team. (2001). ALSPAC—The avon longitudinal study of parents and children. I. Study methodology. *Paediatric and Perinatal Epidemiology, 15*, 74–87.

Gonçalves, M. I., Radzinsky, T. C., Saba da Silva, N., Chiari, B. M., & Consonni, D. (2008). Speech-language and hearing complaints of children and adolescents with brain tumors. *Pediatric Blood & Cancer, 50*, 706–708.

Goodglass, H., & Kaplan, E. (1972). *Boston diagnostic aphasia examination*. Philadelphia: Lea and Febiger.

Goodman, R. (1997). The strengths and difficulties questionnaire: A research note. *Journal of Child Psychology and Psychiatry, 38*, 581–586.

Goodman, R. (1999). The extended version of the strengths and difficulties questionnaire as a guide to child psychiatric caseness and consequent burden. *Journal of Child Psychology and Psychiatry, 40*, 791–799.

Gordon, D. (1990). *Propositional coherence in thought-disordered schizophrenic and non-schizophrenic discourse: A listener's perspective*, MSc dissertation, City University, London

Gordon, R. M. (1986). Folk psychology as simulation. *Mind & Language, 1*, 158–171.

Gorno-Tempini, M. L., Brambati, S. M., Ginex, V., Ogar, J., Dronkers, N. F., Marcone, A., et al. (2008). The logopenic/phonological variant of primary progressive aphasia. *Neurology, 71*, 1227–1234.

Grant, C. M., Apperly, I., & Oliver, C. (2007). Is theory of mind understanding impaired in males with fragile X syndrome? *Journal of Abnormal Child Psychology, 35*, 17–28.

Gray, C. (1994). *Comic strip conversations*. Jenison: Jenison Public Schools.

Gray, C. (1995). *Writing social stories with Carol Gray*. Arlington: Future Horizon.

Greenwood, K. E., Morris, R., Sigmundsson, T., Landau, S., & Wykes, T. (2008). Executive functioning in schizophrenia and the relationship with symptom profile and chronicity. *Journal of the International Neuropsychological Society, 14*, 782–792.

Gregory, C., Lough, S., Stone, V., Erzinclioglu, S., Martin, L., Baron-Cohen, S., et al. (2002). Theory of mind in patients with frontal variant frontotemporal dementia and Alzheimer's disease: Theoretical and practical implications. *Brain, 125*, 752–764.

Gregory, J., & Bryan, K. (2011). Speech and language therapy intervention with a group of persistent and prolific young offenders in a non-custodial setting with previously undiagnosed speech, language and communication difficulties. *International Journal of Language & Communication Disorders, 46*, 202–215.

Gresham, F., & Elliot, S. (1990). *Social skills rating system*. Circle Pines: American Guidance Service.

Grice, H. P. (1957). Meaning. *The philosophical review, 66*, 377–388.

Grice, H. P. (1989). *Studies in the way of words*. Cambridge: Harvard University Press.

Griffin, R., Friedman, O., Ween, J., Winner, E., Happé, F., & Brownell, H. (2006). Theory of mind and the right cerebral hemisphere: Refining the scope of impairment. *Laterality, 11*, 195–225.

Griffiths, C. C. B. (2007). Pragmatic abilities in adults with and without dyslexia: A pilot study. *Dyslexia, 13*, 276–296.

Grindrod, C. M., & Baum, S. R. (2005). Hemispheric contributions to lexical ambiguity resolution in a discourse context: Evidence from individuals with unilateral left and right hemisphere lesions. *Brain and Cognition, 57*, 70–83.

Grossman, M., Gross, R. G., Moore, P., Dreyfuss, M., McMillan, C. T., Cook, P. A., et al. (2012). Difficulty processing temporary syntactic ambiguities in Lewy body spectrum disorder. *Brain and Language, 120*, 52–60.

Hale, C. M., & Tager-Flusberg, H. (2005). Brief report: The relationship between discourse deficits and autism symptomatology. *Journal of Autism and Developmental Disorders, 35*, 519–524.

Hall, Dh., Ouyang, B., Lonnquist, E., & Newcombe, J. (2011). Pragmatic communication is impaired in Parkinson's disease. *International Journal of Neuroscience, 121*, 254–256.

Hall, K. A., & O'Connor, D. W. (2004). Correlates of aggressive behaviour in dementia. *International Psychogeriatrics, 16*, 141–158.

Hall, N. E., & Segarra, V. R. (2007). Predicting academic performance in children with language impairment: The role of parent report. *Journal of Communication Disorders, 40*, 82–95.

Halliday, M. A. K., & Hasan, Ra. (1976). *Cohesion in English.* London: Longman.

Halpern, H., & McCartin-Clark, M. (1984). Differential language characteristics in adult aphasic and schizophrenic subjects. *Journal of Communication Disorders, 17*, 289–307.

Hamilton, A. F. de C., Brindley, R., & Frith, U. (2009). Visual perspective taking impairment in children with autistic spectrum disorder. *Cognition, 113*, 37–44.

Hannus, S., Kauppila, T., & Launonen, K. (2009). Increasing prevalence of specific language impairment (SLI) in primary healthcare of a Finnish town, 1989–99. *International Journal of Language & Communication Disorders, 44*, 79–97.

Hanten, G., Li, X., Newsome, M. R., Swank, P., Chapman, S. B., Dennis, M., et al. (2009). Oral reading and expressive language after childhood traumatic brain injury: Trajectory and correlates of change over time. *Topics in Language Disorders, 29*, 236–248.

Happé, F. G. E. (1993). Communicative competence and theory of mind in autism: A test of relevance theory. *Cognition, 48*, 101–119.

Happé, F., Brownell, H., & Winner, E. (1999). Acquired 'theory of mind' impairments following stroke. *Cognition, 70*, 211–240.

Harrow, M., Grossman, L. S., Jobe, T. H., & Herbener, E. S. (2005). Do patients with schizophrenia ever show periods of recovery? A 15-year multi-follow-up study. *Schizophrenia Bulletin, 31*, 723–734.

Harvey, P. D., Davidson, M., Mueser, K. T., Parrella, M., White, L., & Powchik, P. (1997). Social-Adaptive Functioning Evaluation (SAFE): A rating scale for geriatric psychiatric patients. *Schizophrenia Bulletin, 23*, 131–145.

Harvey, R. J., Skelton-Robinson, M., & Rossor, M. N. (2003). The prevalence and causes of dementia in people under the age of 65 years. *Journal of Neurology, Neurosurgery & Psychiatry, 74*, 1206–1209.

Haskins, B. G., & Arturo Silva, J. (2006). Asperger's disorder and criminal behavior: Forensic-psychiatric considerations. *Journal of the American Academy of Psychiatry and the Law, 34*, 374–384.

Hatta, T., Hasegawa, J., & Wanner, P. J. (2004). Differential processing of implicature in individuals with left and right brain damage. *Journal of Clinical and Experimental Neuropsychology, 26*, 667–676.

Havet-Thomassin, V., Allain, P., Etcharry-Bouyx, F., & Le Gall, D. (2006). What about theory of mind after severe brain injury? *Brain Injury, 20*, 83–91.

Hay, E., & Moran, C. (2005). Discourse formulation in children with closed head injury. *American Journal of Speech-Language Pathology, 14*, 324–336.

Hays, S.-J., Niven, B., Godfrey, H., & Linscott, R. (2004). Clinical assessment of pragmatic language impairment: A generalisability study of older people with Alzheimer's disease. *Aphasiology, 18*, 693–714.

Heath, R. L., & Blonder, L. X. (2005). Spontaneous humor among right hemisphere stroke survivors. *Brain and Language, 93*, 267–276.

Heerey, E. A., Capps, L. M., Keltner, D., & Kring, A. M. (2005). Understanding teasing: Lessons from children with autism. *Journal of Abnormal Child Psychology, 33*, 55–68.

Helland, W. A., Helland, T., & Heimann, M. (to appear). Language profiles and mental health problems in children with specific language impairment and children with ADHD. *Journal of Attention Disorders.*

Henry, A., Tourbah, A., Chaunu, M.-P., Rumbach, L., Montreuil, M., & Bakchine, S. (2011). Social cognition impairments in relapsing-remitting multiple sclerosis. *Journal of the International Neuropsychological Society, 17*, 1122–1131.

Henry, J. D., Phillips, L. H., Crawford, J. R., Ietswaart, M., & Summers, F. (2006). Theory of mind following traumatic brain injury: The role of emotion recognition and executive dysfunction. *Neuropsychologia, 44*, 1623–1628.

Henry, L. A., Messer, D. J., & Nash, G. (2012). Executive functioning in children with specific language impairment. *Journal of Child Psychology and Psychiatry, 53*, 37–45.

Henry, M. L., & Gorno-Tempini, M. L. (2010). The logopenic variant of primary progressive aphasia. *Current Opinion in Neurology, 23*, 633–637.

Hilari, K., Needle, J. J., & Harrison, K. L. (2012). What are the important factors in health-related quality of life for people with aphasia? A systematic review. *Archives of Physical Medicine and Rehabilitation, 93*, S86–S95.

Hilari, K., Northcott, S., Roy, P., Marshall, J., Wiggins, R. D., Chataway, J., et al. (2010). Psychological distress after stroke and aphasia: The first six months. *Clinical Rehabilitation, 24*, 181–190.

Hilton, D. A., Ghani, A. C., Conyers, L., Edwards, P., McCardle, L., Ritchie, D., et al. (2004). Prevalence of lymphoreticular prion protein accumulation in UK tissue sample. *Journal of Pathology, 203*, 733–739.

Hinckley, J. J. (2002). Vocational and social outcomes of adults with chronic aphasia. *Journal of Communication Disorders, 35*, 543–560.

Hird, K., & Kirsner, K. (2003). The effect of right cerebral hemisphere damage on collaborative planning in conversation: An analysis of intentional structure. *Clinical Linguistics & Phonetics, 17*, 309–315.

Ho, A. K., Sahakian, B. J., Brown, R. G., Barker, R. A., Hodges, J. R., Ané, M. N., Snowden, J., Thompson, J., Esmonde, T., Gentry, R., Moore, J. W., Bodner, T., & NEST-HD Consortium. (2003). Profile of cognitive progression in early Huntington's disease. *Neurology, 61*, 1702–1706.

Hoey, M. (1991). *Patterns of lexis in text*. Oxford: Oxford University Press.

Hogan, A., Shipley, M., Strazdins, L., Purcell, A., & Baker, E. (2011). Communication and behavioural disorders among children with hearing loss increases risk of mental health disorders. *Australian and New Zealand Journal of Public Health, 35*, 377–383.

Holck, P., Sandberg, A. D., & Nettelbladt, U. (2010). Inferential ability in children with cerebral palsy, spina bifida and pragmatic language impairment. *Research in Developmental Disabilities, 31*, 140–150.

Holland, A. L. (1980). *Communication activities of daily living*. Austin: Pro-Ed.

Holland, A. L. (1991). Pragmatic aspects of intervention in aphasia. *Journal of Neurolinguistics, 6*, 197–211.

Holtgraves, T., & McNamara, P. (2010a). Pragmatic comprehension deficit in Parkinson's disease. *Journal of Clinical and Experimental Neuropsychology, 32*, 388–397.

Holtgraves, Ts., & McNamara, P. (2010b). Parkinson's disease and politeness. *Journal of Language and Social Psychology, 29*, 178–193.

Holwerda, A., van der Klink, J. J. L., Groothoff, J. W., & Brouwer, S. (2012). Predictors for work participation in individuals with autism spectrum disorder: A systematic review. *Journal of Occupational Rehabilitation, 22*, 333–352.

Hong, D., Dunkin, B., & Reiss, A. L. (2011). Psychosocial functioning and social cognitive processing in girls with Turner syndrome. *Journal of Developmental and Behavioral Pediatrics, 32*, 512–20.

Hooker, C., & Park, S. (2002). Emotion processing and its relationship to social functioning in schizophrenia patients. *Psychiatry Research, 112*, 41–50.

Hooper, S. R., Hatton, D., Sideris, J., Sullivan, K., Hammer, J., Schaaf, J., Mirrett, P., Ornstein, P. A., & Bailey, D. B., Jr. (2008). Executive functions in young males with fragile X syndrome in comparison to mental age-matched controls: Baseline findings from a longitudinal study. *Neuropsychology, 22*, 36–47.

Hoppitt, T., Pall, H., Calvert, M., Gill, P., Yao, G., Ramsay, J., et al. (2011). A systematic review of the incidence and prevalence of long-term neurological conditions in the UK. *Neuroepidemiology, 36*, 19–28.

Hoppitt, T., Calvert, M., Pall, H., Rickards, H., & Sackley, C. (2010). Huntington's disease. *The Lancet, 376,* 1463–1464.

Howlin, P., Goode, S., Hutton, J., & Rutter, M. (2004). Adult outcome for children with autism. *Journal of Child Psychology and Psychiatry, 45,* 212–229.

Huang, Y. (2010). What is said. In L. Cummings (Ed.), *The Routledge pragmatics encyclopedia* (pp. 489–491). London: Routledge.

Huizinga, M., & van der Molen, M. W. (2007). Age-group differences in set-switching and set-maintenance on the Wisconsin Card Sorting Task. *Developmental Neuropsychology, 31,* 193–215.

Hulme, C., Goetz, K., Brigstocke, S., Nash, H. M., Lervåg, A., & Snowling, M. J. (2012). The growth of reading skills in children with Down syndrome. *Developmental Science, 15,* 320–329.

Humber, E., & Snow, P. C. (2001). The oral language skills of young offenders: A pilot investigation. *Psychiatry, Psychology and Law, 8,* 1–11.

Hutchins, T. L., & Prelock, P. A. (2006). Using social stories and comic strip conversations to promote socially valid outcomes for children with autism. *Seminars in Speech and Language, 27,* 47–59.

Hutton, S. B., Puri, B. K., Duncan, L. J., Robbins, T. W., Barnes, T. R., & Joyce, E. M. (1998). Executive function in first-episode schizophrenia. *Psychological Medicine, 28,* 463–473.

Ichikawa, H., Takahashi, N., Hieda, S., Ohno, H., & Kawamura, M. (2008). Agraphia in bulbar-onset amyotrophic lateral sclerosis: Not merely a consequence of dementia or aphasia. *Behavioural Neurology, 20,* 91–99.

Iran-Nejad, A., Ortony, A., & Rittenhouse, R. K. (1981). The comprehension of metaphorical uses of English by deaf children. *Journal of Speech and Hearing Research, 24,* 551–556.

Irwin, W. H., Wertz, R. T., & Avent, J. R. (2002). Relationships among language impairment, functional communication, and pragmatic performance in aphasia. *Aphasiology, 16,* 823–835.

Isaki, E., & Turkstra, L. (2000). Communication abilities and work re-entry following traumatic brain injury. *Brain Injury, 14,* 441–453.

Itier, R. J., & Batty, M. (2009). Neural bases of eye and gaze processing: The core of social cognition. *Neuroscience and Biobehavioral Reviews, 33,* 843–863.

Ito, H., Kano, O., & Ikeda, K. (2008). Different variables between patients with left and right hemispheric ischemic stroke. *Journal of Stroke and Cerebrovascular Diseases, 17,* 35–38.

James, R. S., Bishop, D. V. M., Coppin, B., Dalton, P., Aamodt-Leeper, G., Bacarese-Hamilton, M., et al. (1997). Evidence from Turner's syndrome of an imprinted X-linked locus affecting cognitive function. *Nature, 387,* 705–708.

Jaszczolt, K. M. (2005). *Default semantics: Foundations of a compositional theory of acts of communication.* Oxford: Oxford University Press.

Jaszczolt, K. M. (2012). Semantics/pragmatics boundary disputes. In C. Maienborn, K. von Heusinger & P. Portner (eds.), *Semantics: An international handbook of natural language meaning* (2333–2360). Berlin: Mouton de Gruyter.

Jaszczolt, K. M. (2013). Semantics and pragmatics: The boundary issue. In K. von Heusinger, P. Portner, & C. Maienborn (eds.), *Semantics: An international handbook of natural language meaning.* Berlin: Mouton de Gruyter.

Jensen, A. M., Chenery, H. J., & Copland, D. A. (2006). A comparison of picture description abilities in individuals with vascular subcortical lesions and Huntington's disease. *Journal of Communication Disorders, 39,* 62–77.

Jerome, A. C., Fujiki, M., Brinton, B., & James, S. L. (2002). Self-esteem in children with specific language impairment. *Journal of Speech, Language, and Hearing Research, 45,* 700–714.

Joanette, Y., Ferré, P., & Wilson, M. A. (2014). Right hemisphere damage and communication. In L. Cummings (Ed.), *Cambridge handbook of communication disorders* (247–265). Cambridge: Cambridge University Press.

John, A. E., & Mervis, C. B. (2010). Comprehension of the communicative intent behind pointing and gazing gestures by young children with Williams syndrome or Down syndrome. *Journal of Speech, Language, and Hearing Research, 53,* 950–960.

John, A. E., Rowe, M. L., & Mervis, C. B. (2009). Referential communication skills of children with Williams syndrome: Understanding when messages are not adequate. *American Journal on Intellectual and Developmental Disabilities, 114,* 85–99.

Johnston, J. R., Miller, J., & Tallal, P. (2001). Use of cognitive state predicates by language-impaired children. *International Journal of Language & Communication Disorders, 36,* 349–370.

Jones, A. P., Forster, A. S., & Skuse, D. (2007). What do you think you're looking at? Investigating social cognition in young offenders. *Criminal Behaviour and Mental Health, 17,* 101–106.

Kalkut, E. L., Duke Han, S., Lansing, A. E., Holdnack, J. A., & Delis, D. C. (2009). Development of set-shifting ability from late childhood through early adulthood. *Archives of Clinical Neuropsychology, 24,* 565–574.

Kandalaft, M. R., Didehbani, N., Krawczyk, D. C., Allen, T. T., & Chapman, S. B. (2013). Virtual reality social cognition training for young adults with high-functioning autism. *Journal of Autism and Developmental Disorders, 43,* 34–44.

Kaneda, Y., Jayathilak, K., & Meltzer, H. Y. (2009). Determinants of work outcome in schizophrenia and schizoaffective disorder. *Psychiatry Research, 169,* 178–179.

Kanner, L. (1943). Autistic disturbances of affective contact. *Nervous Child, 2,* 217–250.

Kaplan, E., Goodglass, H., & Weintraub, S. (1983). *Boston naming test.* Philadelphia: Lea & Febiger.

Karkhaneh, M., Clark, B., Ospina, M. B., Seida, J. C., Smith, V., & Hartling, L. (2010). Social stories™ to improve social skills in children with autism spectrum disorder: A systematic review. *Autism, 14,* 641–662.

Kasher, A. (1982). Gricean inference revisited. *Philosophica, 29,* 25–44.

Kasher, A. (1984). On the psychological reality of pragmatics. *Journal of Pragmatics, 8,* 539–557.

Kasher, A. (1991a). On the pragmatic modules: A lecture. *Journal of Pragmatics, 16,* 381–397.

Kasher, A. (1991b). Pragmatics and the modularity of mind. In S. Davis (ed.), *Pragmatics: A reader* (567–582). New York: Oxford University Press.

Kasher, A. (1994). Modular speech act theory: Programme and results. In S. L. Tsohatzidis (ed.), *Foundations of speech act theory: Philosophical and linguistic perspectives* (312–322). London and New York: Routledge.

Kasher, A., Batori, G., Soroker, N., Graves, D., & Zaidel, E. (1999). Effects of right- and left-hemisphere damage on understanding conversational implicatures. *Brain and Language, 68,* 566–590.

Kasher, A., & Meilijson, S. (1996). Autism and pragmatics of language. *Incontri Cita Aperta, 4–5,* 37–54.

Kastenbauer, S., & Pfister, H.-W. (2003). Pneumococcal meningitis in adults: Spectrum of complications and prognostic factors in a series of 87 cases. *Brain, 126,* 1015–1025.

Katsos, N., Roqueta, C. A., Estevan, R. A. C., & Cummins, C. (2011). Are children with specific language impairment competent with the pragmatics and logic of quantification? *Cognition, 119,* 45–57.

Katz, M. J., Lipton, R. B., Hall, C. B., Zimmerman, M. E., Sanders, A. E., Verghese, J., et al. (2012). Age-specific and sex-specific prevalence and incidence of mild cognitive impairment, dementia, and Alzheimer dementia in Blacks and Whites: A report from the Einstein Aging Study. *Alzheimer Disease and Associated Disorders, 26,* 335–343.

Keegstra, A. L., Post, W. J., & Goorhuis-Brouwer, S. M. (2010). Behavioural problems in young children with language problems. *International Journal of Pediatric Otorhinolaryngology, 74,* 637–641.

Kertesz, A. (1979). *Aphasia and associated disorders: Taxonomy, Localization and Recovery.* New York: Grune and Stratton.

Kertesz, A., Jesso, S., Harciarek, M., Blair, M., & McMonagle, P. (2010). What is semantic dementia?: A cohort study of diagnostic features and clinical boundaries. *Archives of Neurology, 67,* 483–489.

Kertesz, A., McMonagle, P., Blair, M., Davidson, W., & Munoz, D. G. (2005). The evolution and pathology of frontotemporal dementia. *Brain, 128,* 1996–2005.

Ketelaars, M. P., Cuperus, J., Jansonius, K., & Verhoeven, L. (2010). Pragmatic language impairment and associated behavioural problems. *International Journal of Language & Communication Disorders, 45,* 204–214.

Ketelaars, M. P., Jansonius, K., Cuperus, J., & Verhoeven, L. (2012). Narrative competence and underlying mechanisms in children with pragmatic language impairment. *Applied Psycholinguistics, 33*, 281–303.

Kibby, M. Y., & Cohen, M. J. (2008). Memory functioning in children with reading disabilities and/or attention deficit/hyperactivity disorder: A clinical investigation of their working memory and long-term memory functioning. *Child Neuropsychology, 14*, 525–546.

Kieffer-Renaux, V., Bulteau, C., Grill, J., Kalifa, C., Viguier, D., & Jambaque, I. (2000). Patterns of neuropsychological deficits in children with medulloblastoma according to craniospatial irradiation doses. *Developmental Medicine and Child Neurology, 42*, 741–745.

Kim, O. H., & Kaiser, A. P. (2000). Language characteristics of children with ADHD. *Communication Disorders Quarterly, 21*, 154–165.

Kipps, C. M., & Hodges, J. R. (2006). Theory of mind in frontotemporal dementia. *Social Neuroscience, 1*, 235–244.

Kipps, C. M., Nestor, P. J., Acosta-Cabronero, J., Arnold, R., & Hodges, J. R. (2009). Understanding social dysfunction in the behavioural variant of frontotemporal dementia: The role of emotion and sarcasm processing. *Brain, 132*, 592–603.

Kiuni, N., Haverinen, K., Salmela-Aro, K., Nurmi, J.-E., Savolainen, H., & Holopainen, L. (2011). Students with reading and spelling disabilities: Peer groups and educational attainment in secondary education. *Journal of Learning Disabilities, 44*, 556–569.

Klein-Tasman, B. P., Mervis, C. B., Lord, C., & Phillips, K. D. (2007). Socio-communicative deficits in young children with Williams syndrome: Performance on the Autism Diagnostic Observation Schedule. *Child Neuropsychology, 13*, 444–467.

Klonoff, P. S., Sheperd, J. C., O'Brien, K. P., Chiapello, D. A., & Hodak, J. A. (1990). Rehabilitation and outcome of right-hemisphere stroke patients: Challenges to traditional diagnostic and treatment methods. *Neuropsychology, 4*, 147–163.

Klugman, T. M., & Ross, E. (2002). Perceptions of the impact of speech, language, swallowing, and hearing difficulties on quality of life of a group of South African persons with multiple sclerosis. *Folia Phoniatrica et Logopaedica, 54*, 201–221.

Knibb, J. A., Woollams, A. M., Hodges, J. R., & Patterson, K. (2009). Making sense of progressive non-fluent aphasia: An analysis of conversational speech. *Brain, 132*, 2743–2746.

Koedam, E. L., Van der Flier, W. M., Barkhof, F., Koene, T., Scheltens, P., & Pijnenburg, Yo A. (2010). Clinical characteristics of patients with frontotemporal dementia with and without lobar atrophy on MRI. *Alzheimer Disease and Associated Disorders, 24*, 242–247.

Koedoot, C., Bouwmans, C., Franken, M.-C., & Stolk, Elly. (2011). Quality of life in adults who stutter. *Journal of Communication Disorders, 44*, 429–443.

Koepsell, T. D., Rivara, F. P., Vavilala, M. S., Wang, J., Temkin, N., Jaffe, K. M., et al. (2011). Incidence and descriptive epidemiologic features of traumatic brain injury in King County, Washington. *Pediatrics, 128*, 946–954.

Kohler, B. A., Ward, E., McCarthy, B. J., Schymura, M. J., Ries, L. A. G., Eheman, C., et al. (2011). Annual report to the nation on the status of cancer, 1975–2007, featuring tumors of the brain and other nervous system. *Journal of the National Cancer Institute, 103*, 714–736.

Kokina, A., & Kern, L. (2010). Social Story™ interventions for students with autism spectrum disorders: A meta-analysis. *Journal of Autism and Developmental Disorders, 40*, 812–826.

Kopelowicz, A., Liberman, R. P., & Zarate, R. (2006). Recent advances in social skills training for schizophrenia. *Schizophrenia Bulletin, 32*, S12–S23.

Kristensen, Hanne. (2000). Selective mutism and comorbidity with developmental disorder/delay, anxiety disorder, and elimination disorder. *Journal of the American Academy of Child and Adolescent Psychiatry, 39*, 249–256.

Kristoffersen, K. E. (2008). Speech and language development in cri du chat syndrome: A critical review. *Clinical Linguistics & Phonetics, 22*, 443–457.

Kruck, C. L., Roth, R. M., Kumbhani, S. R., Garlinghouse, M. A., Flashman, L. A., & McAllister, T. W. (2011). Inferential-reasoning impairment in schizophrenia-spectrum disorders. *The Journal of Neuropsychiatry and Clinical Neurosciences, 23*, 211–214.

Ku, J., Han, K., Lee, H. R., Jang, Hee. Jeong., Kim, K. U., Park, S. H., et al. (2007). VR-based conversation training program for patients with schizophrenia: A preliminary clinical trial. *Cyberpsychology & Behavior, 10*, 567–574.

Kuriyan, A. B., Pelham, W. E., Jr, Molina, B. S. G., Waschbusch, D. A., Gnagy, E. M., Sibley, M. H., et al. (2013). Young adult educational and vocational outcomes of children diagnosed with ADHD. *Journal of Abnormal Child Psychology, 41*, 27–41.

Kwok, H. W., Cui, Y., & Li, J. (2011). Perspectives of intellectual disability in the People's Republic of China: Epidemiology, policy, services for children and adults. *Current Opinion in Psychiatry, 24*, 408–412.

Laakso, K., Brunnegård, K., Hartelius, L., & Ahlsén, E. (2000). Assessing high-level language in individuals with multiple sclerosis: A pilot study. *Clinical Linguistics & Phonetics, 14*, 329–349.

Lacour, A., De Seze, J., Revenco, E., Lebrun, C., Masmoudi, K., Vidry, E., et al. (2004). Acute aphasia in multiple sclerosis: A multicenter study of 22 patients. *Neurology, 62*, 974–977.

Lacroix, A., Aguert, M., Dardier, V., Stojanovik, V., & Laval, V. (2010). Idiom comprehension in French-speaking children and adolescents with Williams syndrome. *Research in Developmental Disabilities, 31*, 608–616.

Lake, J. K., Cardy, S., & Humphreys, K. R. (2010). Animacy and word order in individuals with autism spectrum disorders. *Journal of Autism and Developmental Disorders, 40*, 1161–1164.

Lambert, M., & Naber, D. (Eds.). (2011). *Current schizophrenia* (2nd ed.). London: Springer Healthcare Ltd.

Landa, R. J. (2005). Assessment of social communication skills in preschoolers. *Mental Retardation and Developmental Disabilities Research Reviews, 11*, 247–252.

Lanfranchi, S., Jerman, O., Dal Pont, E., Alberti, A., & Vianello, R. (2010). Executive function in adolescents with Down syndrome. *Journal of Intellectual Disability Research, 54*, 308–319.

Langdon, R., Coltheart, M., Ward, P. B., & Catts, S. V. (2002). Disturbed communication in schizophrenia: The role of poor pragmatics and poor mind-reading. *Psychological Medicine, 32*, 1273–1284.

Larson, E. B., Shadlen, M.-F., Li, W., McCormick, W. C., Bowen, J. D., Teri, L., et al. (2004). Survival after initial diagnosis of Alzheimer disease. *Annals of Internal Medicine, 140*, 501–509.

Lawrence, A. D., Hodges, J. R., Rosser, A. E., Kershaw, A., Ffrench-Constant, C., Rubinsztein, D. C., et al. (1998). Evidence for specific cognitive deficits in preclinical Huntington's disease. *Brain, 121*, 1329–1341.

Laws, G., & Bishop, D. V. M. (2004). Pragmatic language impairment and social deficits in Williams syndrome: A comparison with Down's syndrome and specific language impairment. *International Journal of Language & Communication Disorders, 39*, 45–64.

Le Couteur, A., Rutter, M., Lord, C., Rios, P., Robertson, S., Holdgrafer, M., et al. (1989). Autism Diagnostic Interview: A standardised, investigator based instrument. *Journal of Autism and Developmental Disorders, 19*, 363–387.

Leaf, J. B., Oppenheim-Leaf, M. L., Call, N. A., Sheldon, J. B., Sherman, J. A., Taubman, M., et al. (2012). Comparing the teaching interaction procedure to social stories for people with autism. *Journal of Applied Behavior Analysis, 45*, 281–298.

Leblanc, J., De Guise, E., Feyz, M., & Lamoureux, J. (2006). Early prediction of language impairment following traumatic brain injury. *Brain Injury, 20*, 1391–1401.

Lee, J., Quintana, J., Nori, P., & Green, M. F. (2011). Theory of mind in schizophrenia: Exploring neural mechanisms of belief attribution. *Social Neuroscience, 6*, 569–581.

Leh, S. E., Petrides, M., & Strafella, A. P. (2010). The neural circuitry of executive functions in healthy subjects and Parkinson's disease. *Neuropsychopharmacology Reviews, 35*, 70–85.

Lehman Blake, M. T., & Tompkins, C. A. (2001). Predictive inferencing in adults with right hemisphere brain damage. *Journal of Speech, Language, and Hearing Research, 44*, 639–654.

Leinonen, E., & Kerbel, D. (1999). Relevance theory and pragmatic impairment. *International Journal of Language & Communication Disorders, 34*, 367–390.

Leon, A. C., Solomon, D. A., Mueller, T. I., Turvey, C. L., Endicott, J., & Keller, M. B. (1999). The Range of Impaired Functioning Tool (LIFE-RIFT): A brief measure of functional impairment. *Psychological Medicine, 29*, 869–878.

Leonard, M. A., Milich, R., & Lorch, E. P. (2011). The role of pragmatic language use in mediating the relation between hyperactivity and inattention and social skills problems. *Journal of Speech, Language, and Hearing Research, 54*, 567–579.

Lerna, A., Esposito, D., Conson, M., Russo, L., & Massagli, A. (2012). Social-communicative effects of the picture exchange communication system (PECS) in autism spectrum disorders. *International Journal of Language & Communication Disorders, 47*, 609–617.

Lerner, M. D., Haque, O. S., Northrup, E. C., Lawer, L., & Bursztajn, H. J. (2012). Emerging perspectives on adolescents and young adults with high-functioning autism spectrum disorders, violence, and criminal law. *Journal of the American Academy of Psychiatry and the Law, 40*, 177–190.

Levinson, S. C. (2000). *Presumptive meanings: The theory of generalized conversational implicature*. Cambridge: MIT Press.

Levorato, M. C., & Cacciari, C. (2002). The creation of new figurative expressions: Psycholinguistic evidence in Italian children, adolescents and adults. *Journal of Child Language, 29*, 127–150.

Lewis, F. M., & Murdoch, B. E. (2010). Language skills following risk-adapted treatment for medulloblastoma. *Developmental Neurorehabilitation, 13*, 217–224.

Lewis, F. M., & Murdoch, B. E. (2011a). Language outcomes following risk-adapted treatments for tumors located within the posterior fossa. *Journal of Child Neurology, 26*, 440–452.

Lewis, F. M., & Murdoch, B. E. (2011b). Intact language skills and semantic processing speed following the use of fractionated cranial irradiation therapy for the treatment of childhood medulloblastoma: a 4-year follow-up study. *Neurocase, 17*, 332–344.

Lewis, F. M., Woodyatt, G. C., & Murdoch, B. E. (2008). Linguistic and pragmatic language skills in adults with autism spectrum disorder: A pilot study. *Research in Autism Spectrum Disorders, 2*, 176–187.

Leyhe, T., Saur, R., Eschweiler, G. W., & Milian, M. (2011). Impairment in proverb interpretation as an executive function deficit in patients with amnestic mild cognitive impairment and early Alzheimer's disease. *Dementia and Geriatric Cognitive Disorders Extra, 1*, 51–61.

Liddle, B., & Nettle, D. (2006). Higher-order theory of mind and social competence in school-age children. *Journal of Cultural and Evolutionary Psychology, 4*, 231–246.

Linares-Orama, N. (2005). Language-learning disorders and youth incarceration. *Journal of Communication Disorders, 38*, 311–319.

Lincoln, T. M., Mehl, S., Kesting, M.-L., & Rief, W. (2011). Negative symptoms and social cognition: Identifying targets for psychological interventions. *Schizophrenia Bulletin, 37*, S23–S32.

Lind, S. E., & Bowler, D. M. (2010). Impaired performance on see-know tasks amongst children with autism: Evidence of specific difficulties with theory of mind or domain-general task factors? *Journal of Autism and Developmental Disorders, 40*, 479–484.

Lindholm, C., & Wray, A. (2011). Proverbs and formulaic sequences in the language of elderly people with dementia. *Dementia, 10*, 603–623.

Lindsay, G., & Dockrell, J. (2000). The behaviour and self-esteem of children with specific speech and language difficulties. *British Journal of Educational Psychology, 70*, 583–601.

Lindsay, G., Dockrell, J., & Palikara, O. (2010). Self-esteem of adolescents with specific language impairment as they move from compulsory education. *International Journal of Language & Communication Disorders, 45*, 561–571.

Lindsay, G., Dockrell, J. E., & Strand, S. (2007). Longitudinal patterns of behaviour problems in children with specific speech and language difficulties: Child and contextual factors. *British Journal of Educational Psychology, 77*, 811–828.

Linscott, R. J., Knight, R. G., & Godfrey, H. P. (1996). The Profile of Functional Impairment in Communication (PFIC): A measure of communication impairment for clinical use. *Brain Injury, 10*, 397–412.

Lobo, A., Launer, L. J., Fratiglioni, L., Andersen, K., Di Carlo, A., Breteler, M. M., et al. (2000). Prevalence of dementia and major subtypes in Europe: A collaborative study of population-based cohorts. Neurologic Diseases in the Elderly research group. *Neurology, 54*, S4–S9.

Lombardo, M. V., Chakrabarti, B., Bullmore, E. T., Baron-Cohen, S., & The MRC AIMS Consortium. (2011). Specialization of right temporo-parietal junction for mentalizing and its relation to social impairments. *Neuroimage, 56*, 1832–1838.

Long, B., Spencer-Smith, M., Jacobs, R., Mackay, M., Leventer, R., Barnes, C., et al. (2011). Executive function following child stroke: The impact of lesion size. *Developmental Neuropsychology, 36*, 971–987.

Lopez, O. L. (2011). The growing burden of Alzheimer's disease. *American Journal of Managed Care, 17*, S339–S345.

Lord, C., Rutter, M., Di Lavore, P., & Risi, S. (1999). *Autism diagnostic observation schedule.* Los Angeles: Western Psychological Services.

Losh, M., & Capps, L. (2003). Narrative ability in high-functioning children with autism or Asperger's syndrome. *Journal of Autism and Developmental Disorders, 33*, 239–251.

Losh, M., Martin, G. E., Klusek, J., Hogan-Brown, A. L., & Sideris, J. (2012). Social communication and theory of mind in boys with autism and fragile X syndrome. *Frontiers in Psychology, 3*, 1–12.

Lough, S., Kipps, C. M., Treise, C., Watson, P., Blair, J. R., & Hodges, J. R. (2006). Social reasoning, emotion and empathy in frontotemporal dementia. *Neuropsychologia, 44*, 950–958.

Loukusa, S., Leinonen, E., Jussila, K., Mattila, M.-L., Ryder, N., Ebeling, H., et al. (2007a). Answering contextually demanding questions: Pragmatic errors produced by children with Asperger syndrome or high-functioning autism. *Journal of Communication Disorders, 40*, 357–381.

Loukusa, S., Leinonen, E., & Ryder, N. (2007b). Development of pragmatic language comprehension in Finnish-speaking children. *First Language, 27*, 279–296.

Loukusa, S., & Moilanen, I. (2009). Pragmatic inference abilities in individuals with Asperger syndrome or high-functioning autism. A review. *Research in Autism Spectrum Disorders, 3*, 890–904.

Lund, N., & Duchan, J. (1983). *Assessing children's language in naturalistic contexts.* Englewood Cliffs: Prentice Hall.

Lysaker, P. H., Erickson, M. A., Buck, B., Buck, K. D., Olesek, K., Grant, M. L., et al. (2011). Metacognition and social function in schizophrenia: Associations over a period of five months. *Cognitive Neuropsychiatry, 16*, 241–255.

Mabbott, D. J., Barnes, M., Laperriere, N., Landry, S. H., & Bouffet, E. (2007). Neurocognitive function in same-sex twins following focal radiation for medulloblastoma. *Neuro-Oncology, 9*, 460–464.

Macedoni-Lukšič, M., Jereb, B., & L. Todorovski. (2003). Long-term sequelae in children treated for brain tumors: Impairments, disability, and handicap. *Pediatric Hematology–Oncology, 20*, 89–101.

MacKay, G., & Shaw, A. (2004). A comparative study of figurative language in children with autistic spectrum disorders. *Child Language Teaching and Therapy, 20*, 13–32.

Mackay, J., & Mensah, G. (2004). *The atlas of heart disease and stroke.* Geneva: World Health Organization.

Mackenzie, C., & Green, J. (2009). Cognitive-linguistic deficit and speech intelligibility in chronic progressive multiple sclerosis. *International Journal of Language & Communication Disorders, 44*, 401–420.

Mackie, L., & Law, J. (2010). Pragmatic language and the child with emotional/behavioural difficulties (EBD): A pilot study exploring the interaction between behaviour and communication disability. *International Journal of Language & Communication Disorders, 45*, 397–410.

MacPherson, M. K., Huber, J. E., & Snow, D. P. (2011). The intonation-syntax interface in the speech of individuals with Parkinson's disease. *Journal of Speech, Language, and Hearing Research, 54*, 19–32.

Maddrey, A. M., Bergeron, J. A., Lombardo, E. R., McDonald, N. K., Mulne, A. F., Barenberg, P. D., et al. (2005). Neuropsychological performance and quality of life of 10 year survivors of childhood medulloblastoma. *Journal of Neuro-Oncology, 72*, 245–253.

Majorek, K., Wolfkühler, W., Küper, C., Saimeh, N., Juckel, G., & Brüne, M. (2009). "Theory of mind" and executive functioning in forensic patients with schizophrenia. *Journal of Forensic Sciences, 54*, 469–473.

Manassis, K., Tannock, R., Garland, E. J., Minde, K., McInnes, A., & Clark, S. (2007). The sounds of silence: Language, cognition, and anxiety in selective mutism. *Journal of the American Academy of Child and Adolescent Psychiatry, 46*, 1187–1195.

Mäntylä, T., Carelli, M. G., & Forman, H. (2007). Time monitoring and executive functioning in children and adults. *Journal of Experimental Child Psychology, 96*, 1–19.

Mao-Draayer, Y., & Panitch, H. (2004). Alexia without agraphia in multiple sclerosis: Case report with magnetic resonance imaging localization. *Multiple Sclerosis, 10*, 705–707.

Mar, R. A. (2011). The neural bases of social cognition and story comprehension. *Annual Review of Psychology, 62*, 103–134.

Marini, A. (2012). Characteristics of narrative discourse processing after damage to the right hemisphere. *Seminars in Speech and Language, 33*, 68–78.

Marini, A., Carlomagno, S., Caltagirone, C., & Nocentini, U. (2005). The role played by the right hemisphere in the organization of complex textual structures. *Brain and Language, 93*, 46–54.

Marini, A., Galetto, V., Zampieri, E., Vorano, L., Zettin, M., & Carlomagno, S. (2011). Narrative language in traumatic brain injury. *Neuropsychologia, 49*, 2904–2910.

Marini, A., Spoletini, I., Rubino, I. A., Ciuffa, M., Bria, P., Martinotti, G., et al. (2008). The language of schizophrenia: An analysis of micro and macrolinguistic abilities and their neuropsychological correlates. *Schizophrenia Research, 105*, 144–155.

Marmaridou, S. S. A. (2000). *Pragmatic meaning and cognition.* Amsterdam: John Benjamins.

Marmaridou, S. S. A. (2010a). Presupposition. In L. Cummings (Ed.), *The Routledge pragmatics encyclopedia* (pp. 349–353). London: Routledge.

Marmaridou, S. S. A. (2010b). Deixis. In L. Cummings (Ed.), *The Routledge pragmatics encyclopedia* (pp. 101–105). London: Routledge.

Martin, G. E., Klusek, J., Estigarribia, B., & Roberts, J. E. (2009). Language characteristics of individuals with Down syndrome. *Topics in Language Disorders, 29*, 112–132.

Martin, I., & McDonald, S. (2003). Weak coherence, no theory of mind, or executive dysfunction? Solving the puzzle of pragmatic language disorders. *Brain and Language, 85*, 451–466.

Martin, I., & McDonald, S. (2004). An exploration of causes of non-literal language problems in individuals with Asperger syndrome. *Journal of Autism and Developmental Disorders, 34*, 311–328.

Marton, K., Abramoff, B., & Rosenzweig, S. (2005). Social cognition and language in children with specific language impairment (SLI). *Journal of Communication Disorders, 38*, 143–162.

Marton, I., Wiener, J., Rogers, M., Moore, C., & Tannock, R. (2009). Empathy and social perspective taking in children with attention-deficit/hyperactivity disorder. *Journal of Abnormal Child Psychology, 37*, 107–118.

Mateer, C. A. (1999). The rehabilitation of executive disorders. In D. T. Stuss, G. Winocur, & I. Robertson (Eds.), *Cognitive neurorehabilitation* (pp. 314–332). Cambridge: Cambridge University Press.

Mathers, M. E. (2006). Aspects of language in children with ADHD: Applying functional analyses to explore language use. *Journal of Attention Disorders, 9*, 523–533.

Mathias, J. L., Bowden, S. C., Bigler, E. D., & Rosenfeld, J. V. (2007). Is performance on the Wechsler test of adult reading affected by traumatic brain injury? *British Journal of Clinical Psychology, 46*, 457–466.

Matsui, Y., Tanizaki, Y., Arima, H., Yonemoto, K., Doi, Y., Ninomiya, T., et al. (2009). Incidence and survival of dementia in a general population of Japanese elderly: The Hisayama study. *Journal of Neurology, Neurosurgery, and Psychiatry, 80*, 366–370.

Mausbach, B. T., Bowie, C. R., Harvey, P. D., Twamley, E. W., Goldman, S. R., Jeste, D. V., et al. (2008). Usefulness of the UCSD performance-based skills assessment (UPSA) for predicting residential independence in patients with chronic schizophrenia. *Journal of Psychiatric Research, 42*, 320–327.

Mausbach, B. T., Harvey, P. D., Pulver, A. E., Depp, C. A., Wolyniec, P. S., Thornquist, M. H., et al. (2010). Relationship of the Brief UCSD Performance-Based Skills Assessment (UPSA-B) to multiple indicators of functioning in people with schizophrenia and bipolar disorder. *Bipolar Disorders, 12*, 45–55.

Mayer, M. (1969). *Frog, where are you?* New York: Penguin Books.

Maylor, E. A., Moulson, J. M., Muncer, A.-M., & Taylor, L. A. (2002). Does performance on theory of mind tasks decline in old age? *British Journal of Psychology, 93*, 465–485.

Mayr, W. T., Pittock, S. J., McClelland, R. L., Jorgensen, N. W., Noseworthy, J. H., & Rodriguez, M. (2003). Incidence and prevalence of multiple sclerosis in Olmsted County, Minnesota, 1985–2000. *Neurology, 61*, 1373–1377.

Mazumdar, P. K., Chaturvedi, S. K., Sinha, V., & Gopinath, P. S. (1991). Scale for assessment of thought, language and communication in psychotic in-patients. *Psychopathology, 24*, 199–202.

Mazza, M., Di Michele, V., Pollice, R., Casacchia, M., & Roncone, R. (2008). Pragmatic language and theory of mind deficits in people with schizophrenia and their relatives. *Psychopathology, 41*, 254–263.

McAuley, T., Christ, S. E., & White, D. A. (2011). Mapping the development of response inhibition in young children using a modified day-night task. *Developmental Neuropsychology, 36*, 539–551.

McCabe, P. J., Sheard, C., & Code, C. (2008). Communication impairment in the AIDS dementia complex (ADC): A case report. *Journal of Communication Disorders, 41*, 203–222.

McDonald, S. (1999). Exploring the process of inference generation in sarcasm: A review of normal and clinical studies. *Brain and Language, 68*, 486–506.

McDonald, S. (2000). Exploring the cognitive basis of right-hemisphere pragmatic language disorders. *Brain and Language, 75*, 82–107.

McDonald, S., & Flanagan, S. (2004). Social perception deficits after traumatic brain injury: Interaction between emotion recognition, mentalizing ability, and social communication. *Neuropsychology, 18*, 572–579.

McDonald, S., Flanagan, S., Rollins, J., & Kinch, J. (2003). TASIT: A new clinical tool for assessing social perception after traumatic brain injury. *Journal of Head Trauma Rehabilitation, 18*, 219–238.

McDonald, S., Tate, R., Togher, L., Bornhofen, C., Long, E., Gertler, P., et al. (2008). Social skills treatment for people with severe, chronic acquired brain injuries: A multicenter trial. *Archives of Physical Medicine and Rehabilitation, 89*, 1648–1659.

McGrath, J. J., Saha, S., Chant, D., & Welham, J. (2008). Schizophrenia: A concise overview of incidence, prevalence, and mortality. *Epidemiologic Reviews, 30*, 67–76.

McGregor, K. K., Berns, A. J., Owen, A. J., Michels, S. A., Duff, D., Bahnsen, A. J., et al. (2012). Associations between syntax and the lexicon among children with or without ASD and language impairment. *Journal of Autism and Developmental Disorders, 42*, 35–47.

McGuinness, B., Barrett, S. L., Craig, D., Lawson, J., & Passmore, A. P. (2010). Executive functioning in Alzheimer's disease and vascular dementia. *International Journal of Geriatric Psychiatry, 25*, 562–568.

McInnes, A., Fung, D., Manassis, K., Fiksenbaum, L., & Tannock, R. (2004). Narrative skills in children with selective mutism: An exploratory study. *American Journal of Speech-Language Pathology, 13*, 304–315.

McInnes, A., Humphries, T., Hogg-Johnson, S., & Tannock, R. (2003). Listening comprehension and working memory are impaired in attention-deficit hyperactivity disorder irrespective of language impairment. *Journal of Abnormal Child Psychology, 31*, 427–443.

McKinlay, A., Dalrymple-Alford, J. C., Grace, R. C., & Roger, D. (2009). The effect of attentional set-shifting, working memory, and processing speed on pragmatic language functioning in Parkinson's disease. *European Journal of Cognitive Psychology, 21*, 330–346.

McKinney, P. A. (2004). Brain tumours: Incidence, survival, and aetiology. *Journal of Neurology, Neurosurgery & Psychiatry, 75*, ii12–ii17.

McMurtray, A., Clark, D. G., Christine, D., & Mendez, M. F. (2006). Early-onset dementia: Frequency and causes compared to late-onset dementia. *Dementia and Geriatric Cognitive Disorders, 21*, 59–64.

McNamara, P., & Durso, R. (2003). Pragmatic communication skills in patients with Parkinson's disease. *Brain and Language, 84*, 414–423.

McNamara, P., Holtgraves, T., Durso, R., & Harris, E. (2010). Social cognition of indirect speech: Evidence from Parkinson's disease. *Journal of Neurolinguistics, 23*, 162–171.

McTear, M. F. (1985) Pragmatic disorders: A case study of conversational disability. *British Journal of Disorders of Communication, 20*, 129–142.

McWilliams, J., & Schmitter-Edgecombe, M. (2008). Semantic memory organization during the early stage of recovery from traumatic brain injury. *Brain Injury, 22*, 243–253.

Mechling, L. C., Pridgen, L. S., & Cronin, B. A. (2005). Computer-based video instruction to teach students with intellectual disabilities to verbally respond to questions and make purchases in fast food restaurants. *Education and Training in Developmental Disabilities, 40*, 47–59.

Mei, C., & Morgan, A. T. (2011). Incidence of mutism, dysarthria and dysphagia associated with childhood posterior fossa tumour. *Child's Nervous System, 27*, 1129–36.

Meilijson, S. R., Kasher, A., & Elizur, A. (2004). Language performance in chronic schizophrenia: A pragmatic approach. *Journal of Speech, Language, and Hearing Research, 47*, 695–713.

Meini, C. (2010). Modularity of mind thesis. In L. Cummings (ed.), *The Routledge pragmatics encyclopedia* (pp. 275–278). London: Routledge.

Menghini, D., Addona, F., Costanzo, F., & Vicari, S. (2010). Executive functions in individuals with Williams syndrome. *Journal of Intellectual Disability Research, 54*, 418–432.

Mentis, M., Briggs-Whittaker, J., & Gramigna, G. D. (1995). Discourse topic management in senile dementia of the Alzheimer's type. *Journal of Speech and Hearing Research, 38*, 1054–1066.

Mervis, C. B., & John, A. E. (2010). Cognitive and behavioral characteristics of children with Williams syndrome: Implications for intervention approaches. *American Journal of Medical Genetics Part C: Seminars in Medical Genetics, 154C*, 229–248.

Meteyard, L., & Patterson, K. (2009). The relation between content and structure in language production: An analysis of speech errors in semantic dementia. *Brain and Language, 110*, 121–134.

Milders, M., Ietswaart, M., Crawford, J. R., & Currie, D. (2006). Impairments in theory of mind shortly after traumatic brain injury and at 1-year follow-up. *Neuropsychology, 20*, 400–408.

Milders, M., Ietswaart, M., Crawford, J. R., & Currie, D. (2008). Social behavior following traumatic brain injury and its association with emotion recognition, understanding of intentions, and cognitive flexibility. *Journal of the International Neuropsychological Society, 14*, 318–326.

Miller, C. A. (2001). False belief understanding in children with specific language impairment. *Journal of Communication Disorders, 34*, 73–86.

Miller, C. A. (2004). False belief and sentence complement performance in children with specific language impairment. *International Journal of Language & Communication Disorders, 39*, 191–213.

Millichap, J. G. (2008). Etiologic classification of attention-deficit/hyperactivity disorder. *Pediatrics, 121*, e358–e365.

Minter, M., Hobson, R. P., & Bishop, M. (1998). Congenital visual impairment and 'theory of mind'. *British Journal of Developmental Psychology, 16*, 183–196.

Mirian, D., Walter Heinrichs, R., & McDermid Vaz, S. (2011). Exploring logical reasoning abilities in schizophrenia patients. *Schizophrenia Research, 127*, 178–180.

Miyake, A., Friedman, N. P., Emerson, M. J., Witzki, A. H., Howerter, A., & Wager, T. D. (2000). The unity and diversity of executive functions and their contributions to complex "frontal lobe" tasks: A latent variable analysis. *Cognitive Psychology, 41*, 49–100.

Mo, S., Su, Y., Chan, R. C. K., & Liu, J. (2008). Comprehension of metaphor and irony in schizophrenia during remission: The role of theory of mind and IQ. *Psychiatry Research, 157*, 21–29.

Monetta, L., Grindrod, C. M., & Pell, M. D. (2009). Irony comprehension and theory of mind deficits in patients with Parkinson's disease. *Cortex, 45*, 972–981.

Monetta, L., & Pell, M. D. (2007). Effects of verbal working memory deficits on metaphor comprehension in patients with Parkinson's disease. *Brain and Language, 101*, 80–89.

Montag, C., Dziobek, I., Richter, I. S., Neuhaus, K., Lehmann, A., Sylla, R., et al. (2011). Different aspects of theory of mind in paranoid schizophrenia: Evidence from a video-based assessment. *Psychiatry Research, 186*, 203–209.

Moody, K. C., Holzer, C. E., Roman, M. J., Paulsen, K. A., Freeman, D. H., Haynes, M., et al. (2000). Prevalence of dyslexia among Texas prison inmates. *Texas Medicine, 96*, 69–75.

Moran, C., & Gillon, G. (2004). Language and memory profiles of adolescents with traumatic brain injury. *Brain Injury, 18*, 273–288.

Moran, C., & Gillon, G. (2005). Inference comprehension of adolescents with traumatic brain injury: A working memory hypothesis. *Brain Injury, 19*, 743–751.

Morgan, A. T., Mageandran, S. D., & Mei, C. (2010). Incidence and clinical presentation of dysarthria and dysphagia in the acute setting following paediatric traumatic brain injury. *Child: Care, Health and Development, 36*, 44–53.

Morgan, A. T., Sell, D., Ryan, M., Raynsford, E., & Hayward, R. (2008). Pre and post-surgical dysphagia outcome associated with posterior fossa tumour in children. *Journal of Neuro-Oncology, 87*, 347–354.

Mouridsen, S. E. (2012). Current status of research on autism spectrum disorders and offending. *Research in Autism Spectrum Disorders, 6*, 79–86.

Muir, C., O'Callaghan, M. J., Bor, W., Najman, J. M., & Williams, G. M. (2011). Speech concerns at 5 years and adult educational and mental health outcomes. *Journal of Paediatrics and Child Health, 47*, 423–428.

Mukand, J. A., Blackinton, D. D., Crincoli, M. G., Lee, J. J., & Santos, B. B. (2001). Incidence of neurologic deficits and rehabilitation of patients with brain tumors. *American Journal of Physical Medicine & Rehabilitation, 80*, 346–350.

Mulhern, R. K., Merchant, T. E., Gajjar, A., Reddick, W. E., & Kun, L. E. (2004). Late neurocognitive sequelae in survivors of brain tumours in childhood. *The Lancet Oncology, 5*, 399–408.

Muller, F., Simion, A., Reviriego, E., Galera, C., Mazaux, J.-M., Barat, M., et al. (2010). Exploring theory of mind after severe traumatic brain injury. *Cortex, 46*, 1088–1099.

Müller, U., Liebermann-Finestone, D. P., Carpendale, J. I. M., Hammond, S. I., & Bibok, M. B. (2012). Knowing minds, controlling actions: The developmental relations between theory of mind and executive function from 2 to 4 years of age. *Journal of Experimental Child Psychology, 111*, 331–348.

Munroe-Blum, H., Collins, E., McCleary, L., & Nuttall, S. The social dysfunction index for patients with schizophrenia and related disorders. *Schizophrenia Research 20*:211-219.

Murdock, L. C., Cost, H. C., & Tieso, C. (2007). Measurement of social communication skills of children with autism spectrum disorders during interactions with typical peers. *Focus on Autism and Other Developmental Disabilities, 22*, 160–172.

Murray, L. L. (2000). Spoken language production in Huntington's and Parkinson's diseases. *Journal of Speech, Language, and Hearing Research, 43*, 1350–1366.

Myers, P. S. (1979). Profiles of communication deficits in patients with right cerebral hemisphere damage: implications for diagnosis and treatment. *Clinical aphasiology conference* (pp. 38–46). Phoenix: BRK Publishers.

Naess, H., Hammersvik, L., & Skeie, G. O. (2009). Aphasia among young patients with ischaemic stroke on long-term follow-up. *Journal of Stroke and Cerebrovascular Diseases, 18*, 247–250.

Naigles, L. R., Kelty, E., Jaffery, R., & Fein, D. (2011). Abstractness and continuity in the syntactic development of young children with autism. *Autism Research, 4*, 422–437.

Najam, N., Tarter, R. E., & Kirisci, L. (1997). Language deficits in children at high risk for drug abuse. *Journal of Child & Adolescent Substance Abuse, 6*, 69–80.

Nass, R., Boyce, L., Leventhal, F., Levine, B., Allen, J., Maxfield, C., et al. (2000). Acquired aphasia in children after surgical resection of left-thalamic tumors. *Developmental Medicine and Child Neurology, 42*, 580–590.

National Institutes of Health. (2008). *NIH develops Down syndrome research plan*. Retrieved from www.nih.gov/news/health/jan2008/nichd-22.htm

Naylor, L., & van Herwegen, J. (2012). The production of figurative language in typically developing children and Williams syndrome. *Research in Developmental Disabilities, 33*, 711–716.

Newbury, D. F., & Monaco, A. P. (2010). Genetic advances in the study of speech and language disorders. *Neuron, 68*, 309–320.

Newcomer, P. L., & Hammill, D. D. (1991). *Test of language development—primary* (2nd ed.). Austin: Pro-Ed.

Nicolle, S., & Clark, B. (1999). Experimental pragmatics and what is said: A response to Gibbs and Moise. *Cognition, 69*, 337–354.

Niklasson, L., & Gillberg, C. (2010). The neuropsychology of 22q11 deletion syndrome. A neuropsychiatric study of 100 individuals. *Research in Developmental Disabilities, 31*, 185–194.

Nippold, M. A., Ward-Lonergan, J. M., & Fanning, J. L. (2005). Persuasive writing in children, adolescents, and adults: A study of syntactic, semantic, and pragmatic development. *Language, Speech, and Hearing Services in Schools, 36*, 125–138.

Nocentini, U., Pasqualetti, P., Bonavita, S., Buccafusca, M., De Caro, M. F., Farina, D., et al. (2006). Cognitive dysfunction in patients with relapsing-remitting multiple sclerosis. *Multiple Sclerosis, 12*, 77–87.

Norbury, C. F., Griffiths, H., & Nation, K. (2010). Sound before meaning: Word learning in autistic disorders. *Neuropsychologia, 48*, 4012–4019.

Northcott, S., & Hilari, K. (2011). Why do people lose their friends after a stroke? *International Journal of Language & Communication Disorders, 46*, 524–534.

Noveck, I. A., & Posada, A. (2003). Characterizing the time course of an implicature: An evoked potentials study. *Brain and Language, 85*, 203–210.

Numminen, H. J. (2011). The incidence of traumatic brain injury in an adult population—how to classify mild cases? *European Journal of Neurology, 18*, 460–464.

O'Brien, G., & Pearson, J. (2004). Autism and learning disability. *Autism, 8*, 125–140.

Okanda, M., Moriguchi, Y., & Itakura, S. (2010). Language and cognitive shifting: Evidence from young monolingual and bilingual children. *Psychological Reports, 107*, 68–78.

Olvera, R. L., Semrud-Clikeman, M., Pliszka, S. R., & O'Donnell, L. (2005). Neuropsychological deficits in adolescents with conduct disorder and comorbid bipolar disorder: A pilot study. *Bipolar Disorders, 7*, 57–67.

Onishi, K. H., Baillargeon, R., & Leslie, A. M. (2007). 15-month-old infants detect violations in pretend scenarios. *Acta Psychologica, 124*, 106–128.

Orjada, S. A. (2007). *Impliciture processing after right hemisphere damage*. PhD thesis, University of Arizona.

Ozdemir, S. (2008). The effectiveness of social stories on decreasing disruptive behaviors of children with autism: Three case studies. *Journal of Autism and Developmental Disorders, 38*, 1689–1696.

Palmerini, F., & Bogousslavsky, J. (2012). Right hemisphere syndromes. *Frontiers of Neurology and Neuroscience, 30*, 61–64.

Papagno, C. (2001). Comprehension of metaphors and idioms in patients with Alzheimer's disease: A longitudinal study. *Brain, 124*, 1450–1460.

Papagno, C., & Caporali, A. (2007). Testing idiom comprehension in aphasic patients: The effects of task and idiom type. *Brain and Language, 100*, 208–220.

Papagno, C., Curti, R., Rizzo, S., Crippa, F., & Colombo, M. R. (2006). Is the right hemisphere involved in idiom comprehension? A neuropsychological study. *Neuropsychology, 20*, 598–606.

Papagno, C., Lucchelli, F., Muggia, S., & Rizzo, S. (2003). Idiom comprehension in Alzheimer's disease: The role of the central executive. *Brain, 126*, 2419–2430.

Papagno, C., Tabossi, P., Colombo, M. R., & Zampetti, P. (2004). Idiom comprehension in aphasic patients. *Brain and Language, 89*, 226–234.

Papagno, C., & Vallar, G. (2001). Understanding metaphors and idioms: A single-case neuropsychological study in a person with Down syndrome. *Journal of the International Neuropsychological Society, 7*, 516–527.

Park, K. W., Kim, H. S., Cheon, S.-M., Cha, J.-K., Kim, S.-H., & Kim, J. W. (2011a). Dementia with Lewy bodies versus Alzheimer's disease and Parkinson's disease dementia: A comparison of cognitive profiles. *Journal of Clinical Neurology, 7*, 19–24.

Park, K.-M., Ku, J., Choi, S.-H., Jang, H.-J., Park, J.-Y., Kim, S. I., et al. (2011). A virtual reality application in role-plays of social skills training for schizophrenia: A randomized, controlled trial. *Psychiatry Research, 189*, 166–172.

Patterson, T. L., Goldman, S., McKibbin, C. L., Hughs, T., & Jeste, D. V. (2001a). UCSD Performance-Based Skills Assessment: Development of a new measure of everyday functioning for severely mentally ill adults. *Schizophrenia Bulletin, 27*, 235–245.

Patterson, T. L., Moscona, S., McKibbin, C. L., Davidson, K., & Jeste, D. V. (2001b). Social skills performance assessment among older patients with schizophrenia. *Schizophrenia Research, 48*, 351–360.

Pei, J., Job, J., Kully-Martens, K., & Rasmussen, C. (2011). Executive function and memory in children with fetal alcohol spectrum disorder. *Child Neuropsychology, 17*, 290–309.

Pelc, K., Kornreich, C., Foisy, M.-L., & Dan, B. (2006). Recognition of emotional facial expressions in attention-deficit hyperactivity disorder. *Pediatric Neurology, 35*, 93–97.

Pellicano, E., & Neil Macrae, C. (2009). Mutual eye gaze facilitates person categorization for typically developing children, but not for children with autism. *Psychonomic Bulletin & Review, 16*, 1094–1099.

Penn, C., & Cleary, J. (1988). Compensatory strategies in the language of closed head-injured patients. *Brain Injury, 2*, 3–17.

Peppé, S., McCann, J., Gibbon, F., O'Hare, A., & Rutherford, M. (2007). Receptive and expressive prosodic ability in children with high-functioning autism. *Journal of Speech, Language, and Hearing Research, 50*, 1015–1028.

Perkins, L., Whitworth, A., & Lesser, R. (1998). Conversing in dementia: A conversation analytic approach. *Journal of Neurolinguistics, 11*, 33–53.

Perlini, C., Marini, A., Garzitto, M., Isola, M., Cerruti, S., Marinelli, V., et al. (2012). Linguistic production and syntactic comprehension in schizophrenia and bipolar disorder. *Acta Psychiatrica Scandinavica, 126*, 363–376.

Pexman, P. M., Rostad, K. R., McMorris, C. A., Climie, E. A., Stowkowy, J., & Glenwright, M. R. (2011). Processing of ironic language in children with high-functioning autism spectrum disorders. *Journal of Autism and Developmental Disorders, 41*, 1097–1112.

Phelps-Terasaki, D., & Phelps-Gunn, T. (1992). *Test of pragmatic language.* San Antonio: Psychological Corporation.

Phillips, L. H., Bull, R., Allen, R., Insch, P., Burr, K., & Ogg, W. (2011). Lifespan aging and belief reasoning: Influences of executive function and social cue decoding. *Cognition, 120*, 236–247.

Phillips, L. H., Scott, C., Henry, J. D., Mowat, D., Stephen Bell, J. (2010). Emotion perception in Alzheimer's disease and mood disorder in old age. *Psychology and Aging, 25*, 38–47.

Philofsky, A., Fidler, D. J., & Hepburn, S. (2007). Pragmatic language profiles of school-age children with autism spectrum disorders and Williams syndrome. *American Journal of Speech-Language Pathology, 16*, 368–380.

Pijnacker, J., Hagoort, P., Buitelaar, J., Teunisse, J.-P., & Geurts, B. (2009). Pragmatic inferences in high-functioning adults with autism and Asperger syndrome. *Journal of Autism and Developmental Disorders, 39*, 607–618.

Polanczyk, G., Silva de Lima, M., Lessa Horta, B., Biederman, J., & Augusto Rohde, L. (2007). The worldwide prevalence of ADHD: A systematic review and metaregression analysis. *American Journal of Psychiatry, 164*, 942–948.

Polimeni, J. O., Campbell, D. W., Gill, D., Sawatzky, B. L., & Reiss, J. P. (2010). Diminished humour perception in schizophrenia: Relationship to social and cognitive functioning. *Journal of Psychiatric Research, 44*, 434–440.

Polite, E. J., Leonard, L. B., & Roberts, F. D. (2011). The use of definite and indefinite articles by children with specific language impairment. *International Journal of Speech-Language Pathology, 13*, 291–300.

Pollack, I. F. (2011). Multidisciplinary management of childhood brain tumors: A review of outcomes, recent advances, and challenges. *Journal of Neurosurgery. Pediatrics, 8*, 135–148.

Povlishock, J. T., & Katz, D. I. (2005). Update of neuropathology and neurological recovery after traumatic brain injury. *Journal of Head Trauma Rehabilitation, 20*, 76–94.

Premack, D., & Woodruff, G. (1978). Does the chimpanzee have a "theory of mind"? *Behavioral and Brain Sciences, 1*, 515–526.

Price, J. R., Roberts, J. E., Hennon, E. A., Berni, M. C., Anderson, K. L., & Sideris, J. (2008). Syntactic complexity during conversation of boys with fragile X syndrome and Down syndrome. *Journal of Speech, Language, and Hearing Research, 51*, 3–15.

Prinz, P. M. (1980). A note on requesting strategies in adult aphasics. *Journal of Communication Disorders, 13*, 65–73.

Prizant, B. M., & Duchan, J. F. (1981). The functions of immediate echolalia in autistic children. *Journal of Speech and Hearing Disorders, 46*, 241–249.

Prizant, B. M., & Rydell, P. J. (1984). Analysis of functions of delayed echolalia in autistic children. *Journal of Speech and Hearing Research, 27*, 183–192.

Proctor, T., & Beail, N. (2007). Empathy and theory of mind in offenders with intellectual disability. *Journal of Intellectual & Developmental Disability, 32*, 82–93.

Prutting, C. A., & Kirchner, D. M. (1987). A clinical appraisal of the pragmatic aspects of language. *Journal of Speech and Hearing Disorders, 52*, 105–119.

Purdy, M. H. (2002). Executive function ability in persons with aphasia. *Aphasiology, 16*, 549–557.

Quinsey, V. L., Harris, G. T., Rice, M. E., & Cormier, C. A. (1998). *Violent offenders: Appraising and managing risk.* Washington, DC: American Psychological Association.

Quirmbach, L. M., Lincoln, A. J., Feinberg-Gizzo, M. J., Ingersoll, B. R., & Andrews, S. M. (2009). Social stories: Mechanisms of effectiveness in increasing game play skills in children diagnosed with autism spectrum disorder using a pretest posttest repeated measures randomized control group design. *Journal of Autism and Developmental Disorders, 39*, 299–321.

Raaphorst, J., de Visser, M., van Tol, M.-J., Linssen, W. H. J. P., van der Kooi, A. J., de Haan, R. J., et al. (2011). Cognitive dysfunction in lower motor neuron disease: Executive and memory deficits in progressive muscular atrophy. *Journal of Neurology, Neurosurgery, and Psychiatry, 82*, 170–175.

Rainville, C., Giroire, J.-M., Periot, M., Cuny, El., & Mazaux, J.-M. (2003). The impact of right subcortical lesions on executive functions and spatio-cognitive abilities: A case study. *Neurocase, 9*, 356–367.

Rapp, A. M., & Wild, B. (2011). Nonliteral language in Alzheimer dementia: A review. *Journal of the International Neuropsychological Society, 17*, 207–218.

Rasmussen, C., Wyper, K., & Talwar, V. (2009). The relation between theory of mind and executive functions in children with fetal alcohol spectrum disorders. *Canadian Journal of Clinical Pharmacology, 16*, e370–380.

Rassiga, C., Lucchelli, F., Crippa, F., & Papago, C. (2009). Ambiguous idiom comprehension in Alzheimer's disease. *Journal of Clinical and Experimental Neuropsychology, 31*, 402–411.

Rautanen, M., & Lauerma, H. (2011). Imprisonment and diagnostic delay among male offenders with schizophrenia. *Criminal Behaviour and Mental Health, 21*, 259–264.

Reck, S. G., & Hund, A. M. (2011). Sustained attention and age predict inhibitory control during early childhood. *Journal of Experimental Child Psychology, 108*, 504–512.

Reichow, B., & Sabornie, E. J. (2009). Brief report: Increasing verbal greeting initiations for a student with autism via a social story intervention. *Journal of Autism and Developmental Disorders, 39*, 1740–1743.

Reichow, B., Steiner, A. M., & Volkmar, F. (2012). Social skills groups for people aged 6 to 21 with autism spectrum disorders (ASD). *Cochrane Database of Systematic Reviews*, Issue 7. Art. No.: CD008511. doi:10.1002/14651858.CD008511.pub2.

Reilly, J., & Peelle, J. E. (2008). Effects of semantic impairment on language processing in semantic dementia. *Seminars in Speech and Language, 29*, 32–43.

Reilly, J., Rodriguez, A. D., Lamy, M., & Neils-Strunjas, J. (2010). Cognition, language, and clinical pathological features of non-Alzheimer's dementias: An overview. *Journal of Communication Disorders, 43*, 438–452.

Reiner, A., Dragatsis, I., & Dietrich, P. (2011). Genetics and neuropathology of Huntington's disease. *International Review of Neurobiology, 98*, 325–372.

Reisberg, B., Ferris, S. H., de Leon, M. J., & Crook, T. (1982). The Global Deterioration Scale for assessment of primary degenerative dementia. *American Journal of Psychiatry, 139*, 1136–1139.

Renfrew, C. E. (1997). *Bus story test: A test of narrative speech*. Bicester: Winslow.

Renvoize, E., Hanson, M., & Dale, M. (2011). Prevalence and causes of young onset dementia in an English health district. *International Journal of Geriatric Psychiatry, 26*, 106–107.

Reynhout, G., & Carter, M. (2006). Social stories™ for children with disabilities. *Journal of Autism and Developmental Disorders, 36*, 445–469.

Ribi, K., Reilly, C., Landolt, M. A., Alber, F. D., Boltshauser, E., & Grotzer, M. A. (2005). Outcome of medulloblastoma in children: long-term complications and quality of life. *Neuropediatrics, 36*, 357–365.

Riby, D. M., Doherty-Sneddon, G., & Bruce, V. (2008). Exploring face perception in disorders of development: Evidence from Williams syndrome and autism. *Journal of Neuropsychology, 2*, 47–64.

Richardson, J., & Joughin, C. (2002). *Parent training programmes for the management of young children with conduct disorders*. London: The Royal College of Psychiatrists.

Riches, N. G., Loucas, T., Baird, G., Charman, T., & Simonoff, E. (2010). Sentence repetition in children with specific language impairment and autism: A study of linguistic factors affecting recall. *International Journal of Language and Communication Disorders, 45*, 47–60.

Richter, S., Schoch, B., Kaiser, O., Groetschel, H., Hein-Kropp, C., Maschke, M., et al. (2005). Children and adolescents with chronic cerebellar lesions show no clinically relevant signs of aphasia or neglect. *Journal of Neurophysiology, 94*, 4108–4120.

Rinaldi, M. C., Marangolo, P., & Baldassarri, F. (2004). Metaphor comprehension in right brain-damaged patients with visuo-verbal and verbal material: A dissociation (re)considered. *Cortex, 40*, 479–490.

Ringman, J. M., Kwon, E., Flores, D. L., Rotko, C., Mendez, M. F., & Lu, P. (2010). The use of profanity during letter fluency tasks in frontotemporal dementia and Alzheimer disease. *Cognitive and Behavioral Neurology, 23*, 159–164.

Ripley, K., & Yuill, N. (2005). Patterns of language impairment and behaviour in boys excluded from school. *British Journal of Educational Psychology, 75*, 37–50.

Riva, D., & Giorgi, C. (2000). The cerebellum contributes to higher functions during development: evidence from a series of children surgically treated for posterior fossa tumours. *Brain, 123*, 1051–1061.

Roberstson, J. M., Tanguay, P. E., L'Ecuyer, S., Sims, A., & Waltrip, C. (1999). Domains of social communication handicap in autism spectrum disorder. *Journal of the American Academy of Child & Adolescent Psychiatry, 38*, 738–745.

Roberts-South, A., Findlater, K., Strong, M. J., & Orange, J. B. (2012). Longitudinal changes in discourse production in amyotrophic lateral sclerosis. *Seminars in Speech and Language, 33*, 79–94.

Robinson, S., Goddard, L., Dritschel, B., Wisley, M., & Howlin, P. (2009). Executive functions in children with autism spectrum disorders. *Brain and Cognition, 71*, 362–368.

Rockers, K., Ousley, O., Sutton, T., Schoenberg, E., Coleman, K., Walker, E., et al. (2009). Performance on the modified card sorting test and its relation to psychopathology in adolescents and young adults with 22q11.2 deletion syndrome. *Journal of Intellectual Disability Research, 53*, 665–676.

Rogalski, E., Cobia, D., Harrison, T. M., Wieneke, C., Thompson, C. K., Weintraub, S., et al. (2011b). Anatomy of language impairments in primary progressive aphasia. *Journal of Neuroscience, 31*, 3344–3350.

Rogalski, E., Cobia, D., Harrison, T. M., Wieneke, C., Weintraub, S., & Mesulam, M. M. (2011a). Progression of language decline and cortical atrophy in subtypes of primary progressive aphasia. *Neurology, 76*, 1804–1810.

Rohrer, J. D., Rossor, M. N., & Warren, J. D. (2010). Syndromes of nonfluent primary progressive aphasia: A clinical and neurolinguistic analysis. *Neurology, 75*, 603–610.

Rohrer, J. D., Sauter, D., Scott, S., Rossor, M. N., & Warren, J. D. (2012). Receptive prosody in nonfluent primary progressive aphasias. *Cortex, 48*, 308–316.

Rossell, S. L., & David, A. S. (2006). Are semantic deficits in schizophrenia due to problems with access or storage? *Schizophrenia Research, 82*, 121–134.

Roujeau, T., Di Rocco, F., Dufour, C., Bourdeaut, F., Puget, S., Rose, C. S., et al. (2011). Shall we treat hydrocephalus associated to brain stem glioma in children? *Child's Nervous System, 27*, 1735–1739.

Rousseaux, M., Vérigneaux, C., & Kozlowski, O. (2010a). An analysis of communication in conversation after severe traumatic brain injury. *European Journal of Neurology, 17*, 922–929.

Rousseaux, M., Daveluy, W., & Kozlowski, O. (2010b). Communication in conversation in stroke patients. *Journal of Neurology, 257*, 1099–1107.

Rousseaux, M., Sève, A., Vallet, M., Pasquier, F., & Mackowiak-Cordoliani, M. A. (2010c). An analysis of communication in conversation in patients with dementia. *Neuropsychologia, 48*, 3884–3890.

Rowan, L. E., Leonard, L. B., Chapman, K., & Weiss, A. L. (1983). Performative and presuppositional skills in language-disordered and normal children. *Journal of Speech and Hearing Research, 26*, 97–106.

Ruffman, T., Slade, L., & Crowe, E. (2002). The relation between children's and mother's mental state language and theory-of-mind understanding. *Child Development, 73*, 734–751.

Rumpf, A.-L., Kamp-Becker, I., Becker, K., & Kauschke, C. (2012). Narrative competence and internal state language of children with Asperger syndrome and ADHD. *Research in Developmental Disabilities, 33*, 1395–1407.

Russell, R. L. (2007). Social communication impairments: Pragmatics. *Pediatric Clinics of North America, 54*, 483–506.

Rust, J., & Smith, A. (2006). How should the effectiveness of Social stories to modify the behaviour of children on the autistic spectrum be tested? Lessons from the literature. *Autism, 10*, 125–138.

Rutherford, M. D., Baron-Cohen, S., & Wheelwright, S. (2002). Reading the mind in the voice: A study with normal adults and adults with Asperger syndrome and high functioning autism. *Journal of Autism and Developmental Disorders, 32*, 189–194.

Rutter, M., Bailey, A., & Lord, C. (2003). *The social communication questionnaire (SCQ)*. Los Angeles: Western Psychological Services.

Rybarova, D. (2007). *Frontal mechanisms in language pragmatics: Neuropsychological and electrophysiological evidence*. PhD thesis, University of Arizona.

Ryder, N., & Leinonen, E. (2003). Use of context in question answering by 3-, 4- and 5-year-old children. *Journal of Psycholinguistic Research, 32*, 397–415.

Ryder, N., Leinonen, E., & Schulz, J. (2008). Cognitive approach to assessing pragmatic language comprehension in children with specific language impairment. *International Journal of Language & Communication Disorders, 43*, 427–447.

Sadiq, F. A., Slator, L., Skuse, D., Law, J., Gillberg, C., & Minnis, H. (2012). Social use of language in children with reactive attachment disorder and autism spectrum disorders. *European Child & Adolescent Psychiatry, 21*, 267–276.

Sailor, K. M., Zimmerman, M. E., & Sanders, A. E. (2011). Differential impacts of age of acquisition on letter and semantic fluency in Alzheimer's disease patients and healthy older adults. *Quarterly Journal of Experimental Psychology, 64*, 2383–2391.

Saldert, C., Fors, A., Ströberg, S., & Hartelius, L. (2010). Comprehension of complex discourse in different stages of Huntington's disease. *International Journal of Language & Communication Disorders, 45*, 656–669.

Saldert, C., & Hartelius, L. (2011). Echolalia or functional repetition in conversation—a case study of an individual with Huntington's disease. *Disability and Rehabilitation, 33*, 253–260.

Saltzman, J., Strauss, E., Hunter, M., & Archibald, S. (2000). Theory of mind and executive functions in normal human aging and Parkinson's disease. *Journal of the International Neuropsychological Society, 6*, 781–788.

Sanger, D. D., Creswell, J. W., Dworak, J., & Schultz, L. (2000). Cultural analysis of communication behaviors among juveniles in a correctional facility. *Journal of Communication Disorders, 33*, 31–57.

Sanger, D., Maag, J. W., & Spilker, A. (2006). Communication and behavioral considerations in planning programs for female juvenile delinquents. *Journal of Correctional Education, 57*, 108–125.

Sanger, D. D., Moore-Brown, B. J., Magnuson, G., & Svoboda, N. (2001). Prevalence of language problems among adolescent delinquents: A closer look. *Communication Disorders Quarterly, 23*, 17–26.

Sanger, D. D., Moore-Brown, B. J., Montgomery, J. K., & Larson, V. L. (2002). Service delivery framework for adolescents with communication problems who are involved in violence. *Journal of Communication Disorders, 35*, 293–303.

Sanger, D. D., Moore-Brown, B. J., Montgomery, J., Rezac, C., & Keller, H. (2003). Female incarcerated adolescents with language problems talk about their own communication behaviors and learning. *Journal of Communication Disorders, 36*, 465–486.

Santangelo, G., Vitale, C., Trojano, L., Errico, D., Amboni, M., Barbarulo, A. M., et al. (2012). Neuropsychological correlates of theory of mind in patients with early Parkinson's disease. *Movement Disorders, 27*, 98–105.

Santos, A., & Deruelle, C. (2009). Verbal peaks and visual valleys in theory of mind ability in Williams syndrome. *Journal of Autism and Developmental Disorders, 39*, 651–659.

Sanz, J. H., Lipkin, P., Rosenbaum, K., & Mahone, E. M. (2010). Developmental profile and trajectory of neuropsychological skills in a child with Kabuki syndrome: Implications for assessment of syndromes associated with intellectual disability. *The Clinical Neuropsychologist, 24*, 1181–1192.

Sarno, M. T. (1969). *Functional communication profile*. New York: Institute for Rehabilitation Medicine, NYU Medical Center.

Sartori, L., Becchio, C., Bara, B. G., & Castiello, U. (2009). Does the intention to communicate affect action kinematics? *Consciousness and Cognition, 18*, 766–772.

Scattone, D., Wilczynski, S. M., Edwards, R. P., & Rabian, B. (2002). Decreasing disruptive behaviors of children with autism using social stories. *Journal of Autism and Developmental Disorders, 32*, 535–543.

Scharfstein, L. A., Beidel, D. C., Sims, V. K., & Finnell, L. R. (2011). Social skills deficits and vocal characteristics of children with social phobia or Asperger's disorder: A comparative study. *Journal of Abnormal Child Psychology, 39*, 865–875.

Scheibel, R. S., Newsome, M. R., Wilde, E. A., McClelland, M. M., Hanten, G., Krawczyk, D. C., et al. (2011). Brain activation during a social attribution task in adolescents with moderate to severe traumatic brain injury. *Social Neuroscience, 6*, 582–598.

Schelletter, C., & Leinonen, E. (2003). Normal and language-impaired children's use of reference: Syntactic versus pragmatic processing. *Clinical Linguistics & Phonetics, 17*, 335–343.

Schenkel, L. S., Spaulding, W. D., & Silverstein, S. M. (2005). Poor premorbid social functioning and theory of mind deficit in schizophrenia: Evidence of reduced context processing? *Journal of Psychiatric Research, 39*, 499–508.

Schiffer, S. R. (1972). *Meaning*. Oxford: Clarendon Press.

Schmidt, K. S., Gallo, J. L., Ferri, C., Giovannetti, T., Sestito, N., Libon, D. J., et al. (2005). The neuropsychological profile of alcohol-related dementia suggests cortical and subcortical pathology. *Dementia and Geriatric Cognitive Disorders, 20*, 286–291.

Schoemaker, K., Bunte, T., Wiebe, S. A., Espy, K. A., Deković, M., & Matthys, W. (2012). Executive function deficits in preschool children with ADHD and DBD. *Journal of Child Psychology and Psychiatry, 53*, 111–119.

Schoen, E., Paul, R., & Chawarska, K. (2011). Phonology and vocal behavior in toddlers with autism spectrum disorders. *Autism Research, 4*, 177–188.

Schürhoff, F., Golmard, J.-L., Szöke, A., Bellivier, F., Berthier, A., Méary, A., et al. (2004). Admixture analysis of age at onset in schizophrenia. *Schizophrenia Research, 71*, 35–41.

Schweizer, T. A., Levine, B., Rewilak, D., O'Connor, C., Turner, G., Alexander, M. P., et al. (2008). Rehabilitation of executive functioning after focal damage to the cerebellum. *Neurorehabilitation & Neural Repair, 22*, 72–77.

Scott-Phillips, T. C. (2010). Social cognition. In L. Cummings (Ed.), *The Routledge pragmatics encyclopedia* (pp. 442–444). London: Routledge.

Searle, J. R. (1969). *Speech acts: An essay in the philosophy of language.* Cambridge: Cambridge University Press.

Searle, J. R. (1979). *Expression and meaning: Studies in the theory of speech acts.* Cambridge: Cambridge University Press.

Sebastian, C. L., Fontaine, N. M., Bird, G., Blakemore, S.-J., De Brito, S. A., McCrory, E. J., et al. (2012). Neural processing associated with cognitive and affective theory of mind in adolescents and adults. *Social Cognitive and Affective Neuroscience, 7*, 53–63.

Segal, G. (1996). The modularity of theory of mind. In P. Carruthers & P. K. Smith (Eds.), *Theories of theories of mind* (pp. 141–157). Cambridge: Cambridge University Press.

Semkovska, M. (2010). Agrammatism in a case of formal thought disorder: Beyond intellectual decline and working memory deficit. *Neurocase, 16*, 37–49.

SENaPS Central Area Team. (2005). *Promoting positive behaviour for children with social communication and behavioural difficulties.* Essex: Essex County Council.

Sepelyak, K., Crinion, J., Molitoris, J., Epstein-Peterson, Z., Bann, M., Davis, C., et al. (2011). Patterns of breakdown in spelling in primary progressive aphasia. *Cortex, 47*, 342–352.

Sepulcre, J., Peraita, H., Goñi, J., Arrondo, G., Martincorena, I., Duque, B., et al. (2011). Lexical access changes in patients with multiple sclerosis: A two-year follow-up study. *Journal of Clinical and Experimental Neuropsychology, 33*, 169–175.

Shamay-Tsoory, S. G., Tomer, R., & Aharon-Peretz, J. (2005). The neuroanatomical basis of understanding sarcasm and its relationship to social cognition. *Neuropsychology, 19*, 288–300.

Shany-Ur, T., Poorzand, P., Grossman, S. N., Growdon, M. E., Jang, J. Y., Ketelle, R. S., et al. (2012). Comprehension of insincere communication in neurodegenerative disease: Lies, sarcasm, and theory of mind. *Cortex, 48*, 1329–1341.

Shin, M., Besser, L. M., Kucik, J. E., Lu, C., Siffel, C., Correa, A., & The Congenital Anomaly Multistate Prevalence and Survival (CAMPS) Collaborative. (2009). Prevalence of Down syndrome among children and adolescents in 10 regions of the United States. *Pediatrics, 124*, 1565–1571.

Silver, H., Goodman, C., Knoll, G., & Isakov, V. (2004). Brief emotion training improves recognition of facial emotions in chronic schizophrenia. A pilot study. *Psychiatry Research, 128*, 147–154.

Silvestre, N., Ramspott, A., & Pareto, I. D. (2007). Conversational skills in a semistructured interview and self-concept in deaf students. *Journal of Deaf Studies and Deaf Education, 12*, 38–54.

Simmons-Mackie, N., & Damico, J. S. (1996). Accounting for handicaps in aphasia: Communicative assessment from an authentic social perspective. *Disability and Rehabilitation, 18*, 540–549.

Simpson, J., & John Done, D. (2004). Analogical reasoning in schizophrenic delusions. *European Psychiatry, 19*, 344–348.

Sitzer, D. I., Twamley, E. W., Patterson, T. L., & Jeste, D. V. (2008). Multivariate predictors of social skills performance in middle-aged and older outpatients with schizophrenia spectrum disorders. *Psychological Medicine, 38*, 755–763.

Skarakis, E., & Greenfield, P. M. (1982). The role of new and old information in the verbal expression of language-disordered children. *Journal of Speech and Hearing Research, 25*, 462–467.

Skuse, D. H., Mandy, W. P. L., & Scourfield, J. (2005). Measuring autistic traits: Heritability, reliability and validity of the Social and Communication Disorders Checklist. *British Journal of Psychiatry, 187*, 568–572.

Skuse, D. H., Mandy, W., Steer, C., Miller, L. L., Goodman, R., Lawrence, K., et al. (2009). Social communication competence and functional adaptation in a general population of children: Preliminary evidence for sex-by-verbal IQ differential risk. *Journal of the American Academy of Child & Adolescent Psychiatry, 48*, 128–137.

Snow, P. C., Douglas, J., & Ponsford, J. (1998). Conversational discourse abilities following severe traumatic brain injury: A follow-up study. *Brain Injury, 12*, 911–935.

Snow, P. C., & Powell, M. B. (2004). Developmental language disorders and adolescent risk: A public-health advocacy role for speech pathologists? *Advances in Speech-Language Pathology, 6*, 221–229.

Snow, P. C., & Powell, M. B. (2005). What's the story? An exploration of narrative language abilities in male juvenile offenders. *Psychology, Crime & Law, 11*, 239–253.

Snow, P. C., & Powell, M. B. (2008). Oral language competence, social skills and high-risk boys: What are juvenile offenders trying to tell us? *Children & Society, 22*, 16–28.

Snow, P. C., & Powell, M. B. (2011). Oral language competence in incarcerated young offenders: Links with offending severity. *International Journal of Speech-Language Pathology, 13*, 480–489.

Snowden, J., Mann, D., & Neary, D. (2002). Distinct neuropsychological characteristics in Creutzfeldt-Jakob disease. *Journal of Neurology, Neurosurgery & Psychiatry, 73*, 686–694.

Solomon, M., Olsen, E., Niendam, T., Ragland, J. D., Yoon, J., Minzenberg, M., et al. (2011). From lumping to splitting and back again: Atypical social and language development in individuals with clinical-high-risk for psychosis, first episode schizophrenia, and autism spectrum disorders. *Schizophrenia Research, 131*, 146–151.

Solomon, M., Ozonoff, S., Carter, C., & Caplan, R. (2008). Formal thought disorder and the autism spectrum: Relationship with symptoms, executive control, and anxiety. *Journal of Autism and Developmental Disorders, 38*, 1474–1484.

Solomon, O. (2004). Narrative introductions: Discourse competence of children with autistic spectrum disorders. *Discourse Studies, 6*, 253–276.

Sommer, M., Meinhardt, J., Eichenmüller, K., Sodian, B., Döhnel, K., & Hajak, G. (2010). Modulation of the cortical false belief network during development. *Brain Research, 1354*, 123–131.

Song, J.-E., Yang, D.-W., Seo, H.-J., Ha, S.-Y., Park, K.-Y., Kwon, O.-S., et al. (2010). Conduction aphasia as an initial symptom in a patient with Creutzfeldt-Jakob disease. *Journal of Clinical Neuroscience, 17*, 1341–1343.

Soroker, N., Kasher, A., Giora, R., Batori, G., Corn, C., Gil, M., et al. (2005). Processing of basic speech acts following localized brain damage: A new light on the neuroanatomy of language. *Brain and Cognition, 57*, 214–217.

Spanoudis, G., Natsopoulos, D., & Panayiotou, G. (2007). Mental verbs and pragmatic language difficulties. *International Journal of Language & Communication Disorders, 42*, 487–504.

Sparks, A., McDonald, S., Lino, B., O'Donnell, M., & Green, M. J. (2010). Social cognition, empathy and functional outcome in schizophrenia. *Schizophrenia Research, 122*, 172–178.

Sparrow, S. S., Balla, D. A., & Cichetti, D. V. (1984). *Vineland adaptive behaviour scales.* Circle Pines: American Guidance Services.

Speltz, M. L., DeKlyen, M., Calderon, R., Greenberg, M. T., & Fisher, P. A. (1999). Neuropsychological characteristics and test behaviors of boys with early onset conduct problems. *Journal of Abnormal Psychology, 108*, 315–325.

Sperber, D., & Wilson, D. (1987). Précis of relevance: Communication and cognition. *Behavioral and Brain Sciences, 10*, 697–754.

Sperber, D., Cara, F., & Girotto, V. (1995). Relevance theory explains the selection task. *Cognition, 57*, 31–95.

Sperber, D., & Girotto, V. (2002). Use or misuse of the selection task? Rejoinder to Fiddick, Cosmides, and Tooby. *Cognition, 85*, 277–290.

Sperber, D., & Wilson, D. [1986] (1995). *Relevance: Communication and cognition*. Oxford: Blackwell

Sperber, D., & Wilson, D. (2002). Pragmatics, modularity and mind-reading. *Mind & Language, 17*, 3–23.

St Clair, M. C., Pickles, A., Durkin, K., & Conti-Ramsden, G. (2011). A longitudinal study of behavioral, emotional and social difficulties in individuals with a history of specific language impairment. *Journal of Communication Disorders, 44*, 186–199.

St Clair-Thompson, H. L., & Gathercole, S. E. (2006). Executive functions and achievements in school: Shifting, updating, inhibition, and working memory. *Quarterly Journal of Experimental Psychology, 59*, 745–759.

Stattin, H., & Klackenberg-Larsson, I. (1993). Early language and intelligence development and their relationships to future criminal behaviour. *Journal of Abnormal Psychology, 102*, 369–378.

Steinhausen, H.-C., Wachter, M., Laimböck, K., & Metzke, C. Wi. (2006). A long-term outcome study of selective mutism in childhood. *Journal of Child Psychology & Psychiatry, 47*, 751–756.

Stoel-Gammon, C. (2001). Down syndrome phonology: Developmental patterns and intervention strategies. *Down's Syndrome Research and Practice, 7*, 93–100.

Stojanovik, V. (2014). Language in genetic syndromes and cognitive modularity. In L. Cummings (Ed.), *The Cambridge handbook of communication disorders* (pp. 541–558). Cambridge: Cambridge University Press, to appear.

Storebø, O. J., Gluud, C., Winkel, P., & Simonsen, E. (2012). Social-skills and parental training plus standard treatment versus standard treatment for children with ADHD—the randomised SOSTRA trial. *PloS One, 7*, e37280.

Struchen, M. A., Pappadis, M. R., Sander, A. M., Burrows, C. S., & Myszka, K. A. (2011). Examining the contribution of social communication abilities and affective/behavioral functioning to social integration outcomes for adults with traumatic brain injury. *Journal of Head Trauma Rehabilitation, 26*, 30–42.

Sturm, V. E., McCarthy, M. E., Yun, I., Madan, A., Yuan, J. W., Holley, S. R., et al. (2011). Mutual gaze in Alzheimer's disease, frontotemporal and semantic dementia. *Social Cognitive and Affective Neuroscience, 6*, 359–367.

Sudhalter, V., & Belser, R. C. (2001). Conversational characteristics of children with fragile X syndrome: Tangential language. *American Journal on Mental Retardation, 106*, 389–400.

Sullivan, K., & Tager-Flusberg, H. (1999). Second-order belief attribution in Williams syndrome: Intact or impaired? *American Journal of Mental Retardation, 104*, 523–532.

Sullivan, K., Winner, E., & Tager-Flusberg, H. (2003). Can adolescents with Williams syndrome tell the difference between lies and jokes? *Developmental Neuropsychology, 23*, 85–103.

Sundheim, S. T. P. V., & Voeller, K. K. S. (2004). Psychiatric implications of language disorders and learning disabilities: Risks and management. *Journal of Child Neurology, 19*, 814–826.

Surian, L., & Siegal, M. (2001). Sources of performance on theory of mind tasks in right hemisphere-damaged patients. *Brain & Language, 78*, 224–232.

Svensson, I., Lundberg, I., & Jacobson, C. (2001). The prevalence of reading and spelling difficulties among inmates of institutions for compulsory care of juvenile delinquents. *Dyslexia, 7*, 62–76.

Swettenham, J. (2000). Teaching theory of mind to individuals with autism. In S. Baron-Cohen, H. Tager-Flusberg, & D. Cohen (eds.), *Understanding other minds: Perspectives from developmental cognitive neuroscience* (pp. 442–458). Oxford: Oxford University Press.

Tadić, V., Pring, L., & Dale, N. (2010). Are language and social communication intact in children with congenital visual impairment at school age? *Journal of Child Psychology and Psychiatry, 51*, 696–705.

Tager-Flusberg, H., Paul, R., & Lord, C. (2005). Language and communication in autism. In F. R. Volkmar, R. Paul, A. Klin, & D. Cohen (eds.), *Handbook of autism and pervasive developmental disorder. Volume 1: Diagnosis, development, neurobiology and behavior* (335–364). Hoboken: Wiley.

Talerico, K. A., Evans, L. K., & Strumpf, N. E. (2002). Mental health correlates of aggression in nursing home residents with dementia. *The Gerontologist, 42*, 169–177.

Tanaka, J. W., Wolf, J. M., Klaiman, C., Koenig, K., Cockburn, J., Herlihy, L. et al. (2012). The perception and identification of facial emotions in individuals with autism spectrum disorders using the *Let's Face It!* Emotion Skills Battery. *Journal of Child Psychology and Psychiatry. 53*, 1259–1267

Tannock, R. (2005). Language and mental health disorders: The case of ADHD. In W. Østreng (Ed.), *Convergence: Interdisciplinary communications 2004/2005* (pp. 45–53). Oslo: Centre for Advanced Study.

Tavano, A., Sponda, S., Fabbro, F., Perlini, C., Rambaldelli, G., Ferro, A., et al. (2008). Specific linguistic and pragmatic deficits in Italian patients with schizophrenia. *Schizophrenia Research, 102*, 53–62.

Teichmann, M., Dupoux, E., Kouider, S., Brugières, P., Boissé, M.-F., Baudic, S., et al. (2005). The role of the striatum in rule application: The model of Huntington's disease at early stage. *Brain, 128*, 1155–1167.

Tényi, T., Herold, R., Szili, I. M., & Trixler, M. (2002). Schizophrenics show a failure in the decoding of violations of conversational implicatures. *Psychopathology, 35*, 25–27.

Terada, S., Sato, S., Honda, H., Kishimoto, Y., Takeda, N., Oshima, E., et al. (2011). Perseverative errors on the Wisconsin Card Sorting Test and brain perfusion imaging in mild Alzheimer's disease. *International Psychogeriatrics, 23*, 1552–1559.

Thagard, E. K., Hilsmier, A. S., & Easterbrooks, S. R. (2011). Pragmatic language in deaf and hard of hearing students: Correlation with success in general education. *American Annals of the Deaf, 155*, 526–534.

Thiemann, K. S., & Goldstein, H. (2001). Social stories, written text cues, and video feedback: Effects on social communication of children with autism. *Journal of Applied Behavior Analysis, 34*, 425–446.

Thoma, P., Hennecke, M., Mandok, T., Wähner, A., Brüne, M., Juckel, G., et al. (2009). Proverb comprehension impairments in schizophrenia are related to executive dysfunction. *Psychiatry Research, 170*, 132–139.

Thomas, M. S., van Duuren, M., Purser, H. R., Mareschal, D., Ansari, D., & Karmiloff-Smith, A. (2010). The development of metaphorical language comprehension in typical development and in Williams syndrome. *Journal of Experimental Child Psychology, 106*, 99–114.

Thomas, P. (1997). What can linguistics tell us about thought disorder? In J. France & N. Muir (Eds.), *Communication and the mentally ill patient: Developmental and linguistic approaches to schizophrenia* (pp. 30–42). London: Jessica Kingsley Publishers.

Thorne, J. C., Coggins, T. E., Olson, H. C., & Astley, S. J. (2007). Exploring the utility of narrative analysis in diagnostic decision making: Picture-bound reference, elaboration, and fetal alcohol spectrum disorders. *Journal of Speech, Language, and Hearing Research, 50*, 459–474.

Titone, D., Ditman, T., Holzman, P. S., Eichenbaum, H., & Levy, D. L. (2004). Transitive inference in schizophrenia: Impairments in relational memory organization. *Schizophrenia Research, 68*, 235–247.

Tomblin, J. B., Records, N. L., Buckwalter, P., Zhang, X., Smith, E., & O'Brien, M. (1997). Prevalence of specific language impairment in kindergarten children. *Journal of Speech, Language, and Hearing Research, 40*, 1245–1260.

Tompkins, C. A., Baumgaertner, A., Lehman, M. T., & Fassbinder, W. (2000). Mechanisms of discourse comprehension impairment after right hemisphere brain damage: Suppression in lexical ambiguity resolution. *Journal of Speech, Language, and Hearing Research, 43*, 62–78.

Tompkins, C. A., Fassbinder, W., Blake, M. L., Baumgaertner, A., & Jayaram, N. (2004). Inference generation during text comprehension by adults with right hemisphere brain damage: Activation failure versus multiple activation. *Journal of Speech, Language, and Hearing Research, 47*, 1380–1395.

Tompkins, C. A., Lehman-Blake, M. T., Baumgaertner, A., & Fassbinder, W. (2001). Mechanisms of discourse comprehension impairment after right hemisphere brain damage: Suppression in inferential ambiguity resolution. *Journal of Speech, Language, and Hearing Research, 44*, 400–415.

Tompkins, C. A., Meigh, K., Scott, A. G., & Lederer, L. G. (2009). Can high-level inferencing be predicted by Discourse Comprehension Test performance in adults with right hemisphere brain damage? *Aphasiology, 23*, 1016–1027.

Tompkins, C. A., Scharp, V. L., Meigh, K. M., & Fassbinder, W. (2008). Coarse coding and discourse comprehension in adults with right hemisphere brain damage. *Aphasiology, 22*, 204–223.

Torralva, T., Roca, M., Gleichgerrcht, E., Bekinschtein, T., & Manes, F. (2009). A neuropsychological battery to detect specific executive and social cognitive impairments in early fronto-temporal dementia. *Brain, 132*, 1299–1309.

Toupin, J., Déry, M., Pauzé, R., Mercier, H., & Fortin, L. (2000). Cognitive and familial contributions to conduct disorder in children. *Journal of Child Psychology and Psychiatry, 41*, 333–344.

Tran, Y., Blumgart, E., & Craig, A. (2011). Subjective distress associated with chronic stuttering. *Journal of Fluency Disorders, 36*, 17–26.

Tsai, Y.-C., Metzger, S., Riess, O., Soehn, A. S., & Nguyen, H. P. (2012). Genetic analysis of polymorphisms in the kalirin gene for association with age-at-onset in European Huntington disease patients. *BMC Medical Genetics, 13*, 48.

Tso, I. F., Mui, M. L., Taylor, S. F., & Deldin, P. J. (2012). Eye-contact perception in schizophrenia: Relationship with symptoms and socioemotional functioning. *Journal of Abnormal Psychology, 121*, 616–627.

Tur, C., Penny, S., Khaleeli, Z., Altmann, D., Cipolotti, L., Ron, M., et al. (2011). Grey matter damage and overall cognitive impairment in primary progressive multiple sclerosis. *Multiple Sclerosis Journal, 17*, 1324–1332.

Turkstra, L. S., McDonald, S., & Kaufmann, P. M. (1996). Assessment of pragmatic communication skills in adolescents after traumatic brain injury. *Brain Injury, 10*, 329–346.

U.S. Department of Education. (2003). *Twenty-fifth annual report to congress on the implementation of the Individuals with disabilities education act*. Washington, DC: U.S. Department of Education.

Urben, S., van der Linden, M., & Barisnikov, K. (2011). Development of the ability to inhibit a prepotent response: Influence of working memory and processing speed. *British Journal of Developmental Psychology, 29*, 981–998.

Utendale, W. T., Hubert, M., Saint-Pierre, A. B., & Hastings, P. D. (2011). Neurocognitive development and externalizing problems: The role of inhibitory control deficits from 4 to 6 years. *Aggressive Behavior, 37*, 476–488.

Vachha, B., & Adams, R. (2003). Language difference in young children with myelomeningocele and shunted hydrocephalus. *Pediatric Neurosurgery, 39*, 184–189.

Valverde, A. H., Jimenez-Escrig, A., Gobernado, J., & Barón, M. (2009). A short neuropsychologic and cognitive evaluation of frontotemporal dementia. *Clinical Neurology and Neurosurgery, 111*, 251–255.

Van Agt, H., Verhoeven, L., van den Brink, G., & de Koning, H. (2011). The impact on socioemotional development and quality of life of language impairment in 8-year-old children. *Developmental Medicine & Child Neurology, 53*, 81–88.

Van Borsel, J., Defloor, T., & Curfs, L. M. G. (2007). Expressive language in persons with Prader-Willi syndrome. *Genetic Counseling, 18*, 17–28

Van Daal, J., Verhoeven, L., van Balkam, H. (2007). Behaviour problems in children with language impairment. *Journal of Child Psychology and Psychiatry, 48*, 1139–1147.

Van Daal, J., Verhoeven, L., & van Balkom, H. (2009). Cognitive predictors of language development in children with specific language impairment (SLI). *International Journal of Language & Communication Disorders, 44*, 639–655.

Van Den Eeden, S. K., Tanner, C. M., Bernstein, A. L., Fross, R. D., Leimpeter, A., Bloch, D. A., et al. (2003). Incidence of Parkinson's disease: Variation by age, gender, and race/ethinicity. *American Journal of Epidemiology, 157*, 1015–1022.

Van der Henst, J.-B. (1999). The mental model theory of spatial reasoning re-examined: The role of relevance in premise order. *British Journal of Psychology, 90*, 73–84.

Van der Henst, J.-B., & Sperber, D. (2004). Testing the cognitive and communicative principles of relevance. In I. Noveck & D. Sperber (eds.), *Experimental pragmatics* (229–279). Basingstoke: Palgrave Macmillan.

Van der Sluis, S., de Jong, P. F., & van der Leij, A. (2007). Executive functioning in children, and its relations with reasoning, reading and arithmetic. *Intelligence, 35,* 427–449.

Van Swieten, J. C., & Rosso, S. M. (2006). Epidemiology of frontotemporal dementia. *Advances in Clinical Neuroscience & Rehabilitation, 6,* 9–10.

Varley, R., Cowell, P. E., Gibson, A., & Romanowski, C. A. (2005). Disconnection agraphia in a case of multiple sclerosis: The isolation of letter movement plans from language. *Neuropsychologia, 43,* 1503–1513.

Viana, A. G., Beidel, D. C., & Rabian, B. (2009). Selective mutism: A review and integration of the last 15 years. *Clinical Psychology Review, 29,* 57–67.

Vivithanaporn, P., John Gill, M., & Power, C. (2011). Impact of current antiretroviral therapies on neuroAIDS. *Expert Review of Anti-Infective Therapy, 9,* 371–374.

Vogel, A. P., Chenery, H. J., Dart, C. M., Doan, B., Tan, M., & Copland, D. A. (2009). Verbal fluency, semantics, context and symptom complexes in schizophrenia. *Journal of Psycholinguistic Research, 38,* 459–473.

Volden, J., Coolican, J., Garon, N., White, J., & Bryson, S. (2009). Brief report: Pragmatic language in autism spectrum disorder: Relationships to measures of ability and disability. *Journal of Autism and Developmental Disorders, 39,* 388–393.

Volicer, L., Van der Steen, J. T., & Frijters, D. H. M. (2009). Modifiable factors related to abusive behaviors in nursing home residents with dementia. *Journal of the American Medical Directors Association, 10,* 617–622.

Von Reichmann, H., Deuschl, G., Riedel, O., Spottke, A., Förstl, H., Henn, F., et al. (2010). The German study on the epidemiology of Parkinson's disease with dementia (GEPAD): More than Parkinson. *MMW Fortschritte der Medizin, 152,* 1–6.

Vuorinen, E., Laine, M., & Rinne, J. (2000). Common pattern of language impairment in vascular dementia and in Alzheimer disease. *Alzheimer Disease and Associated Disorders, 14,* 81–86.

Wadman, R., Botting, N., Durkin, K., & Conti-Ramsden, G. (2011). Changes in emotional health symptoms in adolescents with specific language impairment. *International Journal of Language & Communication Disorders, 46,* 641–656.

Walsh, B., & Smith, A. (2011). Linguistic complexity, speech production, and comprehension in Parkinson's disease: Behavioral and physiological indices. *Journal of Speech, Language, and Hearing Research, 54,* 787–802.

Walter, H., Adenzato, M., Ciaramidaro, A., Enrici, I., Pia, L., & Bara, B. G. (2004). Understanding intentions in social interaction: The role of the anterior paracingulate cortex. *Journal of Cognitive Neuroscience, 16,* 1854–1863.

Walter, H., Ciaramidaro, A., Adenzato, M., Vasic, N., Ardito, R. B., Erk, S., et al. (2009). Dysfunction of the social brain in schizophrenia is modulated by intention type: An fMRI study. *Scan, 4,* 166–176.

Wassenberg, R., Hendriksen, J. G., Hurks, P P. M., Feron, F. J. M., Vles, J. S. H., & Jolles, J. (2010). Speed of language comprehension is impaired in ADHD. Journal of Attention Disorders, 13, 374–385.

Watts, A. J., & Douglas, J. M. (2006). Interpreting facial expression and communication competence following severe traumatic brain injury. *Aphasiology, 20,* 707–722.

Weed, E. (2008). Theory of mind impairment in right hemisphere damage: A review of the evidence. *International Journal of Speech-Language Pathology, 10,* 414–424.

Weed, E., McGregor, W., Nielsen, J. F., Roepstorff, A., & Frith, U. (2010). Theory of mind in adults with right hemisphere damage: What's the story? *Brain and Language, 113,* 65–72.

Weinrich, M., Mccall, D., Boser, K. I., & Virata, T. (2002). Narrative and procedural discourse production by severely aphasic patients. *Neurorehabilitation and Neural Repair, 16,* 249–274.

Weintraub, D., Moberg, P. J., Culbertson, W. C., Duda, J. E., Katz, I. R., & Stern, M. B. (2005). Dimensions of executive function in Parkinson's disease. *Dementia and Geriatric Cognitive Disorders, 20,* 140–144.

Weiss, A. L. (2004). Why we should consider pragmatics when planning treatment for children who stutter. *Language, Speech, and Hearing Services in Schools, 35*, 34–45.

Welland, R. J., Lubinski, R., & Higginbotham, D. J. (2002). Discourse comprehension test performance of elders with dementia of the Alzheimer type. *Journal of Speech, Language, and Hearing Research, 45*, 1175–1187.

Wellman, H. M., & Lagattuta, K. H. (2000). Developing understandings of mind. In S. Baron-Cohen, H. Tager-Flusberg, & D. J. Cohen (Eds.), *Understanding other minds: Perspectives from developmental cognitive neuroscience* (pp. 21–49). New York: Oxford University Press.

Welsh, S. W., Corrigan, F. M., & Scott, M. (1996). Language impairment and aggression in Alzheimer's disease. *International Journal of Geriatric Psychiatry, 11*, 257–261.

Wertz, R. T., Collins, M. J., Weiss, D., Kurtzke, J. F., Friden, T., Brookshire, R. H., et al. (1981). Veterans Administration cooperative study on aphasia: A comparison of individual and group treatment. *Journal of Speech and Hearing Research, 24*, 580–594.

Wetherby, A. M., & Prutting, C. A. (1984). Profiles of communicative and cognitive-social abilities in autistic children. *Journal of Speech and Hearing Research, 27*, 364–377.

Wharton, T. (2010a). Natural and non-natural meaning. In L. Cummings (Ed.), *The Routledge pragmatics encyclopedia* (pp. 285–286). London: Routledge.

Wharton, T. (2010b). (Grice, H. P.) In L. Cummings (ed.), *The Routledge pragmatics encyclopedia* (182–183). London: Routledge.

Whitehouse, A. J. O., & Bishop, D. V. M. (2009). *Communication checklist-adult (CC-A)*. London: Pearson Assessment.

Whitehouse, A. J. O., Watt, H. J., Line, E. A., & Bishop, D. V. M. (2009b). Adult psychosocial outcomes of children with specific language impairment, pragmatic language impairment and autism. *International Journal of Language & Communication Disorders, 44*, 511–528.

Whitehouse, A. J., Line, E. A., Watt, H. J., & Bishop, D. V. (2009a). Qualitative aspects of developmental language impairment relate to language and literacy outcome in adulthood. *International Journal of Language & Communication Disorders, 44*, 489–510.

Whitehouse, A. J. O., Robinson, M., & Zubrick, S. R. (2011). Late talking and the risk for psychosocial problems during childhood and adolescence. *Pediatrics, 128*, e324–e332.

Whiteneck, G. G., Brooks, C. A., Charlifue, S., Gerhart, K. A., Mellick, D., Overholser, D., et al. (1992a). *Guide for use of the CHART*. Englewood: Craig Hospital.

Whiteneck, G. G., Charliefue, M. A., Gerhart, K. A., Overholser, J. D., & Richardson, G. N. (1992b). Quantifying handicap: A new measure of longterm rehabilitation outcomes. *Archives of Physical Medicine and Rehabilitation, 73*, 519–526.

Whitworth, A., Webster, J., & Morris, J. (2014). Acquired aphasia. In L. Cummings (ed.), *Handbook of communication disorders* (436–456). Cambridge: Cambridge University Press.

Wichstrøm, L., Berg-Nielsen, T. S., Angold, A., Egger, H. L., Solheim, E., & Sveen, T. H. (2012). Prevalence of psychiatric disorders in pre-schoolers. *Journal of Child Psychology and Psychiatry, and Allied Disciplines, 53*, 695–705.

Wiebe, S. A., Sheffield, T., Nelson, J. M., Clark, C. A. C., Chevalier, N., & Espy, K. A. (2011). The structure of executive function in 3-year-olds. *Journal of Experimental Child Psychology, 108*, 436–452.

Wiig, E. H., & Secord, W. (1989). *Test of language competence-expanded edition*. San Antonio: The Psychological Corporation.

Wilkinson, I. M., & Graham-White, J. (1980). Psychogeriatric dependency rating scales (PGDRS): A method of assessment for use by nurses. *British Journal of Psychiatry, 137*, 558–565.

Willer, B., Ottenbacher, K. J., & Coad, M. L. (1994). The community integration questionnaire: A comparative examination. *American Journal of Physical Medicine & Rehabilitation, 73*, 103–111.

Willer, B., Rosenthal, M., Kreutzer, J. S., Gordon, W. A., & Rempel, R. (1993). Assessment of community integration following rehabilitation for traumatic brain injury. *Journal of Head Trauma Rehabilitation, 8*, 75–87.

Williams, B. T., Gray, K. M., & Tonge, B. J. (2012). Teaching emotion recognition skills to young children with autism: A randomised controlled trial of an emotion training programme. *Journal of Child Psychology and Psychiatry*, 53, 1268–1276.

Williams, D., & Happé, F. (2010). Representing intentions in self and other: Studies of autism and typical development. *Developmental Science, 13*, 307–319.

Williams, W. H., Mewse, A. J., Tonks, J., Mills, S., Burgess, C. N. W., & Cordan, G. (2010). Traumatic brain injury in a prison population: Prevalence and risk for re-offending. *Brain Injury, 24*, 1184–1188.

Willinger, U., Brunner, E., Diendorfer-Radner, G., Sams, J., Sirsch, U., & Eisenwort, B. (2003). Behaviour in children with language development disorders. *Canadian Journal of Psychiatry, 48*, 607–614.

Wilson, B. M., & Proctor, A. (2002). Written discourse of adolescents with closed head injury. *Brain Injury, 16*, 1011–1024.

Wilson, D. (2005). New directions for research on pragmatics and modularity. *Lingua, 115*, 1129–1146.

Wilson, D. (2010). Relevance theory. In L. Cummings (ed.), *The Routledge pragmatics encyclopedia* (393–399). London: Routledge.

Wilson, D., & Dan, S. (1991). Pragmatics and modularity. In S. Davis (ed.), *Pragmatics: A reader* (pp. 583–595). New York: Oxford University Press.

Wilson, S. M., Henry, M. L., Besbris, M., Ogar, J. M., Dronkers, N. F., Jarrold, W., et al. (2010). Connected speech production in three variants of primary progressive aphasia. *Brain, 133*, 2069–2088.

Wing, L., Leekam, S. R., Libby, S. J., Gould, J., & Larcombe, M. (2002). The diagnostic interview for social and communication disorders: Background, inter-rater reliability and clinical use. *Journal of Child Psychology and Psychiatry, 43*, 307–325.

Winner, E., Brownell, H., Happé, F., Blum, A., & Pincus, D. (1998). Distinguishing lies from jokes: Theory of mind deficits and discourse interpretation in right hemisphere brain-damaged patients. *Brain and Language, 62*, 89–106.

Wong, P. (2010). Selective mutism: A review of etiology, comorbities, and treatment. *Psychiatry (Edgemont), 7*, 23–31.

Woods, S. P., Moore, D. J., Weber, E., & Grant, I. (2009). Cognitive neuropsychology of HIV-associated neurocognitive disorders. *Neuropsychology Review, 19*, 152–168.

World Health Organization. (1993). *International classification of diseases*. Geneva: WHO.

World Health Organization. (2001). *International classification of functioning, disability and health*. Geneva: WHO.

Worrall, L., & Yiu, E. (2000). Effectiveness of functional communication therapy by volunteers for people with aphasia following stroke. *Aphasiology, 14*, 911–924.

Wright, H. H., & Newhoff, M. (2005). Pragmatics. In L. L. LaPointe (Ed.), *Aphasia and related neurogenic language disorders* (pp. 237–248). New York: Thieme.

Yamaguchi, H., Maki, Y., & Yamaguchi, T. (2011). A figurative proverb test for dementia: Rapid detection of disinhibition, excuse and confabulation, causing discommunication. *Psychogeriatrics, 11*, 205–211.

Yaruss, J. S. (2001). Evaluating treatment outcomes for adults who stutter. *Journal of Communication Disorders, 34*, 163–182.

Yirmiya, N., Solomonica-Levi, D., Shulman, C., & Pilowsky, T. (1996). Theory of mind abilities in individuals with autism, Down syndrome, and mental retardation of unknown etiology: The role of age and intelligence. *Journal of Child Psychology and Psychiatry, 37*, 1003–1014.

Yoo, A. J., Romero, J., Hakimelahi, R., Noqueira, R. G., Rabinov, J. D, Pryor, J. C., et al. (2010). Predictors of functional outcome vary by the hemisphere of involvement in major ischemic stroke treated with intra-arterial therapy: A retrospective cohort study. *BMC Neurology, 10*, 25

Yoshimasu, K., Barbaresi, W. J., Colligan, R. C., Killian, J. M., Voigt, R. G., Weaver, A. L., et al. (2010). Gender, attention-deficit/hyperactivity disorder, and reading disability in a population-based birth cohort. *Pediatrics, 126*, e788–e795.

Young, A. R., Beitchman, J. H., Johnson, C., Douglas, L., Atkinson, L., Escobar, M., et al. (2002). Young adult academic outcomes in a longitudinal sample of early identified language impaired and control children. *Journal of Child Psychology and Psychiatry, 43*, 635–645.

Zaccai, J., McCracken, C., & Brayne, C. (2005). A systematic review of prevalence and incidence studies of dementia with Lewy bodies. *Age and Aging, 34*, 561–566.

Zaidel, E., Kasher, A., Soroker, N., & Batori, G. (2002). Effects of right and left hemisphere damage on performance of the "Right Hemisphere Communication Battery". *Brain and Language, 80*, 510–535.

Zandbelt, B. B., van Buuren, M., Kahn, R. S., & Vink, M. (2011). Reduced proactive inhibition in schizophrenia is related to corticostriatal dysfunction and poor working memory. *Biological Psychiatry, 70*, 1151–1158.

Zgaljardic, D. J., & Temple, R. O. (2010). Neuropsychological assessment battery (NAB): Performance in a sample of patients with moderate-to-severe traumatic brain injury. *Applied Neuropsychology, 17*, 283–288.

Index

L. Cummings, *Pragmatic Disorders*, Perspectives in Pragmatics, Philosophy & Psychology 3, DOI: 10.1007/978-94-007-7954-9, © Springer Science+Business Media Dordrecht 2014

Printed in the United States
By Bookmasters